Psychobiological
Foundations of
Psychiatric Care

Psychobiological Foundations of Psychiatric Care

Norman L. Keltner, RN, CRNP, EdD
Associate Professor
School of Nursing
University of Alabama at Birmingham
Birmingham, Alabama

David G. Folks, MD
Professor and Chair
Department of Psychiatry
Creighton University School of Medicine

University of Nebraska College of Medicine
Omaha, Nebraska

Cheryl Ann Palmer, MD
Assistant Professor
Division of Neuropathology and Department of Neurology
University of Alabama at Birmingham
Birmingham, Alabama

Richard E. Powers, MD
Associate Professor of Pathology
University of Alabama at Birmingham

Director, Bureau of Geriatric Psychiatry
Alabama Department of Mental Health and Mental Retardation
Tuscaloosa, Alabama

with 127 full-color illustrations

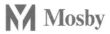

St. Louis Baltimore Boston Carlsbad Chicago Minneapolis New York Philadelphia Portland
London Milan Sydney Tokyo Toronto

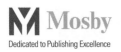

Dedicated to Publishing Excellence

A Times Mirror
Company

Vice President and Publisher: Nancy L. Coon
Editor: Jeff Burnham
Developmental Editor: Linda Caldwell; Jeff Downing
Project Manager: Deborah L. Vogel
Production Editor: Jodi Willard
Designer: Pati Pye
Manufacturing Manager: Linda Ierardi

A NOTE TO THE READER:

The authors and publisher have made every attempt to check dosages and pharmacological and nursing content for accuracy. Because the science of pharmacology is continually advancing, our knowledge base continues to expand. Therefore we recommend that the reader always check product information for changes in dosage or administration before administering any medication. This is particularly important with new or rarely used drugs.

Printed in the United States of America
Composition by Graphic World, Inc.
Lithography/color film by Graphic World, Inc.
Printing/binding by RR Donnelley & Sons Company

Mosby–Year Book, Inc.
11830 Westline Industrial Drive
St. Louis, Missouri 63146

Library of Congress Cataloging in Publication Data

Psychobiological foundations of psychiatric care / Norman L. Keltner
    . . . [et al.]—1st ed.
        p.   cm.
    Includes bibliographical references and index.
    ISBN 0-8151-5658-8 (pbk.)
    1. Neuropsychiatry.   I. Keltner, Norman L.
    [DNLM: 1. Mental Disorders—physiopathology.   2. Neuropsychology.
3. Brain—physiopathology.   WM 140 P974 1997]
RC341. P893   1997
616.8'5—dc21
DNLM/DLC
for Library of Congress   97-262
                                                                                            CIP

97 98 99 00 01/9 8 7 6 5 4 3 2 1

about the authors
Norman L. Keltner

Dr. Keltner is associate professor of nursing at the University of Alabama at Birmingham. In this capacity he teaches psychiatric and community mental health nursing. Dr. Keltner received his Associate Degree in Nursing from Delta College in Stockton, California. After serving as a warrant officer during the Vietnam War, he returned to school to earn both a BSN and an MSN (in psychiatric nursing) from Fresno State University. He received his EdD from the University of San Francisco. He is certified as a gerontological nurse practitioner.

Dr. Keltner began working as a psychiatric nurse in 1966 at Stockton State Hospital and worked in several capacities at that facility over a span of 15 years. He began his teaching career at the University of Wyoming and has also taught at Baylor University and California State University at Bakersfield. Dr. Keltner is the coauthor of *Psychiatric Nursing* and *Psychotropic Drugs*, has contributed to other textbooks, and has written numerous journal articles.

Dr. Keltner is a member of the American Nurses Association, the American Psychiatric Nurses Association, and the National Alliance for the Mentally Ill. Dr. Keltner was a member of the ANA task force on psychopharmacology, which produced the *Psychiatric Mental Health Nursing Psychopharmacology Project*. His clinical and research interests focus on the treatment of individuals with chronic mental illness.

Dr. Keltner grew up in Manteca, California and considers the Central Valley region of that state to be his home. He is married to the former Bette J. Rusk of Stockton, California. They have three children, Sarah, Amanda, and Alexander.

David G. Folks

Dr. Folks is professor and chair, Department of Psychiatry at Creighton University and University of Nebraska Medical Center. Dr. Folks received his medical degree from Oklahoma University and trained at Vanderbilt University. He is board certified in psychiatry and has added qualifications in geriatrics. Dr. Folks is active in the American Psychiatric Association and with the American Board of Psychiatry and Neurology. He participated in the development of the *Diagnostic and Statistical Manual of Mental Disorders,* fourth edition, and he is coauthor of *Psychotropic Drugs.* He has published more than 100 articles, chapters, and abstracts and has participated in several funded research projects involving anxiety and mood disorders, Alzheimer's disease, and other age-related problems. He is married to Diane Baker Folks, a nurse, and they have seven children ranging from 1 to 25 years of age.

Cheryl Ann Palmer

Dr. Palmer is an assistant professor of pathology and neurology at the University of Alabama at Birmingham. She is board certified in both neurology and neuropathology and has a joint appointment in the Department of Neurology and the Division of Neuropathology. Dr. Palmer's clinical practice involves both diagnostic surgical and autopsy neuropathology, as well as consultation on hospitalized patients with neurological problems.

After graduating as valedictorian from her hometown high school in Charleroi, Pennsylvania, Dr. Palmer graduated from the University of Pittsburgh with a BS in pharmacy and practiced as a licensed pharmacist for 5 years before entering medical school. She earned her medical degree at West Virginia University in Morgantown, West Virginia. At the University of Utah in Salt Lake City, she completed 7 years of postgraduate medical education, including both internal medicine and pathology internships, a neurology residency, and a neuropathology fellowship.

Since her appointment at the University of Alabama at Birmingham in 1993, Dr. Palmer has presented clinical research projects and has delivered lectures at both national and international conferences. She has also written numerous scientific articles, mostly in the field of neuro-oncology.

Dr. Palmer is a member of various neurological associations (American Academy of Neurology and Society for Neuro-Oncology) and neuropathological associations (American Association of Neuropathologists, International Society of Neuropathology, and the Society for Experimental Neuropathology [SENP]). She also serves as the treasurer for the SENP. Her most recent recognition was the 1996 University of Alabama at Birmingham Department of Neurology award for "Best Teaching Faculty."

Richard E. Powers

Dr. Powers is a geriatric psychiatrist and neuropathologist. He trained at the University of Kentucky in Lexington and at the Johns Hopkins Hospital in Baltimore, Maryland. He is currently associate professor of pathology at the University of Alabama at Birmingham and serves as interim clinical director at Mary Starke Harper Geriatric Psychiatry Center. Dr. Powers is the director of geriatric psychiatry for the Department of Mental Health for the state of Alabama and is the director of the University of Alabama Brain Resource Program. He also serves as chairman of the Alabama Joint Legislative Study Committee on Alzheimer's Disease.

Dr. Powers was born and raised in Boston, Massachusetts. He is a graduate of Boston College and presently resides in Birmingham, Alabama.

preface

Although the human brain is treated with great respect and some mystical fear, the distinction between brain, mind, and soul is often blurred by the general public and health care providers alike. This blurring occurs because individuals with brain disorders often remain physically healthy and do not demonstrate outward signs of physical impairment. Further confusion arises because of consequent behavioral and psychiatric symptoms that appear "intentional." Hence, the brain-mind-soul continuum is often discussed but is rarely understood.

To illustrate, consider the presentation of a rose to a loved one. The brain, a physical organ, examines the rose and identifies it as a flower. The mind interprets this present by synthesizing the sensory information (i.e., smell and sight) and the context of the rose. The soul is moved by the symbolism of the flower's beauty and the meaning of the present to the beloved individual.

Scientists continue to attempt to understand the function of the brain and the mind, but defining the brain-mind continuum remains elusive. The public, on the other hand, makes judgments about behaviors of patients with mental illness that infer a disorder of the soul rather than of the brain or mind. For example, the elderly Alzheimer victim who struggles during bathing may be viewed as stubborn or mean rather than as demented or confused. The young person with schizophrenia who does not bathe or work is viewed as lazy rather than as psychotic and disorganized. These judgments imply a disorder of the soul rather than of the brain or mind, and they provoke strong emotions in the health care worker, family, or public.

The human brain and intellect can be conceptualized using the personal computer (PC) as a model. The typical PC has four major components: the hard disk, the workstation, the systems program, and the data entry/transmission system. The human intellect also has four similar components or neuronal systems that are located in distinct brain regions. The human "hard disk" consists of the cortical neurons in the cerebral hemispheres and is the repository of long-term memories. The human "workstation" uses conscious and subconscious thought that is partially processed in the temporal lobe. Most acquired information must pass through the temporal lobe, especially the hippocampus and the entorhinal cortex, to enter storage in the hard disk (i.e., the cortex). The system programs of a typical PC set the speed and parameters with which the computer runs. In human brains, these functions are served by the brainstem nuclei, including the locus ceruleus and the raphe neurons, which set the firing rates in the cerebral cortex. Most new human information enters through our five special senses (the "data entry" system) and is encoded in primary sensory cortices and processed in association cortices.

Specific neuropsychiatric disorders result from the dysfunction of these distinct neuronal systems. Mental retardation and dementia are disorders of the hard disk (i.e., failure of the cerebral cortex to store or retrieve information). Disorders of the workstation include an inability to organize conscious thoughts (e.g., thought disorder or paranoia) or to distinguish stored memories from new sensory perceptions (e.g., hallucinations). Schizophrenia is an example of workstation malfunction. Dysregulation of brainstem nuclei causes system acceleration or deceleration, which results in mania or depression, a system program disorder. For example, a patient with bipolar disorder remains intellectually normal and sensorially competent despite elation, depression, or psychosis. Disorders of the data entry/transmission system include conditions such as blindness and deafness, in which patients are unable to access sensory information. Psychiatric complications can arise from such disorders (e.g., visually impaired individuals are predisposed to visual hallucinations).

Neuropsychiatric disorders appear confusing because compartmentalization of function allows one system to operate properly while other systems fail. Patients with schizophrenia remain intellectually intact but are unable to think clearly or suppress hallucinations. Patients with Alzheimer's disease retain many cognitive functions but cannot load new information into the hard disk. Patients with mania seem intellectually bright but are unable to control their thoughts. These confusing symptoms result from alterations in the structure and function of the human brain and mind.

This book is expressly written to explain important neuroanatomical functions and concepts to health care professionals. This explanation is facilitated by efforts to define neurological, cognitive, and psychiatric symptoms of common brain disorders. We, as health care professionals, should not confuse brain-mind malfunction with disorders of the soul.

Norman L. Keltner
David G. Folks
Cheryl Ann Palmer
Richard E. Powers

acknowledgments

There are many different levels of texts. In the pages of this book we are able to share with our readers the results of many years of study in the areas of neuropathology, neurobiology, and neuropsychiatry. We believe that presenting our own original source material provides a definitive, authoritative, and current resource for our readers.

To obtain the most current findings in the field, we occasionally have had to rely on some of our colleagues to provide materials from their research, and we are honored to have their work in our publication. We especially want to thank the following individuals from the University of Alabama at Birmingham:

Frank G. Gilliam, MD, Department of Neurology

Ruben I. Kuzniecky, MD, Department of Neurology

Van B. Wadlington, MD, Department of Radiology

We also wish to thank Deanah Alexander, RN, CS, MSN for reviewing the text; and Libby Teichmiller, BSN, for the vivid and detailed illustrations she provided for this text.

Norman L. Keltner
David G. Folks
Cheryl Ann Palmer
Richard E. Powers

contents in brief

contents

p a r t 2 **Biogenesis and Clinical Management of Mental Disorders**

Appendixes

Psychobiological
Foundations of
Psychiatric Care

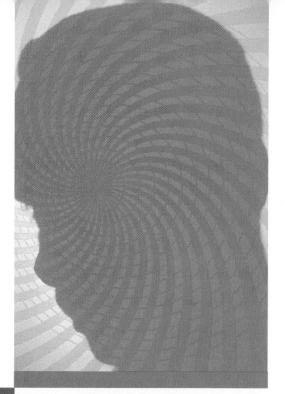

part

1 ——

Psychobiological Bases

Macroscopic Anatomy of the Brain

The human nervous system is composed of two separate but connected divisions. The **central nervous system (CNS)** is composed of the cerebral hemispheres, diencephalic structures, brainstem, cerebellum, and spinal cord, all of which are encased by the dura mater and, in some areas, bone. The **peripheral nervous system (PNS)** contains both the peripheral nerves and the cranial nerves just outside of the brainstem, where they take on peripheral myelin.

Because of their brainstem origin, cranial nerves are discussed as part of the CNS. The neuroanatomy of the CNS is discussed first and in more detail. A brief discussion of brain development is helpful to better understand the functioning and geography of the adult CNS. An understanding of the vascular system is essential in the study of brain neuroanatomy, and the different localizations of the vascular territories are significant in entities such as stroke. Therefore a discussion of the vascular system concludes the chapter.

Central Nervous System
Brain Development

The nervous system develops from the dorsal ectoderm of the embryo; brain cells are derived from "neuroectoderm," the outer layer of ectoderm similar to the cells that eventually become epidermis, or the covering of the skin. The **neural plate** is the first evidence of a developing nervous system and appears on the sixteenth day of fetal development. The neural plate deepens during the next 2 days to form the **neural groove**, which continues to proliferate. By the end of the third week, the two edges of the neural groove meet to form the **neural tube**. This fusion begins in the center and proceeds rostrally (toward the head) and caudally (toward the feet); the two ends close between the twenty-fourth and twenty-sixth day of fetal development.

Growth and development occur to the greatest extent in the rostral portion of the neural tube, which eventually develops into the brain; the remainder of the neural tube becomes the spinal cord. The rostral end of the neural tube forms three primary vesicles at the end of the fourth week of fetal life: the **prosencephalon** (forebrain), the **mesencephalon** (midbrain), and the **rhombencephalon** (hindbrain). By the fifth week, the first and third vesicles each change into two swellings so that there are five secondary vesicles: the **telencephalon** and **diencephalon** (from the prosencephalon), the mesencephalon, and the **metencephalon** and **myelencephalon** (from the rhombencephalon). The further development of these secondary vesicles into the mature brain is presented in Table 1.1. Errors at any step in this development may result in some form of congenital malformation of varying degrees of severity. From this point the brain continues to mature, forming gyri and sulci. The immature fetal brain (Figure 1.1) is fairly smooth, but all of the expected gyri and sulci are formed by the time of birth.

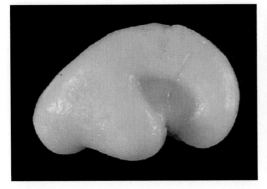
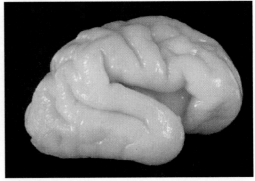

figure 1.1   Immature fetal brain at two different gestational ages. **A,** 20 weeks. **B,** 34 weeks. In contrast to the smooth brain surface of the younger fetus, the brain surface of the older fetus has numerous sulci and gyri. *(Courtesy Dr. Richard E. Powers, Director, University of Alabama at Birmingham Brain Resource Program.)*

table 1.1
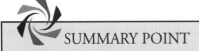
Brain Maturation from the Brain Vesicles

PRIMARY VESICLE	SECONDARY VESICLE	MATURE BRAIN
Prosencephalon	Telencephalon	Cerebral hemispheres
	Diencephalon	Thalamus, epithalamus, hypothalamus, and subthalamus
Mesencephalon	Mesencephalon	Midbrain
Rhombencephalon	Metencephalon	Pons and cerebellum
	Myelencephalon	Medulla

SUMMARY POINT

Neural plate (16th day) ⇒ neural groove (18th day) ⇒ neural tube (21st day) ⇒ tube closes (26th day)

Dura and Leptomeninges

Three layers of meninges cover the surface of the CNS: the **dura mater**, the **arachnoid**, and the **pia mater**. The dura mater is a thick, tough covering that serves as the outer covering and often directly underlies bone (Figure 1.2). The layers of dura mater are usually fused, except where they contain the venous sinuses, which are discussed later in this chapter. One of the dural projections is the **falx cerebri**, which is located in the interhemispheric fissure between the right and left hemispheres. The posterior leaflet of the dura mater is the **tentorium cerebelli**, which lies above the cerebellum, separates the occipital lobe from the cerebellum, and constitutes the border into the **posterior fossa,** which contains the cerebellum and brainstem. The dura is separated from the arachnoid (from the root word of *spiderweb*) by the **subdural space**, which normally contains only minute amounts of cerebrospinal fluid (CSF).

The arachnoid is a thin, glistening, translucent membrane covering the surface of the brain. It does not dip into the sulci or fissures except to follow the falx cerebri and the tentorium cerebelli.

The numerous **arachnoid granulations,** which are located over the convexities and near the falx cerebri on both hemispheres, project into the superior sagittal sinus (p. 31) and are responsible for resorption of CSF. The arachnoid membrane is attached to the pia mater via the arachnoid trabeculae. It is separated from the pia mater by the **subarachnoid space**, which contains numerous brain blood vessels and considerable amounts of CSF.

The pia mater is an even thinner connective tissue membrane that completely covers the CNS. It extends into the sulci and fissures and around the blood vessels in the brain. The arachnoid and pia mater together are known as the **leptomeninges**.

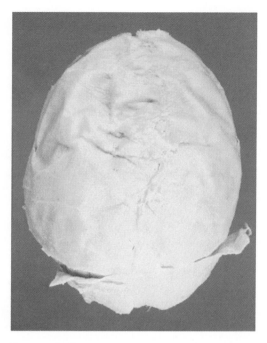

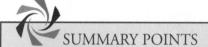
SUMMARY POINTS

1. Three layers: dura mater, arachnoid, pia mater
2. Two dural projections: falx cerebri, tentorium cerebelli
3. Arachnoid granulations resorb CSF

figure 1.2   Intact dura mater as viewed from the top of the head. *(Courtesy Dr. Richard E. Powers, Director, University of Alabama at Birmingham Brain Resource Program.)*

Cerebral Hemispheres

The surfaces of the cerebral hemispheres contain many fissures and sulci that divide the cerebrum into the following lobes or areas: **frontal, temporal, parietal, occipital, insular,** and **limbic** (Figure 1.3). **Fissures** tend to be deeper than **sulci** and are visible earlier in brain development. The portions of the brain that lie between the sulci are called **gyri** (singular *gyrus*). Some gyri are fairly constant in placement, but others are more variable among human brains.

The left and right cerebral hemispheres are separated by the deep **interhemispheric fissure**. The **Sylvian** (or lateral) **fissure** separates the temporal lobe from the frontal and parietal lobes (Figure 1.3, *E*). The **central sulcus** arises in the midline of the superior surface of the brain and separates the frontal lobe from the parietal lobe.

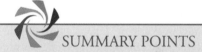
SUMMARY POINTS

1. Brain has six areas/lobes
2. Fissures (deeper) and sulci divide gyri

Frontal Lobe

The frontal lobe extends from the frontal pole of the brain (the frontal tip) to the central sulcus. The major areas of the frontal lobe include the following:

- ***Precentral gyrus.*** This is the primary motor area that serves as the origination of the corticospinal tract. Consisting mostly of large neurons called *Betz's cells* (see Chapter 2), this cortex controls voluntary movement of skeletal

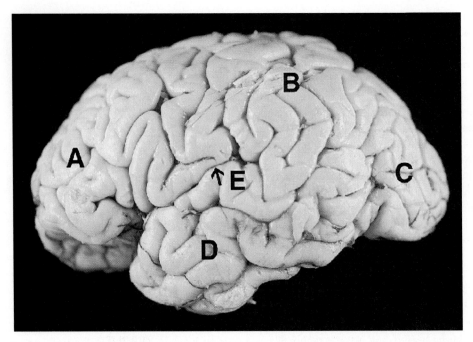

figure 1.3   Lateral view of the brain, with the leptomeninges and vessels removed. **A,** Frontal lobe. **B,** Parietal lobe. **C,** Occipital lobe. **D,** Temporal lobe. **E,** Sylvian fissure. *(Courtesy Dr. Richard E. Powers, Director, University of Alabama at Birmingham Brain Resource Program.)*

muscle on the opposite side of the body. Lesions in this area can cause contralateral (opposite side) weakness or "kinetic apraxia"—a loss of fine motor control. Discrete regions are mapped out for various muscle groups (somatotopic organization).

- **Superior frontal gyrus.** This portion of the frontal lobe contains the supplementary motor area, which is an adjunct to the primary motor system.
- **Middle frontal gyrus.** This portion of the frontal lobe contains the frontal eye fields, which are thought to play a role in voluntary eye movements.
- **Inferior frontal gyrus.** This frontal lobe gyrus includes the pars orbitale, pars triangularis, and pars opercularis. Lesions here in the dominant hemisphere can cause Broca's dysphasia or aphasia.

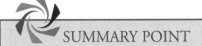

SUMMARY POINT

Frontal lobe ⇒ primary and supplementary motor, eye movements, language, cognition, personality

Parietal Lobe

The parietal lobe extends posteriorly from the central sulcus to the parieto-occipital fissure, which divides it from the occipital lobe. The major areas of the parietal lobe include the following:

- **Postcentral gyrus.** This portion of the parietal lobe is the primary sensory area, with the gustatory sense located in the most ventral portion. Called the "somatesthetic" area, this region also receives touch and proprioceptive information (the realization of where the limbs are located in space) from the opposite side of the body. Irritative lesions in the postcentral gyrus can cause contralateral sensation abnormalities or a complete loss of sensation. Paresthesias are tingling feelings indicative of sensory abnormalities.

- *Superior parietal lobule.*
- *Inferior parietal lobule.* Lesions in the inferior parietal lobule of the dominant lobe cause Gerstmann's syndrome. This syndrome consists of finger agnosia, right-left confusion, **agraphia** (the inability to write), and acalculia. The inferior parietal lobule is subdivided into the following two areas:
  - *Supramarginal gyrus.* A dominant hemisphere lesion in this area causes ideomotor apraxia, in which patients know what they want to do but cannot perform the movement.
  - *Angular gyrus.* A dominant hemisphere lesion in this area causes **alexia** (the inability to read) with agraphia.

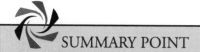

SUMMARY POINT

Parietal lobe ⇒ sensation, taste, praxis, reading, writing

Temporal Lobe

The temporal lobe lies below the Sylvian fissure and extends back to the level of the parieto-occipital fissure on the medial surface of the hemisphere, which divides it from the occipital lobe. The major areas in the temporal lobe include the following:

- *Superior temporal gyrus.* The superior temporal gyrus consists of Wernicke's area. Lesions here in the dominant hemisphere cause Wernicke's dysphasia.
- *Middle temporal gyrus.*
- *Inferior temporal gyrus.*
- *Transverse gyri of Heschl.* These gyri form the primary auditory area. Loss of function in this region can cause the perception of buzzing

or roaring sounds. Bilateral loss of function in this area can cause deafness.

- *Parahippocampal gyrus and uncus.* These structures form the primary olfactory area and are also part of the limbic system (Figure 1.4, *F* and *G*).

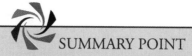

SUMMARY POINT

Temporal lobe ⇒ hearing, sense of smell, speech center

Occipital Lobe

The occipital lobe is located posterior to the frontal and temporal lobes behind the parieto-occipital fissure. The occipital lobe itself is divided by the **calcarine sulcus**. The cortex bordering this sulcus on both sides is the primary visual cortex and is also called the **calcarine cortex**. Irritative lesions of this region can provoke visual hallucinations, such as a perception of flashing lights, or the loss of sight in various fields of vision.

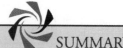

SUMMARY POINT

Occipital lobe ⇒ primary and associated visual cortices

Insula

The insula can be seen only when the temporal and frontal lobes are separated on their exterior aspect. The insula lies deep inside the Sylvian fissure and contains several gyri and sulci.

Limbic System

The limbic system is an area rather than a specific lobe and consists of the large cortical convolutions and other grey matter structures on the mesial aspect of the hemispheres. The cortical components that belong functionally to the limbic

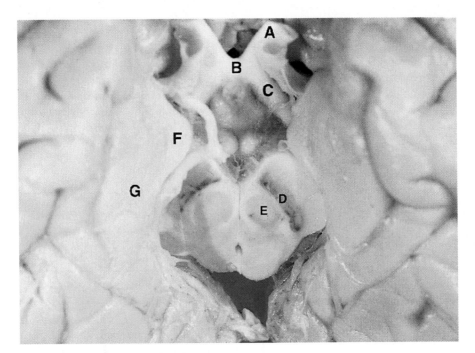

figure 1.4   External view of the brain from the ventral surface. **A,** Optic nerve. **B,** Optic chiasm. **C,** Optic tract. **D,** Substantia nigra. **E,** Red nucleus. **F,** Uncus. **G,** Parahippocampal gyrus. *(Courtesy Dr. Richard E. Powers, Director, University of Alabama at Birmingham Brain Resource Program.)*

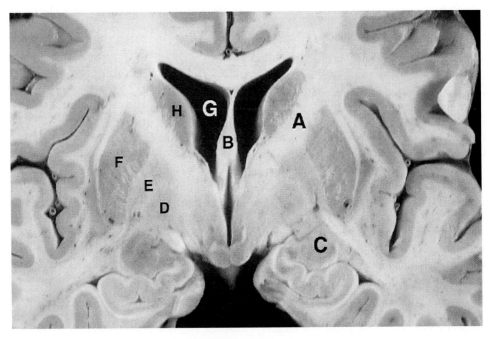

figure 1.5   Coronal section of the brain at the level of the basal ganglia. **A,** Internal capsule. **B,** Fornix. **C,** Amygdala. **D,** Globus pallidus interna. **E,** Globus pallidus externa. **F,** Putamen. **G,** Lateral ventricle. **H,** Caudate nucleus. *(Courtesy Dr. Cheryl A. Palmer, Division of Neuropathology, University of Alabama at Birmingham.).*

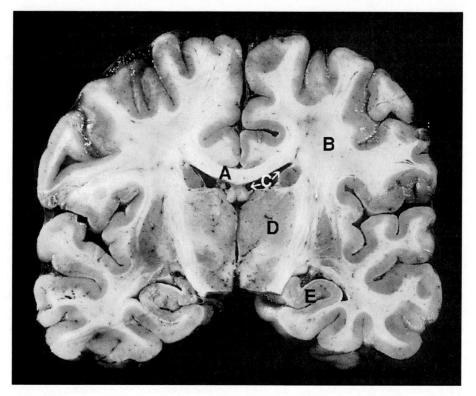

figure 1.6 Coronal section of the brain at the level of the thalamus. **A,** Corpus callosum. **B,** Centrum semiovale. **C,** Lateral ventricle. **D,** Thalamus. **E,** Hippocampus. *(Courtesy Dr. Cheryl A. Palmer, Division of Neuropathology, University of Alabama at Birmingham.)*

system include the cingulate, parahippocampal, and subcallosal gyri. Also included in the limbic system are the fornix, the hippocampal formation, and the amygdala. As can be seen with a microscope, much of the limbic system has different cytoarchitecture than the neocortex of the brain. The most primitive cortex in this area is the archicortex, which has only three layers of neurons instead of the normal six layers in the neocortex.

Current research suggests that the basic functions of the limbic system contribute both to the continuation of the species and to the preservation of the specific individual. These basic functions include feeding behavior, aggression, the expression of emotion, and the autonomic, behavioral, and endocrinological aspects of sexual response. Olfaction plays a role in triggering these types of behaviors.

The **amygdala** (Figure 1.5, *C*) underlies the uncus in the dorsomedial portion of the temporal lobe. It appears to be concerned with visceral, endocrine, and behavioral functions. Input to the amygdala includes olfactory data from the temporal lobe and lateral olfactory tract. Bilateral lesions may cause an increase in aggressive and assaultive behavior. The amygdala also plays an important role in food and water intake.

The **hippocampus** (Figure 1.6, *E*) is a primitive cortical structure that extends the length of the floor of the inferior horn of the lateral ventricle and becomes continuous with the fornix below the splenium of the corpus callosum. For the purposes of study, the hippocampus has been divided into five different sections: **cornu ammonis (CA) 1, CA2, CA3, CA4,** and the **dentate gyrus**. The hippocampus shows the histologic features of an archicortex with three layers: dendrite, pyramidal cell, and axonal.

The dentate gyrus receives its input from the overlying **subiculum** and the adjacent temporal cortex. The granule cells of the dentate gyrus send axons (mossy fibers) to the pyramidal cells of the hippocampus, mostly to the CA3 region. These cells in turn project to the **fornix** (see Figure 1.5, *B*), which is a major efferent pathway; it is an arched white fiber tract that extends from the hippocampal formation to the diencephalon.

The hippocampus is involved in converting short-term memory (up to 60 minutes) to long-term memory (several days or more). The anatomic substrate for long-term memory probably includes the temporal lobes. Patients with a bilateral loss of hippocampal function demonstrate anterograde amnesia, in which events before the loss are retained but no new long-term memories can be established. A person with retrograde amnesia would not be able to make sense of a book because of an inability to remember the plot. This lack of memory is also present in patients with any type of bilateral interruption of the fornices.

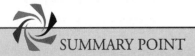

SUMMARY POINT

Limbic system ⇒ feeding, emotion, sexual behavior, aggression, memory

White Matter

The white matter of the adult cerebral hemispheres contains myelinated nerve fibers of many sizes, as well as many neuroglia (mostly oligodendrocytes, which are discussed in Chapter 2). The majority of the white matter in the hemispheres is contained in the centrum semiovale (see Figure 1.6, *B*). There are three types of white matter fibers: **projection fibers, association fibers,** and **commissural** (transverse) **fibers.**

Projection Fibers

Projection fibers connect distant loci with the cortex and form the corona radiata. The corona radiata includes the **internal capsule** and the **optic radiations**.

The internal capsule (see Figure 1.5, *A*) is a broad band of myelinated fibers that separate the lentiform nuclei from the medial caudate nucleus and the thalamus. It consists of an anterior limb, a posterior limb, a retrolenticular portion, and a sublenticular portion. In a horizontal section of the brain the internal capsule has a V-shaped appearance, with the **genu** ("bent knee") pointing medially. The anterior limb of the internal capsule contains fibers primarily from the thalamus, including the thalamocortical radiations and the corticothalamic tract. It also contains the frontopontine tract, which runs from the frontal lobe to the pons, as well as fibers traveling between the caudate and the putamen. The posterior limb of the capsule contains the corticospinal and corticobulbar tracts.

Association Fibers

The association fibers connect regions of the same hemisphere with each other. There are three main subdivisions:

- **Short association fibers.** These fibers consist of the "U fibers," which lie directly under the neocortex and connect adjacent gyri.
- **Long association fibers.** These fibers connect more widely separated areas and consist of three important components. The **uncinate fasciculus** connects the orbital frontal gyri with the anterior temporal lobe. The **arcuate fasciculus** connects the superior and middle frontal gyri with the temporal lobe. Lesions to the arcuate fasciculus in the dominant hemisphere cause a conduction aphasia. The **cingulum**, a white matter band within the cingulate gyrus, connects the frontoparietal areas with the temporal lobe.
- **Extreme and external capsules.**

Commissural Fibers

The commissural fibers connect the right and left hemispheres and consist of three primary structures. The **corpus callosum** (see Figure 1.6, *A*) is a large myelinated bundle of fibers. It generally arises from parts of the neocortex and travels to the corresponding neocortex in the other hemisphere. It is the largest white matter commissure connecting the right and left hemispheres. As with many structures in the brain, the corpus callosum is **C**-shaped. The anterior curved portion is the genu, the middle portion stretching from anterior to posterior is known as the **body**, and the most posterior portion is called the **splenium** of the corpus callosum, which overlies the midbrain. The **anterior commissure**, in its anterior portion, connects the olfactory structures bilaterally; in its posterior portion it connects the middle and inferior temporal gyri. The **posterior commissure** lies below the pineal gland (p. 14).

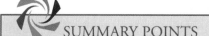

SUMMARY POINTS

1. Projection fibers (internal capsule, optic radiations) ⇒ connect distant loci in same hemisphere
2. Association fibers ⇒ connect the same hemisphere
3. Commissural fibers (corpus callosum, commissures) ⇒ connect two hemispheres

Basal Ganglia and Associated Nuclei

The basal ganglia are subcortical nuclear masses derived from the prosencephalon. The terminology can be quite confusing: the **corpus striatum** includes the caudate nucleus, putamen, and globus pallidus. The **striatum** includes the caudate nucleus and putamen, and the **lentiform nuclei** include the putamen and globus pallidus.

- *Putamen.* Lying lateral to and just below the insular cortex, the putamen is the most lateral portion of the basal ganglia and the largest nucleus in the group (see Figure 1.5, *F*).
- *Globus pallidus.* Medial to the putamen, the globus pallidus is smaller and triangular. The numerous myelinated fibers that travel here make the globus pallidus appear lighter in color than the caudate nucleus or putamen. A

medullary lamina divides the globus pallidus into two areas: the **globus pallidus interna** and the **globus pallidus externa** (see Figure 1.5, *D* and *E*).
- *Caudate nucleus.* The caudate head protrudes into the anterior horn of the lateral ventricle. The tail is **C**-shaped, found near the lateral wall of the lateral ventricle, and terminates near the amygdala (see Figure 1.5, *H*).

Basal Ganglia Connections

Afferent input to the corpus striatum comes from the corticostriate tract, thalamostriate tract (originating in the centromedian nucleus), nigrostriatal tract, and subthalamopallidal tract. Efferent fibers include the striatonigral tract, pallidosubthalamic tract, ansa lenticularis, pallidothalamic tract, and pallidotegmental tract.

Basal Ganglia Function

The function of the corpus striatum (loosely referred to as the **extrapyramidal system**) is to integrate automatic movements such as postural adjustments, defensive reactions, and feeding. Most of the fibers in the corpus striatum are topographically arranged. Because it is also involved with muscle tone regulation, bilateral lesions in the corpus striatum cause bradykinesias, dyskinesias, chorea, tremors, and athetosis. Unilateral lesions of the corpus striatum are often asymptomatic.

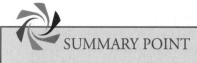

SUMMARY POINT

Basal ganglia dysfunction ⇒ movement disorders (see Chapter 13)

Diencephalon

The diencephalon is part of the cerebrum and includes the **thalamus, geniculate bodies, hypothalamus, subthalamic nuclei, epithalamus** (which includes the pineal gland and the habenula), and the **nucleus basalis of Meynert.**

Thalamus

Each half of the brain contains a thalamus (see Figure 1.6, *D*), which is separated by and surrounds the third ventricle. All sensory input except olfaction is modulated in the thalamus. In many people a connection between the two thalami (called the **massa intermedia**) bridges the third ventricle. The massa intermedia has no known neurologic function.

The thalamus is divided into five groups of nuclei. The **anterior nuclear group** is composed of several components. The largest nucleus of the group is the anteroventral nucleus, which receives the mamillothalamic tract and some fibers from the fornix. It projects to the cingulate gyrus via the anterior limb of the internal capsule.

The **midline nuclear group** is located just beneath the third ventricular lining. This group connects with the hypothalamus and may be concerned with visceral activities. One of the larger nuclei of this group is the centromedian nucleus. It receives impulses from the reticular activating system in the brainstem and from the cerebellar dentate and fastigial nuclei. Efferent fibers from the centromedian nucleus project to the putamen and caudate nucleus.

The **medial nuclear group** contains several components. The largest nucleus in the medial nuclear group is the dorsomedial nucleus, which receives afferent impulses from the amygdala and projects to the frontal cortex. This nucleus may mediate affective impulses or emotions that contribute to personality characteristics.

The **lateral nuclear group** contains six separate subdivisions, which include the following:
- *Reticular nucleus.*
- *Ventral anterior nucleus (VA).* Afferent fibers to the VA arise from the globus pallidus and substantia nigra. Efferent fibers from the VA are proposed to diffusely project to the anterior insula and the frontal cortex.
- *Ventral lateral nucleus (VL).* The VL obtains its afferent input from the cerebellum (dentate nucleus), globus pallidus, and substantia nigra. The efferent fibers from the VL project somatotopically to the precentral gyrus.
- *Dorsolateral nucleus.* Afferent input to the

dorsolateral nucleus is unknown. Efferent fibers from the dorsolateral nucleus project to the cingulate gyrus and parietal lobe.
- *Ventral posterolateral nucleus (VPL).* The VPL is an important sensory relay station. The afferent input of the VPL comes primarily from the medial lemniscus, the spinothalamic tract, and the trigeminal tract. The VPL projects somatotopically to the postcentral gyrus of the parietal lobe, which is involved with sensation.
- *Ventral posteromedial nucleus (VPM).* Afferent input to the VPM comes from the trigeminothalamic tract (from the head and face). Efferent VPM connections involve the postcentral gyrus and may mediate the sensation of taste.

The **posterior nuclear group** includes the pulvinar nucleus, the medial geniculate bodies, and the lateral geniculate bodies. The **pulvinar nucleus** is the largest of the thalamic nuclei and receives input from other thalamic nuclei and from the medial and lateral geniculate bodies. It projects to the posterior parietal and temporal lobes.

Geniculate Bodies

The **lateral geniculate body (LGB)** is a part of the visual pathway. It receives most of its input from the optic tract and sends most of its efferent fibers to the visual cortex in the occipital lobe. On the other hand, the **medial geniculate body (MGB)** lies lateral to the midbrain and beneath the pulvinar nucleus, and it is part of the auditory pathway. It receives afferent input from the lateral lemniscus and inferior colliculus, and it sends efferent fibers to the temporal lobe cortex.

SUMMARY POINTS

1. Thalamus contains five nuclear groups
2. Thalamus mediates all sensory input except olfaction, including hearing, taste, vision

Hypothalamus

The **hypothalamus** lies slightly anterior and caudal to the thalamus and forms the floor and lower walls of the third ventricle. Limiting borders include the optic chiasm, the tuber cinereum and the infundibulum, and the mamillary bodies, which lie between the cerebral peduncles.

The hypothalamus is composed of several divisions. The most anterior region of the hypothalamus is called the **supraoptic portion** because of its position directly above the optic chiasm. The supraoptic portion contains the supraoptic nucleus and the paraventricular nucleus. The **tuberal portion,** directly above the tuber cinereum, contains the ventromedial, dorsomedial, and arcuate nuclei. The third division is the **mamillary portion,** which is the posterior extent of the hypothalamus and contains the posterior nucleus and several mamillary nuclei.

Afferent connections to the hypothalamus include fibers from the paraolfactory area, the basal ganglia, the thalamus, and the fornix. Efferent output from the hypothalamus includes the hypothalamicohypophysial tract, which runs from the supraoptic and paraventricular nuclei to the neurohypophysis (the posterior pituitary gland); the mamillotegmental tract from the mamillary nuclei to the anterior thalamic nuclei; and the tuberohypophysial tract, which travels from the tuberal portion of the hypothalamus to the posterior pituitary gland.

Although small in volume, the importance of the hypothalamus is immense in human brains. The functions of the hypothalamus are as follows:

- *Eating.* The hypothalamus controls eating behavior via a "satiety center" in the ventromedial nucleus and a "feeding center" in the lateral hypothalamus. Damage to the feeding center results in anorexia, whereas damage to the satiety center causes hyperphagia and obesity.
- *Temperature.* Stimulation of various regions of the hypothalamus results in loss, conservation, or production of body heat. The set-point of the hypothalamic thermostat is just below 37° C. Fever is the result of an upward regulation of the set-point.
- *Emotional expression.* The hypothalamus is also concerned with the expressions of rage, sexual behavior, pleasure, and fear, all of which occur by fairly unexplored mechanisms.
- *Autonomic system.* The dorsomedial and posterolateral regions of the hypothalamus act as a catecholamine activating region (sympathetic system); the anterior region functions as a parasympathetic activating system.
- *Water balance.* The hypothalamus influences the expression of vasopressin in the posterior pituitary gland. Emotion, pain, stress, or any increase in blood osmolarity alters the secretion of vasopressin. The lack of vasopressin secretion causes polydipsia (increased thirst) or polyuria (increased urine production).
- *Circadian rhythm.* Many body functions have a cyclical influence or a circadian (day-to-day) rhythm, including corticosteroid levels, temperature, and oxygen consumption. The supraoptic nucleus functions as a clock with a 25-hour cycle. Lesions in this nucleus eliminate the circadian cycles.
- *Anterior pituitary function.* The hypothalamus strongly influences secretions of the adenohypophysis by releasing or inhibiting hormones carried by the portohypophysial vascular system. Many endocrine functions are regulated in this manner, including sexual behavior, thyroid and adrenal cortex secretions, growth, and reproduction.

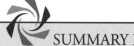

SUMMARY POINT

Hypothalamic functions ⇒ eating, temperature regulation, emotion, autonomics, water balance, circadian rhythm, pituitary function

Subthalamic Nucleus

The subthalamic nucleus is shaped like a thick, biconvex lens. It is dorsolateral to the upper end of the substantia nigra and extends posteriorly to the lateral aspect of the red nucleus. The subthalamic nucleus has many connections with the basal ganglia. Discrete lesions (which are usually hemorrhagic) cause contralateral hemiballismus, which is a violent, forceful, and persistent choreiform movement, usually of the upper extremity.

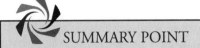

SUMMARY POINT

Subthalamic dysfunction ⇒ hemiballismus

Epithalamus

The epithalamus consists of the **habenular commissure** (Figure 1.7, *A*) and the **pineal gland** (Figure 1.8, *B*). The habenular system has anatomic connections to the thalamus and midbrain, but its clinical function is unknown. The pineal gland is a midline mass that lies between the superior colliculi at the top of the midbrain. The pineal gland secretes melatonin, which is involved in the regulation of human day-night cycles.

The clinical correlations of the epithalamus are largely unknown. The most common pathological reactions in the pineal gland are neoplastic processes. Tumors that prefer the midline of the brain are most common here and include primary pineal neoplasms and germ cell tumors. A mass in the pineal gland causes symptoms known as Parinaud's syndrome, which consists of an inability to gaze upward as a result of pressure on the collicular plate in the midbrain.

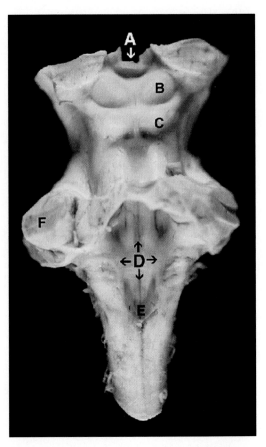

figure 1.7   Brainstem from its ventral aspect. **A,** Habenula. **B,** Superior colliculus. **C,** Inferior colliculus. **D,** Fourth ventricle. **E,** Obex. **F,** Middle cerebellar peduncle. *(Courtesy Dr. Richard E. Powers, Director, University of Alabama at Birmingham Brain Resource Program.)*

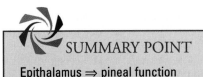

SUMMARY POINT

Epithalamus ⇒ pineal function

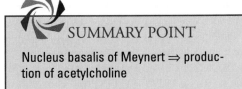

SUMMARY POINT

Nucleus basalis of Meynert ⇒ production of acetylcholine

Nucleus Basalis of Meynert

The nucleus basalis of Meynert is located bilaterally and directly beneath the anterior commissure. It is the major brain site for the production of acetylcholine and projects diffusely to the cerebral cortex.

Cerebellum

The cerebellum is involved with the coordination of somatic muscle activity, regulation of muscle tone, and maintenance of equilibrium. Although it receives sensory input from all types of

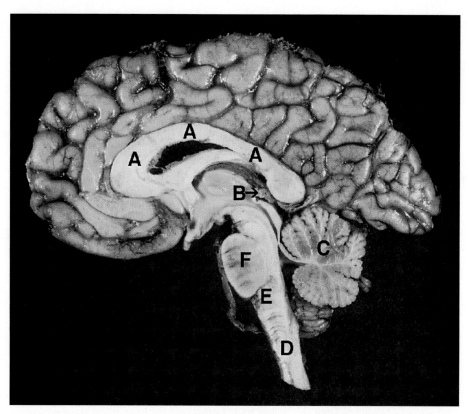

figure 1.8   Sagittal view of the brain in its midsection. **A,** Corpus callosum (genu, body, and sple-nium). **B,** Pineal gland. **C,** Vermis of the cerebellum. **D,** Spinal cord. **E,** Medulla. **F,** Pons. *(Courtesy Dr. Cheryl A. Palmer, Division of Neuropathology, University of Alabama at Birmingham.)*

receptors, it is not especially concerned with sensory perception.

The cerebellum (Figure 1.9) overlies the posterior aspect of the pons and extends laterally underneath the tentorium to fill the largest part of the posterior fossa. It consists of two lateral hemispheres and a midline vermis. Fissures divide the cerebellar surface into lobes: the primary fissure is the posterior boundary of the anterior lobe; the posterior lobe lies between the primary fissure and the posterolateral fissure and is the largest subdivision of the cerebellum. The flocculonodular lobule is rostral to the posterolateral fissure and consists of the nodulus and the paired flocculi.

All parts of the cerebellar cortex project to the deep **cerebellar nuclei**, which consist of the dentate, emboliform, fastigial, and globose nuclei.

The **dentate nucleus** is the largest of the deep cerebellar nuclei. It lies in the white matter close to the vermis. In cross section it resembles the convolutions of the inferior olivary nuclei. The **emboliform nucleus** is a wedge-shaped grey mass close to the hilum of the dentate nucleus. The **fastigial nucleus** is the most medial of the deep cerebellar nuclei and lies near the midline in the roof of the fourth ventricle. This nucleus also receives some vestibular fibers from the vestibular nuclei. The **globose nuclei** consist of one or more rounded grey masses between the fastigial and emboliform nuclei.

The anterior and posterior vermis project primarily to the fastigial nucleus. The paravermal cortex projects to ipsilateral globose and emboliform nuclei. The lateral hemispheres project

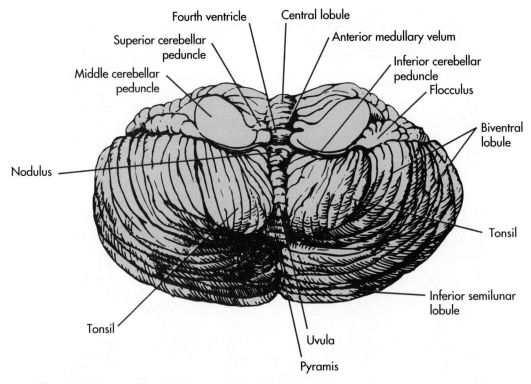

figure 1.9   External cerebellum and its various structures. *(From Waxman SG:* Correlative neuroanatomy, *ed 23, Stanford, Conn, 1991, Appleton & Lange.)*

primarily to the dentate nuclei, and the paraflocculus projects primarily to the caudal fastigial nucleus.

The **cerebellar peduncles** (Figure 1.9) consist of inferior (connects with the medulla), middle (connects with the pons), and superior (connects to the midbrain) portions.

The **inferior cerebellar peduncle** is primarily concerned with connections to the vestibular nuclei and spinal cord. Its components are also known as the "restiform" and the "juxtarestiform" bodies. Afferent input includes the posterior spinocerebellar tract, which conveys information from stretch receptors in the lower extremities. The cuneocerebellar fibers come from the cuneate nucleus in the medulla and convey information from the stretch receptors of the upper extremities. The reticulocerebellar fibers enter to convey primarily tactile impulses. The olivocerebellar fibers are the largest inferior cerebellar peduncle tract; they arise from the contralateral inferior oli-

vary nucleus in the medulla, are assumed to monitor the activity of interneurons, and may be part of a reflex arc. Efferent projections from the fastigial nuclei go to the vestibular nuclei; a small portion go to the thalamic nuclei. Projections from the flocculonodular area also use the inferior cerebellar peduncle to travel to the vestibular nuclei.

The **middle cerebellar peduncle** (Figure 1.9) is also known as the *brachium pontis* and is the largest of the three cerebellar peduncles. The greatest afferent contribution to the middle cerebellar peduncle comes from the pontocerebellar fibers, which convey impulses from the cortex to the cerebellum by way of the pontine nuclei.

The **superior cerebellar peduncle** (Figure 1.9) is also known as the *brachium conjunctivum* and sends impulses to the thalamus and spinal cord, with relays in the red nuclei. Three important afferent tracts lie in the superior cerebellar peduncle. The anterior spinocerebellar tract conveys impulses from stretch receptors, the trigeminocerebellar tract conveys stretch receptor information from the masticatory muscles, and the tectocerebellar fibers originate from the colliculi in the midbrain. Efferent output includes fibers from the dentate, emboliform, and globose nuclei, which travel to the upper pons and decussate (cross to the other side) at the level of the inferior colliculus. Most of these fibers end in the contralateral red nucleus in the midbrain. Information from the dentate neurons ultimately passes to the contralateral motor cortex via the thalamic nuclei.

Clinical correlations in the cerebellum are the result of fairly precise anatomic localization. The cerebellum provides information for gradual alterations of muscle tension for proper maintenance of equilibrium and posture, and it ensures the smooth and orderly sequence of muscle contractions that characterize skilled voluntary movements. Three rules of thumb can be used when evaluating pathological processes in the cerebellum: (1) cerebellar lesions produce ipsilateral disturbances, (2) cerebellar disturbances usually coexist with other related phenomena (i.e., primary degenerative disorders), and (3) extensive cerebellar lesions can cause minimal symptoms (except for lesions involving the deep nuclei) and nonprogressive pathological processes can show a gradual attenuation of symptoms over time.

Lesions in the hemispheres and dentate nuclei primarily affect skilled voluntary movements: hypotonia, in which muscles are easily fatigued; dyssynergia, in which the range, force, direction, or amplitude of muscle contractions are inappropriate; intention tremors; ataxia; nystagmus; and speech disturbances.

SUMMARY POINTS

1. Cerebellum and its deep nuclei mediate muscle coordination, tone, and equilibrium
2. Cerebellar dysfunction produces ipsilateral symptoms

Brainstem

Although physically occupying only a small volume of the CNS, the brainstem performs many functions that are necessary for life itself. In addition, all of the ascending and descending tracts between the cerebral cortices and the spinal cord and cerebellum pass through the brainstem; some of the tracts originate in various levels of the brainstem. Ten of the twelve cranial nerve nuclei originate in the brainstem.

Midbrain

The external anatomy of the midbrain is fairly uncomplicated. The midbrain extends from the pons to the mamillary bodies. Its dorsal surface contains four rounded elevations, the paired **inferior** and **superior colliculi** (see Figure 1.7, *B* and *C*). The colliculi form the "tectum" of the midbrain. The inferior colliculus is a relay nucleus along the auditory pathway; the superior colliculus is involved with voluntary control of ocular movements. The lateral surface of the midbrain is composed primarily of the **cerebral peduncles** (Figure 1.10, *D*).

With a cut section, some of the many internal structures of the midbrain may be seen. The portion of midbrain underlying the tectum is called the tegmentum. Below the colliculi the midbrain's portion of the ventricular system, the cerebral aqueduct, is found (Figure 1.10, *B*). Two cranial nerve nuclei lie in the tegmentum of the midbrain: the oculomotor nucleus (III) and the trochlear nucleus (IV). The paired **red nuclei** are rounded grey matter structures seen below the midbrain tectum. The red nucleus receives input from the cerebellum and sends fibers to the thalamus and spinal cord by the rubrospinal tract. The pigmented regions of the **substantia nigra** directly overlie the cerebral peduncles and are seen bilaterally (Figure 1.10, *C*). The substantia nigra receives afferent fibers from the cortex and basal ganglia; the efferent pathways from the substantia nigra are dopaminergic tracts to the basal ganglia. The cerebral peduncles (Figure 1.10, *D*) are densely myelinated white matter tracts that extend from both sides of the ventral surface of the midbrain. Tracts included in the cerebral peduncles are the corticospinal, corticobulbar, and corticopontine pathways.

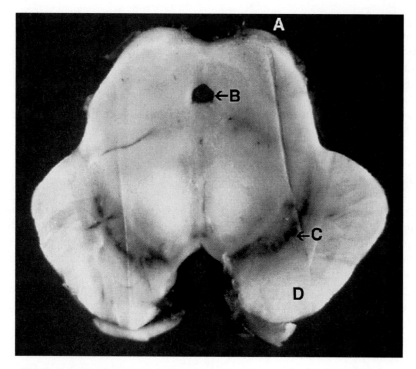

figure 1.10   Axial section of the midbrain. **A,** Superior colliculus. **B,** Cerebral aqueduct. **C,** Substantia nigra. **D,** Cerebral peduncles. *(Courtesy Dr. Cheryl A. Palmer, Division of Neuropathology, University of Alabama at Birmingham.)*

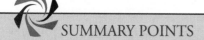

SUMMARY POINTS

1. Midbrain tectum: superior colliculi (vision) and inferior colliculi (hearing)
2. Midbrain tegmentum: substantia nigra, red nucleus, cranial nerve III nucleus, cranial nerve IV nucleus, cerebral peduncles

Pons

Externally, the pons consists of two distinctly different areas, the **basal pons** (basis pontis) and the **dorsal pons**. The pons itself is approximately 2.5 cm long, and the basilar sulcus runs along the ventral surface. The pons merges laterally with the middle cerebellar peduncles; the exit of cranial nerve V marks the transition site.

A sectioning of the pons demonstrates more of the basis pontis, which is located on the ventral surface and contains the pontine nuclei (Figure 1.11). These nuclei synapse with fibers from the ipsilateral cerebral cortex and serve as a large relay station to provide a connection between the cortex and the cerebellum. The basis pontis also contains the fiber bundles of the corticospinal tracts.

The dorsal pons (the pontine tegmentum) contains the fourth ventricle (Figure 1.11, *A*) and the ascending and descending tracts and nuclei of cranial nerves V (the chief sensory nucleus), VI, and VII. In addition, the central tegmental tract (which runs from the thalami to the inferior olivary nuclei), the tectospinal tract (which runs from the midbrain to the cervical spinal cord), and the medial longitudinal fasciculus travel through the pontine tegmentum. A small pigmented nucleus is present bilaterally and is lo-

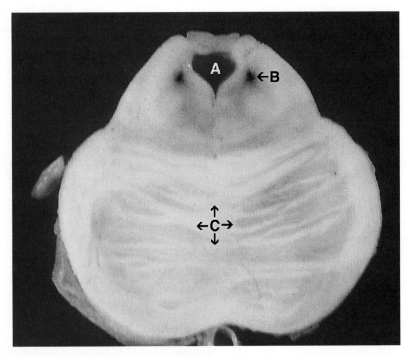

figure 1.11   Axial section of the pons. **A,** Fourth ventricle. **B,** Locus ceruleus. **C,** Basis pontis. *(Courtesy Dr. Cheryl A. Palmer, Division of Neuropathology, University of Alabama at Birmingham.)*

cated at the corners of the fourth ventricle in the pontine tegmentum. The neurons in this nucleus contain neuromelanin; it is called the **locus ceruleus** ("blue place") because the anatomists who named it initially identified it under a small strip of brain parenchyma, where it appeared blue in color (Figure 1.11, *B*). The neurons in the locus ceruleus are the major source of norepinephrine production in the brain (see Chapter 3).

Medulla

The medulla (see Figure 1.8, *E*) is approximately 3 cm in length. The junction of the medulla with the cervical spinal cord is fairly indistinct grossly but occurs at the exit of the first cervical nerve at the level of the foramen magnum. The rostral border with the pons is quite evident. On the ventral side, the ventral median fissure is continuous with that of the spinal cord and is interrupted only by the pyramidal decussation. The lateral border of the pyramids is the bilateral ventrolateral sulci, the point of exit of cranial nerve XII. Lateral to the ventrolateral sulci are the olives, externally marking the position of the inferior olivary nuclei. Just dorsal to the olives are the exits of cranial nerves IX, X, and XI. The fasciculus gracilis and cuneatus continue in the same position as in the spinal cord. On the dorsal aspect of the medulla, the apex of the V-shaped boundary at the inferior portion of the fourth ventricle is called the obex (see Figure 1.7, *E*).

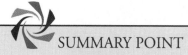

SUMMARY POINT

Medulla ⇒ nuclei of cranial nerves IX, X, XI, and XII; inferior olivary nucleus

Cranial Nerves

Olfactory Nerve (I)

Olfactory cells are found in the epithelium of the nasal cavity and have unmyelinated axons that constitute the olfactory nerves. The olfactory nerves pass through the cribriform plate and enter the olfactory bulb. Impulses from the olfactory bulb traverse down the olfactory tract to the olfactory areas in the cerebral cortex.

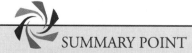

SUMMARY POINT

Cranial nerve I ⇒ neurons in nasal cavity; responsible for olfaction

Optic Nerve (II)

Fibers originating from ganglion cell neurons in the right halves of both retinas traverse through the bilateral optic nerves and partially cross in the optic chiasm (see Figure 1.4, *A, B,* and *C*). The output from the optic chiasm is referred to as the optic tracts, which terminate in the right LGB. Impulses are then transmitted to the visual cortex in the right hemisphere. A contralateral projection also exists. Therefore the left visual field is represented in the right LGB and in the right hemisphere of the visual cortex, and vice versa. The upper half of the visual field is represented in the lateral portion of the LGB and in the visual cortex below the calcarine sulcus; the lower half of the visual field is represented in the medial portion of the LGB and in the visual cortex above the calcarine sulcus.

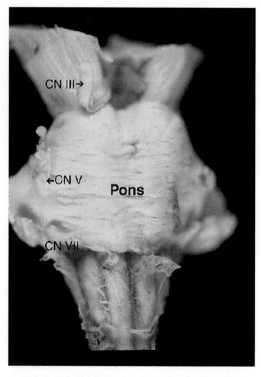

figure 1.12   Brainstem from its dorsal aspect and some of the exit sites of the cranial nerves. *(Courtesy Dr. Richard E. Powers, Director, University of Alabama at Birmingham Brain Resource Program.)*

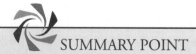

SUMMARY POINT

Cranial nerve II ⇒ neurons in retina; responsible for vision

Oculomotor Nerve (III)

The oculomotor nucleus is situated in the periaqueductal grey matter of the midbrain, ventral to the aqueduct at the level of the superior colliculus. Myelinated axons curve ventrally through the tegmentum; many pass through the red nucleus. The nerve emerges along the sides of the interpeduncular fossa (Figure 1.12). Fibers are both crossed and uncrossed. The Edinger-Westphal nucleus is dorsal to the rostral two thirds of the oculomotor nucleus. These fibers accompany other oculomotor fibers into the lateral wall of the cavernous sinus, leaving the cranial cavity via the superior orbital fissure. The nerve then enters the orbit, where it terminates on the ciliary ganglion.

Lesions of cranial nerve III cause paralysis of all extraocular muscles except the superior oblique and the lateral rectus. This paralysis causes lateral strabismus because of the unopposed action of the lateral rectus; it also causes ptosis because of the cranial nerve III innervation of the levator palpebrae. Interruption of the parasympathetic fibers from the Edinger-Westphal nucleus (e.g., by anticholinergic drugs) causes mydriasis and a lack of pupillary constriction to light.

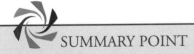

SUMMARY POINT

Cranial nerve III ⇒ neurons in midbrain; responsible for eye movement

Trochlear Nerve (IV)

The trochlear nerve innervates the superior oblique muscle and is the only completely crossed cranial nerve. The trochlear nucleus is immediately caudal to the oculomotor nucleus at the level of the inferior colliculus in the midbrain. The trochlear nerve is the only cranial nerve to emerge from the dorsal aspect of the brainstem. Small nerve fiber bundles curve around the periaqueductal grey and decussate with the opposite side fibers. This slender nerve emerges caudally to the inferior colliculus and continues in the lateral wall of the cavernous sinus. It enters the orbit via the superior orbital fissure. The superior oblique muscle is then supplied by crossed fibers.

The function of the superior oblique muscle is to rotate and depress the eyeball. Paralysis of cranial nerve IV causes vertical diplopia, in which the two images are on top of each other; vertical diplopia is maximal when the eye is directed downward and inward. Isolated lesions of this nerve are rare. Patients may complain of difficulty reading or walking down stairs.

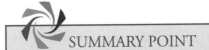

SUMMARY POINT

Cranial nerve IV ⇒ neurons in midbrain; responsible for eye movement

Trigeminal Nerve (V)

The trigeminal nerve (see Figure 1.12) is the principal sensory nerve of the head and is the motor nerve for the muscles of mastication. Several nuclei are integrated into the trigeminal system, including the chief sensory nucleus, the spinal nucleus of the trigeminal nerve, the mesencephalic nucleus, and the motor nucleus.

The sensory portion of the trigeminal nerve has cell bodies that are primarily in the trigeminal (semilunar or gasserian) ganglion. The trigeminal ganglion is located in the dura mater lateral to the cavernous sinus, which is anatomically called Meckel's cave. The projections of these neurons form branches of V_1 (**ophthalmic**), V_2 (**maxillary**), and V_3 (**mandibular**). Cranial nerve V_1 enters the cranial vault through the superior orbital fissure. Fibers of cranial nerve V_2 traverse the foramen rotundum in the skull base. Sensory fibers of cranial nerve V_3, as well as the motor fibers, pass through the foramen ovale, which is also in the skull base. The trigeminal nerve is responsible for sensation from the skin of the face, forehead, and scalp back to the vertex (the top of the skull), the oral and nasal mucosa, the paranasal sinuses, and the teeth. It also contributes sensory fibers to most of the dura mater. Some axons that arise from the trigeminal ganglion enter the pons and terminate in the chief sensory nucleus in the dorsolateral pons. These afferents mediate light touch and travel to the thalamus. Other axons that arise from the trigeminal ganglion and mediate pain and temperature information turn caudally after entering the pons and form the spinal trigeminal tract. Some of these axons travel down to spinal cord segment C3 and intermingle with the dorsolateral tract of Lissauer (discussed more fully in the spinal cord section). Efferent fibers from the sensory trigeminal nuclei are primarily directed to the thalamus via the ventral trigeminothalamic tract. This tract mediates the efferent portion of the corneal reflex.

The motor nucleus of the trigeminal nerve is situated medially to the chief sensory nucleus in the pons. The motor root is the bulk of the V_3 branch. The motor nucleus receives afferents from the corticobulbar tract and has reflex connections with the spinal tract of the trigeminal nerve. It innervates most of the muscles of mastication, as well as the tensor tympani muscle of the middle ear.

Numerous clinical correlations occur with lesions in the trigeminal system. **Trigeminal neuralgia** (tic douloureux) is characterized by paroxysms of pain in the areas of one of the divisions. The maxillary division is most commonly affected, followed by the mandibular and, finally, the ophthalmic. The paroxysms are usually set off by mild facial stimulation. Interruption of the motor portions of cranial nerve V by pathological processes causes paralysis and eventual atrophy of the muscles of mastication. The mandible eventually deviates to the affected side secondary to unopposed action of the lateral pterygoid muscle. Additionally, diminished hearing can occur with paralysis of the tensor tympani muscle. Sensory abnormalities can also occur with pathological processes in the sensory portions of cranial nerve V in the distribution of the affected nerve, such as loss of the corneal reflex.

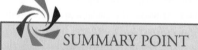

SUMMARY POINT

Cranial nerve V ⇒ neurons in four different nuclei; responsible for facial sensation, corneal reflex, masticatory muscle movement

Abducens Nerve (VI)

The abducens nerve supplies the lateral rectus muscle and is situated beneath the facial colliculus in the floor of the fourth ventricle in the pons. The motor axons pass through the pons and

emerge from the brainstem at the junction of the pons and the pyramid. The nerve passes through the cavernous sinus near the internal carotid artery and exits through the superior orbital fissure.

A palsy of cranial nerve VI is fairly common because of the long intracranial course of the nerve. Convergent strabismus (a deviation of one or both eyes) and diplopia can occur.

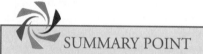

SUMMARY POINT

Cranial nerve VI ⇒ neurons in pons; responsible for eye movement

Facial Nerve (VII)

The facial nerve (see Figure 1.12) contains sensory components of taste and of sensation to part of the external ear, controls lacrimation, and contains motor components supplying the facial muscles of expression. Three separate nuclei are associated with the facial nerve: the facial nucleus and the superior salivatory nucleus (parasympathetic), which are both located in the pons, and the nucleus solitarius in the medulla, which is shared by cranial nerves VII, IX, and X.

The sensory portion of cranial nerve VII is composed of taste buds in the anterior two thirds of the tongue. These taste buds form the peripheral processes of cells in the geniculate ganglion, which lies in the internal auditory meatus. Axons from these cell bodies enter the brainstem via the sensory root of cranial nerve VII (the nervus intermedius) and turn caudally in the tractus solitarius. Ascending fibers from the nucleus solitarius reach the ipsilateral ventral posterior nucleus in the thalamus via the central tegmental tract.

The facial nucleus is located in the caudal third of the pontine tegmentum and accounts for the majority of the motor contribution to the facial nerve. Fibers from this nucleus take an unusual course; they head toward the floor of the fourth ventricle, form a loop over the abducens nucleus, course back through the pons, and exit on the ventral pons. The nerve exits the cranial cavity via the stylomastoid foramen. The frontalis and orbicularis oculi muscles have bilateral facial nerve input, whereas the lower part of the face has only contralateral input.

Therefore total paralysis of half of the face results from a lower motor neuron lesion (i.e., a Bell's palsy) and occurs after the nerve has received its uncrossed fibers. A "central" cranial nerve VII palsy is an upper motor neuron lesion at the level of the brainstem and causes weakness of the muscles of the face below the frontalis and orbicularis oculi muscles.

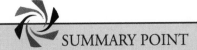

SUMMARY POINT

Cranial nerve VII ⇒ neurons in three different nuclei; responsible for facial movement and some aspects of sensation and taste

Auditory/Vestibulocochlear Nerve (VIII)

The auditory/vestibulocochlear nerve is a complex nerve that arises from the spiral and vestibular ganglia in the labyrinth of the inner ear. The nerve enters the cranial vault through the internal acoustic meatus and then enters the brainstem at the junction of the pons and medulla. The cochlear portion of the nerve, which is concerned with hearing, travels to the two cochlear nuclei, which act as relay nuclei in the auditory pathway. The vestibular portion of the nerve mediates the system of equilibrium and travels to the vestibular nuclear complex, which consists of four nuclei and is situated in the rostral medulla. The vestibular nuclear complex projects to the flocculonodular lobe and the cerebellar nuclei via the inferior cerebellar peduncle.

Dysfunction of cranial nerve VIII causes many different symptoms. Tinnitus, which is characterized by a ringing or roaring in the ear, may be an early sign of peripheral cochlear disease. Deafness in one ear can be caused by impaired sound conduction through the external ear canal and ossicles to the endolymph (conduction deafness). Sensorineural (or nerve) deafness can be caused by the interruption of cochlear nerve fibers from the ear to the brainstem nuclei. A cerebellopontine angle tumor usually diminishes the function of both the vestibular and the cochlear branches.

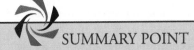

SUMMARY POINT

Cranial nerve VIII ⇒ neurons in medulla; responsible for hearing and equilibrium

Glossopharyngeal Nerve (IX)/Vagus Nerve (X)/Spinal Accessory Nerve (XI)

The glossopharyngeal, vagus, and spinal accessory nerves are considered together because they share common brainstem nuclei, including the nucleus ambiguus, the nucleus solitarius, the inferior salivatory nucleus, and the dorsal nucleus of the vagus (all of which are in the medulla), as well as the spinal accessory nucleus.

The afferent components of cranial nerves IX and X include sensory fibers for taste from the posterior third of the tongue, as well as general sensory afferents for pain, temperature, and touch from the pharynx. Also contained are general visceral afferents from the thoracic viscera, abdominal viscera, and carotid body. Taste fibers, with their cell bodies in the inferior ganglion, terminate in the nucleus solitarius. Fibers from the carotid sinus (IX), and baroreceptors and chemoreceptors in the aortic arch (X), also have their cell bodies in the inferior ganglion and terminate in the nucleus solitarius. Sensation from the pharynx and larynx, with cell bodies in the superior ganglion, travel to the spinal trigeminal tract. This pathway mediates the gag reflex.

Cranial nerves IX, X, and XI provide efferent motor fibers for striated musculature. Cranial nerves IX and X also provide parasympathetic efferents. The nucleus ambiguus is dorsal to the inferior olivary nucleus in the medulla. Fibers exit dorsally and join with other fibers of cranial nerves IX, X, and XI. The nucleus ambiguus supplies muscles of the soft palate, pharynx, larynx, and upper esophagus. Motor neurons of cranial nerve XI supply the trapezius and sternocleido-mastoid muscles and have their cell bodies in the spinal accessory nucleus, which is located in the ventral horn of spinal cord segments C1 to C5. This series of rootlets ascend rostrally and enter the skull base through the foramen magnum. The rootlets merge along the side of the medulla and exit via the jugular foramen to innervate the con-tralateral trapezius and sternocleidomastoid mus-cles.

Fibers in cranial nerves IX and X also accom-modate parasympathetic components. The infe-rior salivatory nucleus contains the origins for some of these fibers. This nucleus supplies the parotid gland. The largest parasympathetic nu-cleus is the dorsal nucleus of the vagus, which ex-tends throughout most of the medulla beneath the floor of the fourth ventricle. Axons from this nucleus supply the abdominal viscera.

Separate and isolated lesions of cranial nerves IX, X, or XI are uncommon. Lesions that can cause destruction of the central nuclei are most commonly of vascular origin. Unilateral lesions of the nucleus ambiguus cause an ipsilateral paralysis of the palate, pharynx, and larynx, with hoarse-ness, respiratory difficulties, and dysphagia. Le-sions of the accessory nerve or nucleus cause con-tralateral weakness of the sternocleidomastoid or trapezius muscles.

SUMMARY POINT

Cranial nerves IX, X, XI ⇒ neurons in nu-merous nuclei in medulla and cervical spinal cord; responsible for taste, gag re-flex, some somatic muscle function, sali-vation, function of autonomic systems

Hypoglossal Nerve (XII)

The hypoglossal nucleus lies between the dorsal nucleus of the vagus and the midline of the medulla. The hypoglossal fibers course ventrally on the lateral edge of the medial lemniscus and emerge along the sulcus between the pyramid and olive; these fibers exit the cranial cavity via the hy-poglossal canal. The hypoglossal nucleus also has central connections with the corticobulbar sys-tem. Cranial nerve XII supplies motor compo-nents to the tongue and several extrinsic muscles.

A unilateral upper motor neuron lesion causes contralateral weakness because the corticobulbar input to the hypoglossal nucleus is primarily crossed. The tongue therefore deviates to the weak side because of unopposed action on the opposite side. A lower motor neuron lesion has the oppo-site effect.

SUMMARY POINT

Cranial nerve XII ⇒ neurons in medulla; responsible for tongue movement

Spinal Cord

Evaluation of the external anatomy of the spinal cord reveals a cylindrical structure that is slightly flattened dorsoventrally. It is protected by vertebrae, ligaments, meninges, and CSF, and it is suspended in the dural sheath by tiny den-ticulate ligaments on each side. The rostral end of the spinal cord is continuous with the medulla at the cervicomedullary junction (see Figure 1.8, D); the caudal end, called the *conus medullaris*, is found in adults at approximately L1 (range T12 to L3). From that level, the cauda equina begins and the cord tapers into the filum terminale, which contains pia mater and neuroglia but has no func-tional significance.

The spinal cord is generally divided function-ally into approximately 30 segments, which corre-late with the 31 pairs of spinal nerves: 8 cervical (C), 12 thoracic (T), 5 lumbar (L), 5 sacral (S), and 1 coccygeal (Figure 1.13). Spinal nerves C1 to C7 leave the spinal canal above the corre-sponding vertebrae. The C8 nerve leaves under-neath the C7 vertebrae. From that point caudally, the spinal nerves exit under their corresponding vertebrae. At each spinal level, the dorsal roots

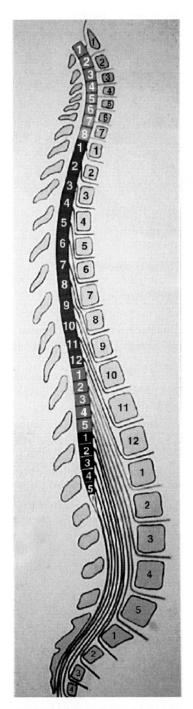

figure 1.13   Levels of the spine, the spinal roots, and their exits. *(From Waxman SG: Correlative neuroanatomy, ed 23, Stanford, Conn, 1991, Appleton & Lange.)*

(which transmit sensory information) and the ventral roots (which transmit motor information) join to form the dorsal root ganglion; the lengths of the roots increase caudally because of the increased distance from the cord segments and the vertebral bodies.

The spinal cord is enlarged in diameter at the cervical region (C4 to T1) for innervation of the upper extremities and from L2 to S3 for innervation of the lower extremities. The surface of the spinal cord is marked by sulci and fissures that define the surface anatomy (Figure 1.14). The ventral (anterior) median fissure contains the anterior spinal artery. The dorsal (posterior) median sulcus separates the right from the left dorsally. The posterolateral sulcus separates the dorsal areas at the midthoracic levels bilaterally; medial to the posterolateral sulcus is the fasciculus gracilis, and lateral to this sulcus is the fasciculus cuneatus. The anterolateral sulcus, in the ventral portion of the spinal cord, marks the exit of the ventral nerve roots.

The grey matter of the spinal cord can be seen in cut sections. In transverse sections, the grey matter of the spinal cord resembles a butterfly (Figure 1.14). It consists of dorsal horns, ventral horns, and an intermediate zone that is sometimes referred to as the grey matter commissure. In levels T1 to L2 there is a small lateral horn. The volume of grey matter changes at various levels of the spinal cord; the ratio between the volume of grey matter and white matter also changes. For example, because the white matter carries information to and from the brain, the volume of white matter is far greater in the cervical cord than in the sacral cord.

The ventral (or anterior) horn is located in front of the central canal. The neurons contained in this structure are referred to as alpha motor neurons, or anterior horn cells. These neurons are the motor neurons that supply information to the ventral roots.

The dorsal horn of the grey matter extends nearly to the posterolateral sulcus, which is slightly lateral to the dorsal intermediate sulcus. This region receives information from the dorsal root. A small bundle of compact fibers known as

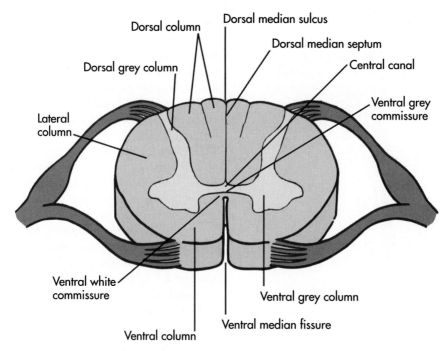

Dorsal median sulcus
Dorsal column
Dorsal median septum
Dorsal grey column
Central canal
Lateral column
Ventral grey commissure
Ventral white commissure
Ventral grey column
Ventral median fissure
Ventral column

figure 1.14   Cross section through the spinal cord and its various structures. *(From Waxman SG: Correlative neuroanatomy, ed 23, Stanford, Conn, 1991, Appleton & Lange.)*

Lissauer's tract, functionally a portion of the pain pathway, lies at the edge of the spinal cord at the end of the dorsal horn.

The grey matter commissure (Figure 1.14) joins the left and right sides of the grey matter of the spinal cord and contains the remnants of the central canal. The intermediolateral grey column is a small lateral projection that is seen between the dorsal and ventral horns. It is present from the T1 through L2 levels and contains neurons that function in the autonomic system.

The white matter of the spinal cord (Figure 1.14) consists of three columns (funiculi): the dorsal column, the lateral funiculus, and the ventral funiculus. The dorsal column carries proprioceptive and vibratory sensation and is located between the posterolateral sulcus and the posterior median sulcus. The lateral funiculus, which carries the major motor pathway (the corticospinal tract), lies between the posterolateral sulcus and the anterolateral sulcus. The ventral funiculus is seen between the anterior median fissure and the anterolateral sulcus.

The central canal of the spinal cord (Figure 1.14) is an extension of the fourth ventricle in the brainstem. Although it is functionally open dur-

ing childhood, it is generally closed in adults.

The dorsal nerve roots (Figure 1.14) enter the spinal cord at the posterolateral sulcus. The ventral nerve roots exit the spinal cord in the anterolateral sulcus, which is lateral to the ventral median fissure.

Many connections are made between the spinal cord and the remainder of the CNS. The afferent sensory fibers enter the spinal cord via the dorsal roots of spinal nerves, and the efferent motor fibers exit via the ventral roots of spinal nerves. This information is transmitted to the brainstem, cerebellum, and thalamus. From the thalamus, this information is transmitted to the cortex, where it becomes part of conscious experience.

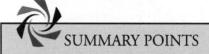

SUMMARY POINTS

1. Spine is divided into 30 segments, with 31 pairs of spinal nerves
2. Ventral horn ⇒ motor function
3. Dorsal horn ⇒ sensory function

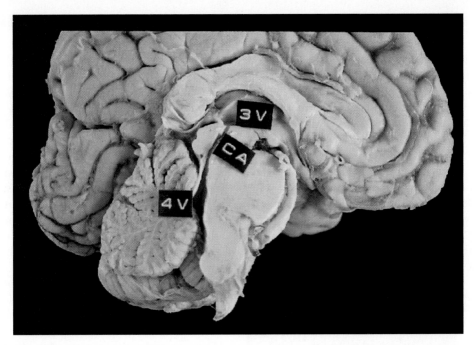

figure 1.15   Sagittal view of the brain, in its midsection. *3v,* Third ventricle; *CA,* cerebral aqueduct; *4v,* fourth ventricle. *(Courtesy Dr. Richard E. Powers, Director, University of Alabama at Birmingham Brain Resource Program.)*

Ventricular System

Within the brain substance is a communicating system of cavities that are lined with ependyma and filled with CSF. These cavities are separated into the two lateral ventricles, the third ventricle, the cerebral aqueduct, and the fourth ventricle.

Lateral Ventricles

The butterfly-shaped lateral ventricles (see Figure 1.5, *G*) are the largest of the ventricles and contain numerous horns. The **frontal** (or anterior) **horn** is in the frontal lobe of the brain. The roof and anterior border of the frontal horn are formed by the corpus callosum. The right and left anterior horns are separated by the **septum pellucidum**, and the floor and lateral wall are formed by the caudate nucleus. The **occipital horn** of the lateral ventricle extends into the occipital lobe. The roof of the occipital horn is also formed by the corpus callosum. The **temporal** (inferior) **horn** of the lateral ventricle is bordered at its roof by the white matter of the temporal lobe. Portions of the medial border are formed by the tail of the

caudate nucleus. The largest portion of the floor is composed of the hippocampal formation. The two lateral ventricles communicate with the third ventricle via the **foramina of Monro**, also known as the intraventricular foramina.

Third Ventricle

The narrow third ventricle (Figure 1.15) is located between the two halves of the diencephalon. Its lateral walls are formed primarily by the thalami, and the lower lateral wall and floor are formed by the hypothalamus.

Cerebral Aqueduct

The slender cerebral aqueduct (see Figures 1.10, *B* and 1.15) is a narrow, curved channel that is located in the midbrain and runs between the posterior third ventricle into the fourth ventricle.

Fourth Ventricle

The floor of the fourth ventricle (see Figure 1.15) is broad in its midportion; it narrows toward the cerebral aqueduct in the midbrain at its superior aspect and in the obex of the medulla at its inferior aspect (see Figure 1.7, *E*). The floor of the fourth ventricle is divided in half by the median sulcus; the sulcus limitans further divides each half into medial and lateral areas. The lateral areas lie above the vestibular nuclei, and the motor nuclei lie beneath the medial areas. A deficiency in the membrane of the roof of the fourth ventricle constitutes the **foramen of Magendie**, which is the principal communication between the ventricular system and the subarachnoid space. The lateral walls of the fourth ventricle contain the **foramina of Luschka**, which are situated at the cerebellopontine angles.

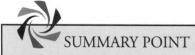

SUMMARY POINTS

1. CSF pathway: lateral ventricle ⇒ foramen of Monro ⇒ third ventricle ⇒ cerebral aqueduct ⇒ fourth ventricle ⇒ foramina of Magendie and Luschka ⇒ subarachnoid space ⇒ arachnoid granulations ⇒ venous sinuses
2. Lateral ventricle: anterior, temporal, occipital horns

Cerebrospinal Fluid

Production

The normal volume of CSF in the adult is approximately 140 mL. In normal conditions, approximately 20 mL/hour is produced and absorbed (approximately 500 mL/day). The majority of CSF is formed by the choroid plexus and involves two distinct processes: filtration through the fenestrated (slit-like openings) capillaries of the choroid plexus, followed by active secretion by the epithelium.

SUMMARY POINT

CSF volume 140 mL; production 20 mL/hr; formed by choroid plexus

Function

The CSF has many functions. One function is to provide physical support for the brain. When suspended in CSF, a 1500-g brain (which normally has a water content of 80%) weighs only 50 g; this difference reflects the specific gravity of the brain and CSF. The CSF is also important in protecting the brain from the acute changes in central venous pressure that are associated with postural and respiratory changes, as well as from alterations in arterial and pulse pressure. In addition, the absence of a lymphatic system in the brain indicates that the products of brain metabolism may be removed by only two routes—capillary blood flow or transfer into the CSF—which allow removal by bulk flow reabsorption or by the choroid plexus. The individual contribution of these two systems is still uncertain.

There is substantial evidence that the CSF serves as an intracerebral transporter to distribute biologically active substances within the CNS. CSF of the third ventricle serves as a path for diffusing releasing factors from cells of origin in the hypothalamus to the effective sites.

The CSF assists in control of the chemical environment of the CNS by contributing to the role of the blood-brain barrier. The CSF helps regulate the composition of the extracellular fluid of the brain in both normal and pathological conditions.

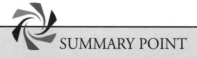

SUMMARY POINT

CSF function ⇒ physical support, transport of nutrients and waste products

Cerebrospinal Fluid Pressure

The pressure level within the right atrium represents the baseline level in measuring the lumbar CSF pressure. The level of CSF pressure is greatly affected by postural influences on central venous pressure: normal values assume that the craniovertebral axis is horizontal. The normal lumbar CSF pressure ranges between 50 mm and 200 mm

table 1.2

CSF Composition Under Normal and Selected Pathological Processes

	NORMAL ADULT	NORMAL NEONATE	PURULENT MENINGITIS	VIRAL MENINGITIS	MULTIPLE SCLEROSIS
Cell count	0-4/mm³	8-9/mm³	↑↑↑	↑	↑ or normal
Protein	20-45 mg/dL	<150 mg/dL	↑↑	↑	↑ or normal
Glucose	45-80 mg/dL	50-90 mg/dL	↓	Normal	Normal

↑, Small increase; ↑↑, moderate increase; ↑↑↑, substantial increase; ↓, decrease.

H₂O in most clinical reports, with an average of approximately 150 mm. This pressure varies with heartbeat and respiration.

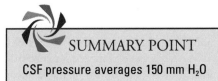

SUMMARY POINT

CSF pressure averages 150 mm H₂O

Appearance

The CSF is normally crystal clear and colorless. In the normal neonate, the CSF is usually xanthochromic (yellow-tinged).

Cellular Content

Normal adult CSF contains no more than 4 lymphocytes or mononuclear cells per cubic mm (Table 1.2). Neutrophils should not be present in normal adult CSF. The normal cell counts are increased in both premature and term neonates; they average 8 to 9 white blood cells per cubic mm.

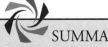

SUMMARY POINT

CSF cellular count ⇒ <4 mononuclear cells; no neutrophils in adults; 8-9 white blood cells in neonates

Proteins

Almost all proteins normally present in CSF are derived from the serum. Protein entry into the CSF from the serum probably depends on pinocytosis across the capillary endothelial cells of the brain and spinal cord. Normal mean total protein in CSF is 35 mg/dL (Table 1.2); the majority consists of albumin. The most widely accepted normal range for CSF protein is between 20 and 45 mg/dL. An increase in CSF protein (up to 150 mg/dL) is generally seen in the normal neonate and is thought to be a result of the immaturity of the blood-brain barrier. Normal levels are reached during the first few months of life. A low lumbar spinal fluid protein, ranging between 3 and 20 mg/dL, occurs normally in young children between 6 months and 2 years of age.

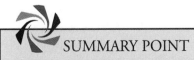

SUMMARY POINT

CSF protein is 20-45 mg/dL in adults; up to 150 mg/dL in neonates

Glucose

The transfer of glucose between blood and CSF, as well as between the blood and brain, depends on carrier transport (facilitated diffusion). The CSF concentration of glucose (Table 1.2) is approximately 60% of the blood glucose in adults in the steady state. The normal range of glucose in

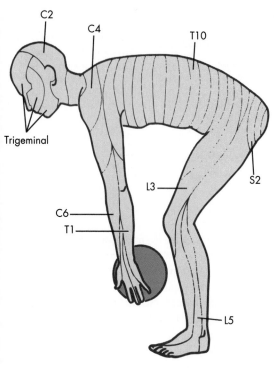

figure 1.16   Different dermatomes innervated by the various spinal nerves. *(From Waxman SG:* Correlative neuroanatomy, *ed 23, Stanford, Conn, 1991, Appleton & Lange.)*

the CSF of adults (with a blood glucose between 70 and 120 mg/dL) is between 45 and 80 mg/dL. In neonates, the glucose level in the CSF more closely approximates the blood glucose level. The need for glucose by the brain is largely supplied by the circulation, not the CSF. The glucose content of the ventricular fluid is usually higher than that of the cisternal fluid, and the glucose content in the latter is slightly higher than that in the lumbar fluid.

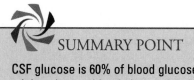

SUMMARY POINT

CSF glucose is 60% of blood glucose in adults; close to blood glucose level in neonates

Peripheral Nervous System

The peripheral nerves anatomically begin at their point of exit from the dura mater.

Sensory Functions

The sensory information carried by the peripheral nerves is organized via a dermatomal system. A *dermatome* is a defined area of the skin that correlates with the level of the spinal nerve. The most rostral dermatome is the portion subserved by the trigeminal nerve, and the remaining segments proceeding caudally are C2 through S5 (Figure 1.16). Because there is some overlap in dermatomal territories, absence of function in a single segment may be difficult to ascertain.

Motor Functions

The motor information carried by the peripheral nerves involves innervations to numerous striated muscle groups. Tables that compile these nerve-muscle groupings can be found in any standard neurology textbook.

Vascular System

Approximately 18% of the total blood volume in the body circulates in the brain and accounts for approximately 2% of the body weight. The blood transports oxygen, nutrients, and other substances necessary for proper functioning of the brain tissues, and it carries away metabolites. Loss of consciousness occurs less than 1 minute after blood flow to the brain has stopped, and irreparable damage to brain tissues can occur within 3 to 5 minutes.

Arterial System

The arterial system of the brain inside the cranial vault is called the **circle of Willis** (Figure 1.17). The circle of Willis shows many normal variations among individuals. As mentioned previously, the arteries course in the subarachnoid space before entering the brain; therefore rupture of a vessel can cause a subarachnoid hemorrhage.

Each major artery supplies a certain territory of the brain; each territory is separated from other territories by boundary zones called *watershed areas.* Separate circulations arise from the internal carotid artery, called the **anterior circulation** of the brain, and from the subclavian arteries, known as the **posterior circulation** of the brain. The major divisions of the anterior circulation are the **internal carotid arteries** and the **anterior** and **middle cerebral arteries**; the major divisions of the posterior circulation are the **posterior cerebral, basilar,** and **vertebral arteries.** Distinct brain territories are subserved by these different arteries. Communicating vessels such as the **anterior communicating** and **posterior communicating arteries** connect various portions of the circulation.

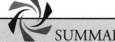

SUMMARY POINTS

1. Internal cerebral artery, anterior cerebral artery, middle cerebral artery ⇒ anterior circulation
2. Posterior cerebral artery, basilar artery, vertebral artery ⇒ posterior circulation

Venous System

The venous drainage of the brain and coverings includes the veins of the brain itself, the dural venous sinuses, the meningeal veins of the dura mater, and the diploic veins between the tables (layers) of the skull. Most of these channels communicate in some fashion with each other. Unlike systemic veins, cerebral veins have no valves and do not accompany the cerebral arteries throughout their course.

The interior of the cerebrum drains into the midline great cerebral vein of Galen, which lies beneath the splenium of the corpus callosum. The internal cerebral veins and the basal veins of Rosenthal drain into the vein of Galen. Some of the veins drain into the sinuses themselves, including the straight sinus, the lateral sinus, and the sagittal sinus. The sinuses form a confluence, which ultimately drains into the internal jugular vein.

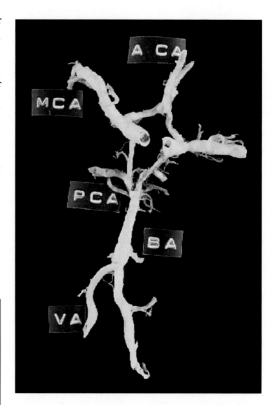

figure 1.17   Circle of Willis, removed from the ventral aspect of the brain. *ACA,* Anterior cerebral artery; *MCA,* middle cerebral artery; *PCA,* posterior cerebral artery; *BA,* basilar artery; *VA,* vertebral artery. *(Courtesy Dr. Richard E. Powers, Director, University of Alabama at Birmingham Brain Resource Program.)*

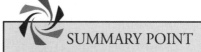

SUMMARY POINT

Veins and dural venous sinuses drain back into systemic circulation via internal jugular vein

BIBLIOGRAPHY

1. Barr ML, Kiernan JA: *The human nervous system: an anatomical viewpoint,* ed 4, Philadelphia, 1983, Harper & Row.
2. Carpenter MB, Sutin J: *Human neuroanatomy,* ed 8, Baltimore, 1983, Williams & Wilkins.
3. deGroot J: *Correlative neuroanatomy,* ed 21, San Mateo, Calif, 1991, Appleton & Lange.

Microscopic Anatomy of the Brain

This chapter focuses on understanding the normal histological characteristics and cellular reactions of the constituents of the central nervous system (CNS). With a recognition of brain substructure, it is hoped that the neuropathology encountered in upcoming chapters will be more easily recognized. The simplest way to present this material is to differentiate the cellular constituents of the CNS.

Pathological expertise has improved enormously in the past few decades as a result of the explosion of new microscopic techniques. Information in the field of **neurocytology** (the study of cells in the nervous system) has been accumulated by varying the staining methods for looking at cells under the microscope. More recently, the development of immunohistochemistry and electron microscopy has enabled detailed study of the subcellular components of cells.

Neurocytological Staining and Microscopic Techniques

Hematoxylin and Eosin

The routine stain in most of pathology, the hematoxylin and eosin (H&E) stain is still the standard baseline view relied on by neuropathologists for basic information. Hematoxylin stains nuclei a bluish-purple color; eosin stains cytoplasm and neuropil (the matrix of the brain) pinkish-red.

Cationic Dyes

Cationic dyes such as cresyl violet and toluidine blue bind to nucleic acids. They therefore assist in the identification of nuclei, nucleoli, and Nissl substance (discussed later in this chapter) in neurons.

Reduced Silver Stains

Reduced silver stains produce deposits of dark colloidal silver in various structures. The most common reduced silver stains in use today include Bielschowsky's, Bodian's, and Seiver-Munger stains. These stains are typically used for the identification of various nervous system cell substructures, including neurofibrillary tangles and axons.

Stains for Myelin

Myelin stains reveal the major fiber tracts, except for the few that consist completely of unmyelinated axons. Stains commonly used to evaluate myelin include Weigert's stain and the Luxol fast blue stain.

Histochemical and Immunocytochemical Methods

Various methods are available (some more so in research laboratories) for localizing substances contained in various subpopulations of all types of cells, including neurons. These substances include neurotransmitters such as norepinephrine, dopamine, and serotonin (see Chapter 3), as well as the enzymes involved in the synthesis or degradation of these neurotransmitters, such as dopamine β-hydroxylase, choline acetyltransferase, and acetylcholinesterase. By colorimetric methods, the presence or absence of various proteins and hormones also can be demonstrated.

Electron Microscopy

Electron microscopy reveals far finer structural detail than light microscopy. Electron density is imparted to the specimen by impregnating it with metal compounds of high atomic number, such as osmium, lead, or uranium. This method enables study of the detailed intracellular structures of neurons and of the specializations existing at their synaptic junctions (see the following sections).

Normal Cellular Histology
Neurons
Neuronal Anatomy

Estimations of the number of neurons in the human cerebral cortex vary widely as a result of the technical difficulties encountered in their enumeration. The numbers range from 2.6 to 14 billion neurons, which indicates that even though exact estimates are unavailable, the actual numbers of cortical neurons are enormous. Neurons assume a great variety of shapes and sizes. This fact makes it difficult to define the morphological characteristics of a typical neuron. Nevertheless, some characteristics are shared by all neurons. The processes (projections) of neurons contain neurofibrils that are composed of thin neurofilaments. The part of the neuron that accepts incoming signals is called the **dendrite**, whereas the portion of the neuron that transmits signals is called the **axon**. Each neuron has only one axon, but differing numbers of dendrites are possible. "Multipolar" neurons have multiple dendrites, "bipolar" neurons have two dendrites, and "unipolar" neurons have only one dendrite.

The portion of the neuron that contains the nucleus is referred to as the **cell body**; the cytoplasm of the cell, not including the processes, is called the **perikaryon**. The active end of a neuron, where neurotransmitters are released, is called the **synaptic terminal**. Large neurons, such as the pyramidal (Betz's) cells of the motor cortex, the Purkinje cells of the cerebellum, and the anterior horn cells of the spinal cord contain large, rounded nuclei with prominent nucleoli (Figure 2.1, *A*). In smaller neurons such as the cerebellar granule cells, the nucleus forms the major constituent of the cell body, and the cytoplasm is nearly invisible (Figure 2.1, *B*).

Perikaryal constituents vary in amount and proportion in different neurons, but most elements are common to all of them. As in other cells that actively synthesize protein, neuronal perikarya are rich in ribosomes, which may be arranged along stacks of membranes in parallel array (the rough endoplasmic reticulum) to form Nissl granules, or **Nissl substance**. One of the functions of Nissl substance, which appears lavender-blue in typical H&E stains, is the synthesis of neurotransmitters essential to proper signal transduction of the neuron. Nissl substance is generally required for the absolute histological identification of neurons under the microscope.

There are two major types of neuronal arrangement in the cortices: **neocortex** (isocortex) and **allocortex** (archicortex). A small transition zone between the two migration patterns is known as **mesocortex** ("middle" cortex). Various regions of neuronal migration and lamination were discovered through comparative neuroanatomy between ancient species such as reptiles and phylogenetically newer species such as humans.

The organization of the cortical layers is called **cytoarchitecture**. The majority of the human cortex consists of neocortex ("new" cortex). The neocortex microscopically contains six layers of neurons, which consist from the outer surface inward of (1) molecular layer, (2) external granular layer, (3) external pyramidal layer, (4) internal granular layer, (5) internal pyramidal layer, and (6) fusiform (multiform) layer. As mentioned in Chapter 1, portions of the limbic lobe are com-

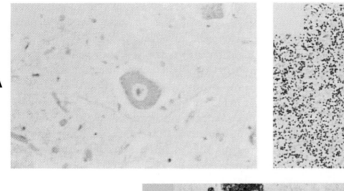

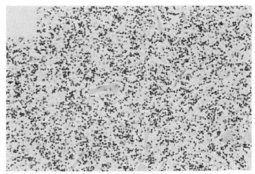

A

B

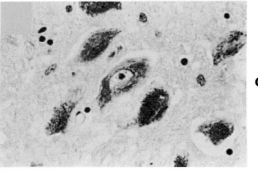

C

figure 2.1   **A,** Anterior horn cell of the spinal cord. It has a large, watery nucleus with a prominent nucleolus and distinctive Nissl substance (H&E stain). **B,** Low-power view of the granular layer of
the cerebellum, filled with small neurons with no visible cytoplasm (H&E stain). **C,** The bright, rich
brown color in the substantia nigra neurons is neuromelanin (H&E stain). *(Courtesy Dr. Cheryl A.
Palmer, Division of Neuropathology, University of Alabama at Birmingham.)*

posed of allocortex ("old" cortex), which consists
of only three neuronal layers.

Several other pigmented substances are normal
components of neurons. **Lipofuschin,** which appears under the microscope as a muddy brownish
color in the cytoplasm of neurons, normally accumulates in greater amounts with increasing age.
Some neurons contain abundant lipofuschin at
early ages such as the third decade of life. For example, olivary neurons and the anterior horn cells
of the spinal cord reveal considerable amounts of
lipofuschin in young adults. Other neurons such
as the Purkinje cells accumulate little lipofuschin
over a lifetime.

Neuromelanin (Figure 2.1, *C*) is found in cells
of the substantia nigra, locus ceruleus, and other
scattered nuclear groups in the brainstem. Neu-

romelanin is synthesized by a different enzymatic
pathway than the melanin that is present in the
skin; therefore albino mammals still possess neuromelanin in their CNS. No neuromelanin is
found in the brain before 5 years of age, and pigmentation is complete only between 20 and 30
years of age.

Artifactual changes are commonly seen histologically in neurons. Postmortem autolysis (the
dissolution of body organs after the time of death)
is less of a problem in the CNS than in other viscera. Autolytic changes that develop after clinical
brain death but while the patient is maintained on
life-support systems may be a major obstacle to
useful histological study. Shrunken dark neurons
are artifactual and are generally caused by pressure
on unfixed brain tissue, such as occurs during

surgical procedures. They have an irregular outline, with dark staining of both the nucleus and cytoplasm. Nissl substance cannot be identified. Perinuclear haloes are thought to be artifacts resulting from shrinkage that occurs during tissue processing.

Neuronal Function

Neurons function as the fundamental sensory and motor unit of nervous tissue in the brain. They are localized to both superficial and deep grey matter. The surface membrane of neurons assumes special importance because of its role in the initiation and propagation of neural impulses. This membrane is semipermeable because it allows some ions to diffuse through it yet restricts others. In the resting state, the membrane is quite permeable to potassium ions, which diffuse from the cytoplasm to the outer surface of the cell membrane. In this way, the outer surface acquires a resting potential. Sudden shifts in ionic concentration that result in an influx of sodium ions cause a reversal of charge and create a local action potential. The axons transmit the electrical impulses that result in action potentials and also transport materials from the perikaryon to the synaptic terminals. Various aspects of neuronal physiology are discussed in greater detail in Chapter 3.

Glial Cells

The terms *neuroglia* or *glial cells* include **astrocytes, oligodendroglia,** and **ependymal cells** because all are derived from similar neuroglial predecessors. Therefore tumors called **gliomas** include astrocytomas (arising from proliferating astrocytes), oligodendrogliomas (proliferating oligodendrocytes), and ependymomas (proliferating ependymal cells). Because the morphological characteristics, functions, and cellular reactions of the various glial cells are completely different, each is discussed separately in the following paragraphs.

Astrocytes

Astrocytes function in many arenas that are still unknown to scientists. Although astrocytes cer-

tainly play a structurally supportive role in the CNS, this is not their only function. During fetal development the radial glia, which are astrocytes, guide migrating neurons to their permanent positions. Electron microscopy also suggests an insulating role for astrocytes because their processes surround and isolate the synaptic surfaces of neurons. Astrocytes are likely to have numerous and poorly understood metabolic roles because they are known to be capable of taking up neurotransmitters. Although phagocytosis in the CNS is usually associated with microglial-macrophage activity, astrocytes also possess some amount of phagocytic capability.

The morphological characteristics of astrocytes formerly were thought to be a key to their function but are now thought to play a smaller role in their cellular differentiation. For many years astrocytes have been classified as **protoplasmic** or **fibrous:** protoplasmic astrocytes were largely confined to grey matter, whereas fibrous astrocytes were thought to be found in white matter. However, recent evidence suggests that these differences may be fairly minimal. Both types of astrocytes have rounded or angular nuclei that are approximately 7 to 10 μm in diameter. The nuclei of these cells contain fine homogeneous chromatin. **Chromatin** is the genetic material in the nucleus and can be arranged differently in different cells. Some cells contain evenly dispersed, fine granular chromatin, whereas others have denser or clumped chromatin material. All astrocytes contain bundles of filaments composed of a protein that has been purified and is known as **glial fibrillary acidic protein (GFAP).** With the use of immunoperoxidase techniques, this protein has become the most reliable method for the histological identification of astrocytes.

Fibrous astrocytes have thick, long processes that often attach to blood vessels. The disposition of astrocytic processes with perivascular end-feet, together with the relative lack of extracellular space in the CNS, forms the basis of the **blood-brain barrier** (see Chapter 3). Protoplasmic astrocytes have abundant short branches that tend to form right angles, thus creating a rounded halo effect around the nucleus. The protoplasmic as-

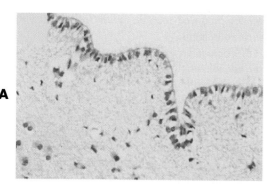

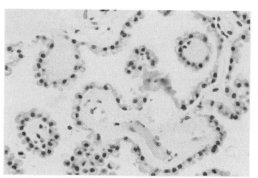

A

B

figure 2.2 **A,** Photograph of the lining of the third ventricle (H&E stain). Ependymal cells are low cuboidal to columnar cells with distinct cilia. **B,** Normal choroid plexus appears as a single row of cuboidal epithelium with a "cobblestone" appearance on its border and a fibrovascular core (H&E stain). *(Courtesy Dr. Cheryl A. Palmer, Division of Neuropathology, University of Alabama at Birmingham.)*

trocytes gather in a satellite fashion around neurons and form clusters around vessels in the grey matter.

Oligodendroglia

Oligodendrocytes function as the myelin-forming cells of the CNS. One oligodendrocyte may produce segments of myelin for as many as 40 different axons.

In oligodendrocytes the morphological characteristics are very similar whether they reside in grey or white matter. In routine H&E–stained sections, oligodendrocytes are seen as small, dark, rounded nuclei that resemble the nuclei of lymphocytes in both size and appearance. Their perikaryon and processes are stainable only with difficulty and not with routine stains. As seen with electron microscopy, the sparse perikaryon contains no glial fibrils and thus is not stained by methods that demonstrate GFAP.

In the white matter, oligodendrocytes are seen mainly as interfascicular glia (parallel groups of cells aligned between various tracts) arranged in longitudinal array, whereas in grey matter they form one type of perineuronal satellite cell. Each oligodendrocyte sends out processes that form internodes on many nearby axons.

There is evidence that oligodendrocytes are derived from the so-called O-2A progenitor cells; they are thought to arise from the subventricular zone and migrate into nearby white and grey matter.

Ependymal Cells

Ependymal cells serve as a barrier between the brain parenchyma and the cerebrospinal fluid (CSF)—the "brain-CSF barrier." The ependymal lining of the ventricles and central canal of the spinal cord is derived from neuroectoderm and may be several cell layers in thickness during fetal development. The appearance of the ependyma varies from place to place within the ventricular system, ranging from low cuboidal to taller columnar cells (Figure 2.2, *A*).

The ventricular surface of the ependyma is normally uninterrupted. Cilia that project from the surface of the ependymal cells originate from the basal bodies. As seen with electron microscopy, the cilia have a characteristic nine pairs of microtubules that surround a central pair of microtubules. Beneath the ependyma there is a layer of "subependymal glia," which are astrocytes that are arranged in compact groups and result in normally abundant glial fibrillary processes.

Microglial Cells

Microglial cells function as the major "scavenger cells" of the brain. They transform to macrophages when a phagocytic response is required. In routinely stained sections, resting microglial cells can be identified by their nuclei, which are rather hyperchromatic and elongated.

Choroid Plexus

A functionally vital cell of the CNS, choroid plexus cells produce the majority of the CSF. As seen under the microscope, the epithelium of the choroid plexus is composed of a single row of cuboidal cells folded into villi (Figure 2.2, B). The ventricular surfaces of these cells have a brush border composed of microvilli. Richly vascularized connective tissue serves as the stalk of the plexus papillae. Calcification of the choroid plexus is a common process and increases with advancing age.

Arachnoid (Meningothelial) Cells

Meningothelial cells (or arachnoidal cap cells) maintain the dura mater, the arachnoid, and the pia mater. Meningothelial cells can proliferate in response to injury to the meninges, forming fibrotic "scar" tissue. In some circumstances they have an ability to be phagocytic. Meningothelial cells contain moderate amounts of cytoplasm, and their nuclei are stereotypically oval with a stippled distribution of chromatin. They are often distributed in small nodules throughout the arachnoid and dura mater.

Pituitary Cells

Because it is intimately involved with CNS function and anatomically located in the cranial vault, the pituitary gland is usually considered part of the CNS. Unlike the **neurohypophysis** (the posterior portion of the pituitary gland), the **adenohypophysis** (the anterior portion of the gland) arises from oral ectoderm during development. Therefore the adenohypophysis retains the typical histological appearance of an endocrine gland composed of cells grouped in cords and follicles. The sinusoidal capillaries form a rich vascular network for the pituitary gland so that the hormones produced may be rapidly transported to their end organs.

Numerous types of pituitary cells are seen in the adenohypophysis, and each produces and secretes various hormones vitally important to endocrinological function. As seen with the routine H&E stain, pituitary cells classically contain abundant cytoplasm of different colorimetric shades. "Chromophobe" cells are so called because they have no affinity for the usual dyes used in histology and therefore have no visible granules with H&E staining. Chromophobe cells are a small fraction of the total cellular population of the pituitary. "Acidophilic" cells have an affinity for acidic stains, whereas "basophils" stain strongly with basic stains. Prior theory suggested that the different cells secreted stereotypical hormones, but that theory has been questioned with the advent of electron microscopy and the discovery that both acidophils and basophils can secrete nearly any sort of neurohormone. The pituitary cell nuclei are oval to round and bland in appearance. In the normal pituitary gland the cells are arranged in nodules and nests separated by septae of connective tissue.

Histological Pathological Responses of Central Nervous System Cells

Neurons

With the possible exception of neurons located in olfactory epithelium, adult mammalian neurons are postmitotic. This simply means that unlike most of the other cells in the body, neurons do not regenerate if they are injured or lost. Once differentiation has been achieved in fetal life, the neuron loses its capacity to synthesize deoxyribonucleic acid (DNA). Various neuronal responses can be identified histologically and are mentioned briefly in the following paragraphs.

Neuronal Ischemia and Cell Death

One of the most common forms of injury to neurons is that caused by hypoxia. Underlying physiological disturbances that produce histological evidence of hypoxia include impaired or arrested blood flow to the brain, reduced oxygen concentration in the blood, and toxic factors. Furthermore, because the neuron depends on glucose as its main metabolic substrate, hypoglycemia can cause similar morphological alterations to the neuron.

The earliest stage of ischemic damage to neurons is microvacuolation of the perikaryon. The majority of vacuoles contain swollen mitochondria. This phenomenon has been seen in animal models after 5 to 15 minutes of hypoxia. Confusion with postmortem autolytic change makes this alteration difficult to see with routine histological tests. In an established ischemic cell change, the neuron is shrunken and its nucleus stains darkly. The cytoplasm becomes markedly eosinophilic, and Nissl substance disperses (Figure 2.3, *A*). The nucleolus may also become eosinophilic.

Neuronophagia

When a necrotic process is very acute, such as is seen in poliomyelitis or encephalitides, the nerve cells undergo rapid death. The nerve cell skeleton is invaded by microglial cells, lymphocytes, or neutrophils and is removed from the brain (Figure 2.3, *B*).

Chromatolysis

Chromatolysis refers to the process in the neuronal cell body that is a reaction to an axonal injury. In sequence, the cell body becomes rounded, and Nissl granules in the central perikaryon disappear and leave only a peripheral rim of cytoplasmic ribonucleic acid (RNA). The nucleus is displaced to the periphery of the cell.

Neurofibrillary Degeneration

A characteristic neuronal abnormality in dementia caused by Alzheimer's disease is the presence of neurofibrillary tangles within the neuronal cytoplasm. These tangles are best demonstrated microscopically by silver impregnation and appear as thickened fibrils—similar to skeins of yarn (Figure 2.3, *C*)—lying parallel to each other or forming an interweaving basketwork. This change

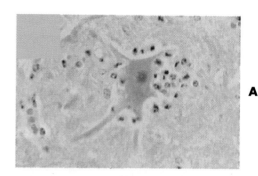

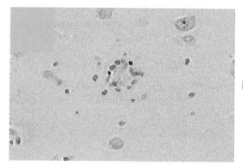

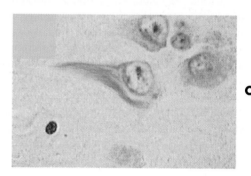

figure 2.3   **A,** Anterior horn cell neuron that is ischemic as a result of hypoxia. Note that the cytoplasm and the nucleolus are eosinophilic, and neuronophagia is commencing (H&E stain). **B,** Neuron is surrounded by lymphocytes and microglial cells, the first stage in neuronophagia (H&E stain). **C,** Hippocampal pyramidal neuron containing a flame-shaped neurofibrillary tangle composed of paired helical filaments that appear as threads of yarn in the cytoplasm (H&E stain). *(Courtesy Dr. Cheryl A. Palmer, Division of Neuropathology, University of Alabama at Birmingham.)*

is prominent in the hippocampal neurons in Alzheimer's disease but is also seen in neocortical neurons.

Neuronal Inclusion Bodies

Pick's disease (see Chapter 10) exemplifies a distinctive type of cortical neuron degeneration, including cellular swelling and **Pick bodies.** These bodies are well-defined, rounded spheres that stain darkly with silver stains (Figure 2.4, *A*). They are likely to be seen in small or medium-sized neurons.

Lafora bodies are rounded concentric bodies with a central basophilic core. They are found in the cytoplasm of neurons in a particular type of myoclonic epilepsy (Figure 2.4, *B*).

Lewy bodies are cytoplasmic inclusions that are seen most often in the neuromelanin-containing pigmented nuclei of the brainstem and are characteristic of Parkinson's disease. They are eosinophilic rounded bodies with a central core and a surrounding pale peripheral rim (Figure 2.4, *C*), and they may be single or multiple.

Nuclear or cytoplasmic inclusions are seen in a number of viral infections of the CNS, including herpes simplex encephalitis, subacute sclerosing panencephalitis, and rabies (Figure 2.4, *D*). Although they may be common findings in viral nervous system diseases, they may be few and far between, and therefore require a prolonged and careful search.

Neuronal Storage Products

One subclass of neurological metabolic diseases involves a hereditary congenital lack of enzymes that function in one specific pathway of metabolism. These diseases are called *storage diseases* because the enzymatic pathway ends when it reaches the missing enzyme step, and the last substance produced cannot be further metabolized. This phenomenon often causes a build-up of that particular substance in various cells of the body. When it occurs in the CNS, the stored substance causes enlargement of neurons, sometimes to a striking degree. These neurons are ballooned, and the nucleus is pushed to one pole of the cell (Figure 2.4, *E*). The cytoplasm appears foamy, and the composition of the storage product sometimes may be identified by staining patterns with various methods.

Neuronal Neoplasia

Although normal neurons are postmitotic and do not divide, chromosomal or other genetic damage (as well as other less-understood processes) causes the normal regulatory systems in all cells, including neurons, to break down. This breakdown causes neoplasia, or the uncontrolled division and replication of cells to form tumors. Brain tumors composed of neoplastic neurons are far less common than astrocytic tumors and oligodendrogliomas, but they are seen occasionally. Various subclasses of these neuronal tumors are recognized, including ganglion cell tumors, neurocytomas, neuroblastomas, and medulloblastomas (Figure 2.4, *F*). Neuronal neoplasms account for less than 5% of all brain tumors.

Glial Cells

Astrocytes

Reactive alterations. Astrocytes show changes in response to almost every type of injury or disease in the CNS. Their reactions may take the form of degeneration, hypertrophy, or hyperplasia. There do not seem to be significant differences between protoplasmic and fibrous astrocytes in their responses to injury. In all progressive reactions abundant glial fibrils are formed; this is called an acute or chronic astrogliosis (Figure 2.5, *A*).

Astrocytes are more resistant to hypoxia than neurons and survive at the margin of lesions inside of which the neurons have died. Degenerative changes in astrocytes include cytoplasmic swelling, the disintegration of their processes into granules, and the appearance of lipid droplets in the cytoplasm.

Hypertrophy and hyperplasia of astrocytes are common findings. The loss of neurons from any cause, such as myelin breakdown or injury to nerve fibers, is followed by an increase in the numbers of astrocytes and, with increasing survival times, a progressive increase in the formation of glial fibrils. Characteristically, gliotic tissue is firmer than normal and tends to appear grey and

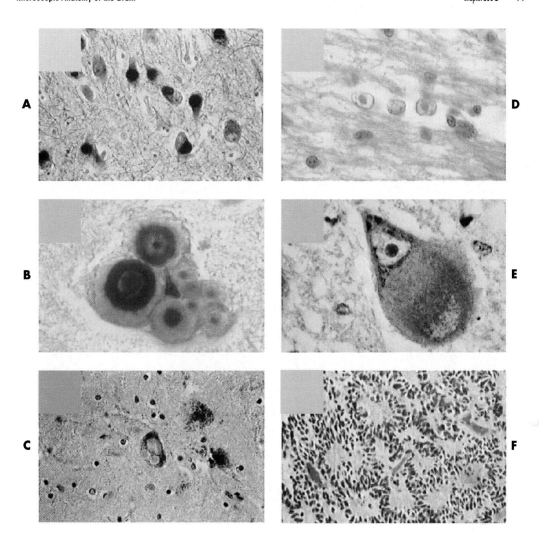

figure 2.4   **A,** Section demonstrating the affinity of Pick bodies for silver. Pick bodies are present in this photograph as rounded, dark inclusion bodies in the cytoplasm of medium-sized neurons (Bielschowsky's stain). **B,** Lafora bodies are single or, in this case, multiple lamellar cytoplasmic inclusions in Lafora's disease, which is associated with myoclonic epilepsy (H&E stain). **C,** Neuron of the substantia nigra, in which several Lewy bodies are seen. Note the white cleared rim around the inclusions, a characteristic feature of Lewy bodies in the brainstem in Parkinson's disease (H&E stain). **D,** Intranuclear inclusions as seen in a case of herpes simplex encephalitis. They are eosinophilic and somewhat glassy-appearing and may be few and far between in these infectious processes (H&E stain). **E,** Neuron engorged with a stored substance, causing rounding of the cell body and compression of the nucleus to one edge of the cell. This particular neuron was found in the brain of a child with San Filippo disease, a neuronal storage disease (H&E stain). **F,** Medulloblastomas, neuronal tumors presumed to arise from the external granular cell layer in the cerebellum, tend to form pseudorosettes, which in this photograph are seen as the cleared regions surrounded by tumor cells (H&E stain). *(Courtesy Dr. Cheryl A. Palmer, Division of Neuropathology, University of Alabama at Birmingham.)*

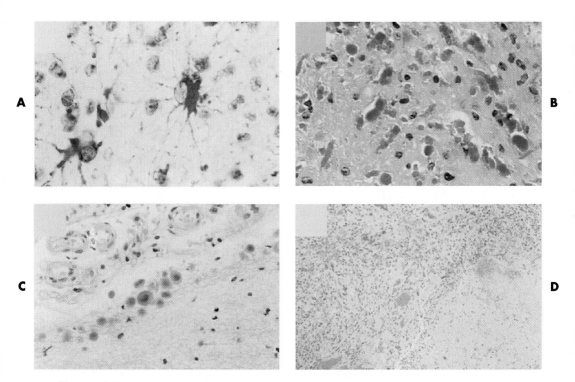

figure 2.5   **A,** The cytoplasmic glial filaments and the spidery processes of the cell can easily be seen in this reactive astrocyte stained with immunohistochemistry for GFAP. **B,** Rosenthal fibers (H&E stain). **C,** Corpora amylacea located in the subpial region (H&E stain). **D,** Glioblastoma multiforme, the most malignant form of astrocytic tumor. It can be identified by the cellularity, pleomorphism, and necrosis seen in this section obtained at surgery from the temporal lobe brain tumor of a 67-year-old man (H&E stain). *(Courtesy Dr. Cheryl A. Palmer, Division of Neuropathology, University of Alabama at Birmingham.)*

translucent. In any neuropathological study, one of the most definite indicators of a CNS abnormality is the finding of excessive numbers of astrocytes. For many years it was considered that astrocytes did not undergo mitosis; this idea is now known to be untrue.

Rosenthal fibers are bodies formed in the perikarya and processes of astrocytes. They appear as refractile, homogeneous, eosinophilic structures that vary greatly in size and may be rounded, oval, or elongated (Figure 2.5, *B*). They are found in a variety of circumstances, including any long-standing intense fibrillary gliosis such as surrounding syringomyelic cavities (clefts in the spinal cord generally caused by trauma) or

noninfiltrating tumors, within slowly growing astrocytomas, and invariably in Alexander's disease.

Corpora amylacea (Figure 2.5, *C*) are spherical bodies with an average diameter of 15 μm. They are often found in the grey matter close to the pia mater or around blood vessels in the white matter. They are more numerous in older persons and are particularly numerous in various degenerative conditions. They contain an amorphous basophilic material, sometimes with a deeper-staining central core. With electron microscopy, they have been shown to be located in the processes of astrocytes and likely represent a degenerative change.

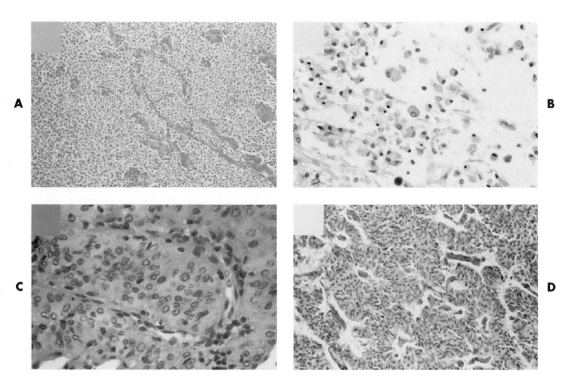

figure 2.6   **A,** Oligodendroglioma that is composed of neoplastic oligodendrocytes and shows a classic cellular tumor of round cells with perinuclear haloes ("fried eggs") and numerous background blood vessels (H&E stain). **B,** Foamy macrophages, transformed from activated microglial cells, are seen in regions that have necrotic material to be transported (H&E stain). **C,** Meningioma composed of nodules of round-to-oval nuclei with a bland chromatin pattern (H&E stain). **D,** Pituitary adenoma that is forming glandlike structures, a pattern commonly seen in adenomas. This tumor produced prolactin (H&E stain). *(Courtesy Dr. Cheryl A. Palmer, Division of Neuropathology, University of Alabama at Birmingham.)*

Neoplastic alterations. Neoplastic transformation of astrocytes gives rise to tumors that by virtue of their clinical and biological diversity overshadow all other primary intracranial neoplasms. Predictable relationships exist among the site and morphological characteristics of the lesions, the age of the patient, and the anticipated clinical course of the disease.

Neoplasms derived from fibrillary astrocytes or their precursors account for nearly all of the astrocytic tumors of the cerebral hemispheres. Astrocytoma, anaplastic astrocytoma, and glioblastoma multiforme (Figure 2.5, *D*) are the three major grades of astrocytic tumors that sequentially exemplify increasing malignant behavior.

Oligodendroglia

Reactive alterations. Little is known about the proliferation of oligodendrocytes for repair or remyelination after injury to myelin sheaths in the CNS. There is evidence that there is a very slow turnover of oligodendrocytes in the normal brain, and a very low percentage of differentiated oligodendrocytes can undergo mitosis.

Neoplastic alterations. Tumors composed of neoplastic oligodendroglial cells (Figure 2.6, *A*) account for approximately 10% to 15% of all gliomas. The neoplasm occurs primarily in adults but may occur in children. Not surprisingly, oligodendrogliomas, which can be either benign or malignant, are predominant in the white matter of the cerebral hemispheres but can also infiltrate the cortex to a great degree.

Demyelination resulting from cell loss. Conditions such as progressive multifocal leukoencephalopathy, which is caused by a virus, fairly selectively destroy oligodendrocytes. In turn, myelin loss occurs. Ongoing studies are in progress in an attempt to determine the amount of remyelination and cellular replacement that occurs in these instances.

Ependymal Cells

Reactive alterations. It seems that mature ependyma has little if any capacity for proliferation and regeneration; once the ventricular surface has been broken, it is probably not reconstituted. Ependymal cells are particularly vulnerable to infections with cytomegalovirus and the mumps virus in patients with acquired immunodeficiency syndrome (AIDS). The most commonly seen pathological change in ependymal cells is granular ependymitis, which may develop after any irritative process but is best known as a characteristic feature of neurosyphilis. The actual mechanism of formation of these granules is unclear.

Neoplastic alterations. Although epithelial in their normal state, ependymal cells are related embryologically to astrocytes and oligodendroglia, and it is this glial heritage that is often expressed when the cells are neoplastically transformed. In other neoplasms, the epithelial potential is retained. As expected, ependymomas show a proclivity for occurring in ventricular chambers and passages. Such intraventricular masses can obstruct the flow of CSF and produce hydrocephalus. Ependymomas can be either benign or malignant, both histologically and prognostically.

Microglial Cells

Reactions to microglial cell injury include an increase in perikaryal size as the cell accumulates products of tissue breakdown and the processes become shortened. The majority of the accumulated products are lipid in nature and are primarily the breakdown products of myelin. These cells are then generally referred to as macrophages.

The conditions under which microglial reactions are found cover the whole gamut of neuropathology, ranging from mild proliferation around chromatolytic neurons, through the removal of degenerating debris, to the ingestion of totally necrotic brain tissue, as is seen in an infarction.

The characteristic lipid phagocyte (Figure 2.6, B) is a spherical cell that is distended by fat droplets and contains a small rounded nucleus near the cell membrane. Many names have been applied to this cell, such as foamy macrophage or gitter cell.

Wallerian Degeneration

The cell body maintains the functional and anatomical integrity of the axon. If the axon is cut, the part distal to the cut degenerates in a phenomenon known as *wallerian degeneration.* Breakdown of the entire arborization of a neuron—which consists of the axon, all of the neuronal dendrites, and axonal branches—inevitably follows the necrosis of the neuronal cell body and its nucleus. Wallerian degeneration in the central and peripheral nervous systems share many similarities. Histological stains can quantitate the amount of myelin debris formed in tract degeneration.

Arachnoid (Meningothelial) Cells

The most common reaction of meningothelial cells is neoplasia. Meningothelial cell tumors (**meningiomas**) are one of the more common tumors to arise in later life (Figure 2.6, *C*); they are uncommon in younger persons. They can arise from any portion of the dura mater or leptomeninges; the most common sites are the parafalcian (over the convexities), sphenoid wing, olfactory groove, optic canal and, occasionally, the posterior fossa. Women are far more susceptible to these types of tumors than are men, possibly because some of the tumors are known to contain progesterone and estrogen receptors. They are most commonly benign, but malignant meningiomas are well-recognized; total surgical excision is usually curative.

Pituitary Cells

Inflammation can occur in pituitary glands in a condition called *lymphocytic hypophysitis.* This condition generally causes failure of hormone secretion. The most common pathological conditions to occur in pituitary glands are microadenomas or macroadenomas (Figure 2.6, *D*). Defined by size, the smaller adenomas usually produce some type of active neurohormone and therefore cause symptoms much earlier than the larger tumors that produce no active hormones (called "null cell" adenomas). The larger pituitary adenomas generally occur with optic chiasm compression and hence visual field defects. The most common substances to be produced by active pituitary adenomas are prolactin and growth hormone.

BIBLIOGRAPHY

1. Barr ML, Kiernan JA: *The human nervous system: an anatomical viewpoint,* ed 4, Philadelphia, 1983, Harper & Row.
2. Carpenter MB, Sutin J: *Human neuroanatomy,* ed 8, Baltimore, 1983, Williams & Wilkins.
3. deGroot J: *Correlative neuroanatomy,* ed 21, San Mateo, Calif, 1991, Appleton & Lange.
4. Junqueira LC, Carneiro J: *Basic histology,* ed 3, Los Altos, Calif, 1980, Lange Medical Publications.

c h a p t e r t h r e e

Chemical Neuroanatomy

Brain function is sustained by cellular metabolism. Products of digestion (i.e., amino acids, fatty acids, and glucose) are absorbed, disseminated, and appropriated by neurons. These products are broken down in the cytoplasm of the neuron.

Cellular metabolism is orchestrated by enzymes. The metabolic processes have many steps, with each step catalyzed by a specific enzyme. For example, glucose is converted to pyruvate in a multistage process of glycolysis. Pyruvate enters the mitochondria, where it is converted to acetyl coenzyme A; acetyl coenzyme A triggers the citric acid cycle. Amino acid neurotransmitters such as glutamate, γ-aminobutyric acid (GABA), and aspartate are products of the citric acid cycle; adenosine triphosphate (ATP), a primary source of energy for cell function, is also a product of this cycle. ATP supplies energy to cells, is instrumental in the storage and transfer of energy, and is used for active transport of molecules. Cellular metabolism therefore contributes the energy essential for the breakdown of amino acids, lipids, and glucose to form cellular structures and for other fundamental cell operations, including the synthesis of enzymes and neurotransmitters.

Cells continuously absorb substances from the extracellular environment and expel substances into that environment. Cellular membranes are semipermeable, allowing the passage of some substances into the cell (e.g., water, glucose, oxygen) and repelling other substances (solutes). Some solutes enter the cell primarily by active transport. Most solutes are electrolytes or ions with a positive charge (cations) or negative charge (anions). Sodium is the principal extracellular cation, and potassium is the principal intracellular cation. Because sodium and potassium carry a positive charge, they are repelled in the lipid bilayer of the cell membrane by calcium, which is also positively charged. Cell depolarization cannot occur unless this repulsion is overcome. Two mechanisms accomplish this task: (1) active transport powered by ATP, and (2) the opening of gated sodium and potassium channels. For example, channels open when acetylcholine attaches to a nicotinic receptor, which allows sodium to enter and potassium to exit the cell. This event results in depolarization of the cell. Cell depolarization, or cell firing, is fundamental to neuronal communication. These processes are discussed in more detail in the following sections.

Neurotransmission

Communication between and among brain areas is achieved by the neuron—the signaling or information transfer unit. The signaling mechanism is a neurochemical process supported by several neurochemical or neurotransmitter systems. Neurochemical systems are linked to every disorder discussed in this text; effective pharmacological treatment of psychobiological disorders is based on the manipulation of these systems. This chapter and Chapters 1 and 2 lay the groundwork for subsequent discussions in Part II of this text.

Neurotransmission is defined as the response that results from communication between a presynaptic neuron and postsynaptic neuron. The communication medium is a neurotransmitter that is released from a presynaptic neuron into a

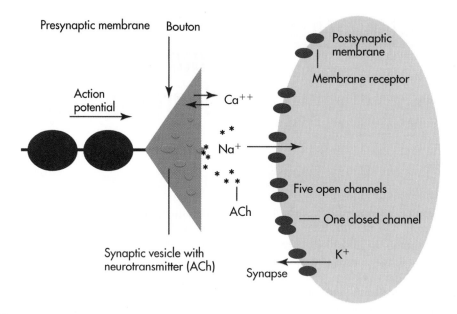

figure 3.1   An action potential opens calcium ion channels and allows Ca^{++} to enter the presynaptic membrane (bouton). The calcium causes vesicles within the bouton to blend with the membrane and release the neurotransmitter acetylcholine (ACh) into the synaptic cleft. Two molecules of ACh bind with an ACh receptor on the membrane of the postsynaptic neuron, which allows sodium (Na^{+}) to enter and potassium (K^{+}) to leave the cell through their respective channel openings. This activity results in neuronal depolarization.

microscopic synaptic space (20 to 30 nm wide) and then binds to a postsynaptic receptor. An individual neuron contains just a few of the many types of discovered neurotransmitters. Only two postsynaptic responses are possible: depolarization (an excitatory response) or hyperpolarization (an inhibitory response). Excitatory responses cause an influx of sodium ions into the neuron, which results in cell depolarization. Inhibition occurs when potassium leaves the cell, chloride enters the cell, or both; this response occurs after their respective ion channel openings have been triggered by a specific neurotransmitter. Although neurotransmitters are referred to as excitatory or inhibitory, it is actually the *receptors* that more directly influence neuronal response.

Action Potentials

It is important to review the concepts of cell excitation and conduction and action potentials be-fore further discussing neurotransmission. For neurotransmission to occur, the presynaptic neuron must send an action potential along its axon to the axonal terminal. Action potentials originate from the axon hillock, which is located at the junction of the cell body and the axon. An action potential can be described as the changes in transmembrane potential that occur during cell depolarization or hyperpolarization. The net flux or transfer of energy across the cell membrane depends on the permeability of the membrane to ions. The axon transmits the action potential in waves of energy to the terminal, where it triggers the opening of calcium channels on the membrane of the synaptic boutons (Figure 3.1). Extracellular calcium enters the bouton, which causes synaptic vesicles containing neurotransmitters to fuse with the bouton's membrane.[11] This mechanism releases the neurotransmitter into the synaptic space by exocytosis. The neurotransmitter distributes across the space and binds to a specific receptor on the membrane of the postsynaptic neuron.

When the neurotransmitter binds with a receptor, ion channels are opened or closed. Because channels are ion-specific, channel opening and closing either allows ions to move into or out of a cell or stops the movement of ions. Sodium (Na^+) and potassium (K^+) ions have a positive charge, and chloride (Cl^-) ions have a negative charge. These specific ions start or stop moving across the postsynaptic membrane; they elicit local changes in the membrane potential and thus launch a new or "downstream" action potential.

A postsynaptic neuron may receive "chemical input" from many presynaptic neurons, some of which release excitatory neurotransmitters and some of which release inhibitory neurotransmitters. Because many receptors accomodate both positive and negative ions, neurons respond to the balance of ionic charges. If more positive ions (e.g., Na^+) flow into the cell, depolarization, or cell firing, results. If more negative ions (e.g., Cl^-) flow into the cell, hyperpolarization occurs.

Receptors

Cellular receptors are protein molecules on the membrane that identify specific, smaller molecules called *ligands* (e.g., neurotransmitters). Two types of receptor systems facilitate neuronal communication: first messenger and second messenger.

First messenger receptors contain a channel through which the ions can pass; the discussion to this point most closely parallels these types of receptors. When a neurotransmitter binds to a first messenger receptor, the receptor channel opens and ions enter. First messenger systems require only a few milliseconds to trigger changes in the cell membrane and are known as a rapid, *direct* form of neurotransmission.[11] Acetylcholine, glutamate, glycine, and GABA act on first messenger receptor systems.

Second messenger systems are *indirect* and relatively slower than first messenger receptor systems. These systems do not cause neuronal excitation or inhibition directly. The receptors activate G-proteins that function in two ways: (1) acting on ion channels to open or close them, and (2) activating small molecules called *second messengers*.[4] These small molecules trigger cellular activities that result in ion channel modification (i.e., the channels open or close), neurotransmitter synthesis, and changes in receptor sensitivity.[9] The monoamines, including dopamine, norepinephrine, and serotonin, act through the second messenger receptor system.

Neurotransmitters

"A neurotransmitter is a chemical that is discharged from a nerve-fiber ending. It reaches and is recognized by a receptor on the surface of a postsynaptic nerve cell or other excitable postjunctional cell and either stimulates or inhibits the second cell."[1] Neurotransmitters can be grouped into four categories: monoamines (or biogenic amines), cholinergics, amino acids, and peptides (or neuropeptides) (Table 3.1). A broader categorization strategy places the first three types of neurotransmitters in a *small amine molecule* grouping. The small amine molecule category has the distinction of being synthesized by cytoplasmic (extranuclear) enzymes, whereas the peptides are produced in the cell body before further processing in the Golgi apparati.[5] In other words, monoamines, acetylcholine, and the amino acids can be created in the synaptic terminals, but the peptides must travel from the cell body down the length of the axon.

Defining Neurotransmitters

Specific criteria have been established to define neurotransmitters. These chemical substances must meet the following model[1]:

1. The neuron contains the enzymes required to synthesize the chemical.
2. The neuron contains the chemical.
3. The neuron releases the chemical when depolarized.
4. The chemical reacts with a specific receptor on a postsynaptic neuron and causes a biological effect.
5. The chemical is somehow inactivated after it is released. Mechanisms of inactivation in-

table 3.1
Neurochemical Systems

NEUROCHEMICAL SYSTEM	NEUROTRANSMITTER	SITE OF SYNTHESIS/ LOCATION	MAJOR PATHWAYS/ EFFERENTS
Monoamine system	Dopamine	Substantia nigra (pars compacta) primarily; also ventral tegmental area, retinal and olfactory interneurons (e.g., amacrine interneurons)	Dopaminergic pathways 1. Nigrostriatal 2. Mesolimbic 3. Mesocortical 4. Tuberoinfundibular
	Norepinephrine	Locus ceruleus in pons	Efferents from locus ceruleus include the following: 1. Thalamus 2. Hypothalamus 3. Entire cortex 4. Hippocampus 5. Basal ganglia 6. Cerebellum and spinal cord
	Serotonin (generally inhibitory)	Raphe nuclei	Efferents from raphe nuclei include the following: 1. Thalamus 2. Hypothalamus 3. Limbic area 4. Basal ganglia 5. Entire cortex
Cholinergic system	Acetylcholine (generally excitatory)	Nucleus basalis of Meynert; septal area	Efferents from cholinergic areas: 1. Cranial nerves III, VII, IX, X 2. Cerebral cortex 3. Hippocampus 4. Hypothalamus
Amino acids	GABA (inhibitory)	Found in most interneuronal circuits	Globus pallidus, cortex, striatum, thalamus, cerebellum, hippocampus, and others
	Glutamate (excitatory)	Synthesized in most neurons	Cortex, striatum, thalamus, motor neurons, spinal cord, hippocampus, cerebellum
Neuropeptides	Enkephalins	Found in hypothalamus, midbrain, spinal cord	Reproduces the action of morphine
	Substance P	Found in periaqueductal grey matter, substantia nigra, amygdala	The primary neurotransmitter for pain

clude reuptake back into the presynaptic terminal or a glial cell, or degradation of the
chemical by an extracellular enzyme.

6. If the chemical is applied exogenously at the
postsynaptic membrane, the effect is the same
as when the presynaptic neuron is stimulated.

Monoamine System

Neurotransmitters containing one amine group
are called monoamines and are synthesized from
amino acids.[6,13] The monoamine system incorpo-
rates an important subcategory—the catecholamines. The two most significant catecholamines
are dopamine and norepinephrine, which are
synthesized from the amino acid tyrosine. Four
enzymes are needed for catecholamine synthesis,
and all are produced intraneuronally: tyrosine
hydroxylase, dopa decarboxylase, dopamine β-
hydroxylase, and phenylethanolamine N-methyl-
transferase. However, not all cells that release catecholamines contain all four enzymes. Neurons
using dopamine do not contain dopamine β-
hydroxylase, and neurons using norepinephrine
do not produce phenylethanolamine N-methyl-
transferase. Catecholamines are also referred to as
adrenergics because they stimulate the sympathetic nervous system. Serotonin, a noncate-
cholamine monoamine, is synthesized from the
amino acid tryptophan.

Monoamines are synthesized primarily in the
brainstem. Moving rostrally, norepinephrine is
synthesized in the locus ceruleus of the pons, serotonin is synthesized in the raphe nuclei of the
pons and midbrain, and dopamine is synthesized
in the substantia nigra pars compacta of the midbrain. Their efferent pathways reach throughout
the central and peripheral nervous systems.

Dopamine

Dopamine is synthesized in the substantia nigra
pars compacta and in the ventral tegmental area in
the midbrain (Figure 3.2). Dopaminergic projections input to the basal ganglia (nigrostriatal
tract), the cortex (mesocortical tract), the limbic structures (mesolimbic tract), and the pituitary gland (tuberoinfundibular tract). Additional

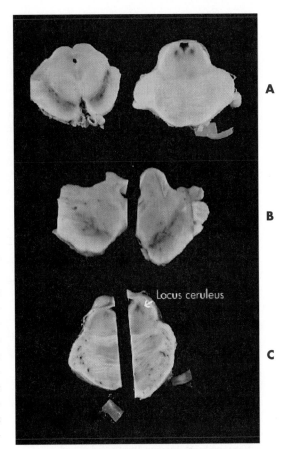

figure 3.2   The effects of aging and disease on
catecholamine centers in the brainstem. **A,** Normal pigment in the substantia nigra *(left)* and locus ceruleus
(right) of a young individual. **B,** Mild age-related loss of
pigment in the brainstem of a normal individual *(right)*
and loss of pigmented neurons in the brainstem of an
individual with parkinsonism *(left)*. **C,** Mild depigmentation of the locus ceruleus in an aged individual *(right)*
and severe depigmentation in parkinsonism *(left)*.
*(Courtesy Dr. Richard E. Powers, Director, University of
Alabama at Birmingham Brain Resource Program.)*

dopaminergic neurons are found in the retina, the
olfactory bulb, and the hypothalamus.[8] There are
five dopamine receptor subtypes (D_1 to D_5) and
many subcategories of those subtypes. (See the
box on p. 52.)

Significant psychiatric and neurological problems stem from failure in this system and are care-

Dopamine synthesis:

Tyrosine ⎯⎯⎯⎯⎯⎯⎯→ Dopa ⎯⎯⎯⎯⎯⎯⎯→ **Dopamine**

        Tyrosine hydroxylase   Dopa decarboxylase

Dopamine metabolism:

Dopamine ⎯⎯⎯⎯⎯⎯⎯→ Norepinephrine

            Dopamine β-hydroxylase

Norepinephrine synthesis:

Tyrosine ⎯⎯⎯⎯⎯⎯→ Dopa ⎯⎯⎯⎯⎯⎯→ Dopamine ⎯⎯⎯⎯⎯⎯→ **Norepinephrine**

     Tyrosine hydroxylase   Dopa decarboxylase   Dopamine β-hydroxylase

Norepinephrine metabolism:

Norepinephrine ⎯⎯⎯⎯⎯⎯⎯⎯→ Epinephrine

            Phenylethanolamine *N*-methyltransferase

fully reviewed in later chapters. For example, excessive levels of dopamine in the mesolimbic area give rise to positive psychotic symptoms (see Chapter 5); inadequate levels of dopamine in the nigrostriatal and mesocortical tracts precipitate movement disorders (see Chapter 13) and negative psychotic symptoms (e.g., anergia, avolition), respectively; and decreased dopamine input in the tuberoinfundibular tract diminishes dopaminergic inhibition of prolactin, which causes an escalation of prolactin-mediated physiological processes (e.g., increased lactation). The dopamine system is also affected by the consumption of drugs of abuse, particularly stimulants (see Chapter 8). Cocaine, for example, affects dopamine uptake in basal ganglia reward centers, which accounts for some of the addictive characteristics of this drug.[3]

Norepinephrine

Norepinephrine (noradrenaline) is synthesized from the amino acid tyrosine. Tyrosine hydroxylase is the rate-limiting step in this process. Synthesis occurs primarily in the locus ceruleus of the

pons (see Figure 3.2). Other brainstem sources of norepinephrine synthesis include the medullary reticular formation, the dorsal motor nucleus of the vagus nerve, and the solitary nucleus.[8] Norepinephrine projections reach to most of the central nervous system (CNS) (mostly from the locus ceruleus) and to the spinal cord (from other norepinephrine synthesis sites). Two types of receptors selectively bind with norepinephrine: *alpha* and *beta* receptors. Both receptors stimulate a second messenger system. Beta receptors, for example, stimulate the adenylate cyclase located on the inner surface of the cell to convert the cellular energy carrier ATP to cyclic adenosine monophosphate (cAMP). cAMP, an important second messenger, sets in motion a number of chemical processes, including changes in ion channels, neurotransmitter synthesis, and changes in receptor sensitivity.[4] (See the box above.)

Norepinephrine drives the sympathetic nervous system. Chemicals stimulating adrenergic receptors (sympathomimetics) increase heart rate and blood pressure. Chemicals that antagonize the

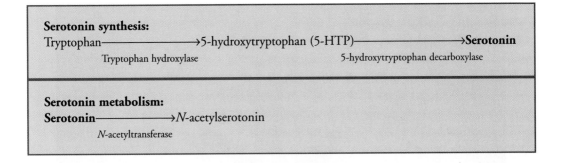

Serotonin synthesis:
Tryptophan————————————→5-hydroxytryptophan (5-HTP)————————————→**Serotonin**
         Tryptophan hydroxylase   5-hydroxytryptophan decarboxylase

Serotonin metabolism:
Serotonin————————————→*N*-acetylserotonin
         N-acetyltransferase

Acetylcholine synthesis:
Acetyl coenzyme A + choline————————————→**Acetylcholine**
                        Choline acetyltransferase

Acetylcholine metabolism:
Acetylcholine————————————→Acetate + choline
                Acetylcholinesterase

sympathetic system have the opposite effect (e.g., hypotension). Most norepinephrine is not degraded enzymatically after release but is inactivated by reuptake into the presynaptic neuron. Norepinephrine can be metabolized by catechol *O*-methyltransferase in the synaptic cleft or by monoamine oxidase in the cell mitochondria or presynaptic terminal after reuptake. Norepinephrine is implicated in mood disorders (see Chapter 6) and anxiety (see Chapter 7).

Serotonin

Serotonin is synthesized in the raphe nuclei near the midline of the brainstem. Serotonin belongs to the chemical family known as the indoles and is referred to as an indolamine. Serotonin is synthesized from the amino acid tryptophan. The rate-limiting step in the synthesis of serotonin is the enzyme tryptophan hydroxylase. Serotonergic efferents from the raphe nuclei project to the thalamus, hypothalamus, limbic areas, basal ganglia, and cortex. Brain imaging studies reveal that serotonin receptors are densely located throughout all six layers of the cortex. Serotonin is involved in the spinal pain pathway, in facilitating motor activity, sleep and wakefulness, and in modulating behavior. Altered serotonin levels are associated with several mental disorders (see Chapters 5 to 8). (See the box at top.)

Cholinergic System
Acetylcholine

Acetylcholine is the neurotransmitter in the cholinergic system. A major site of acetylcholine synthesis in the brain is the nucleus basalis of Meynert, which projects to many areas of the cortex (see Figure 3.3). Acetylcholine is synthesized from neuronal choline and acetyl coenzyme A. Acetylcholine is stored in vesicles at the axonal terminal and is released into the synaptic cleft when the axon is stimulated. The half-life of acetylcholine is measured in milliseconds because it is rapidly degraded by the enzyme acetylcholinesterase. (See the box above.)

There are two types of acetylcholine receptors,

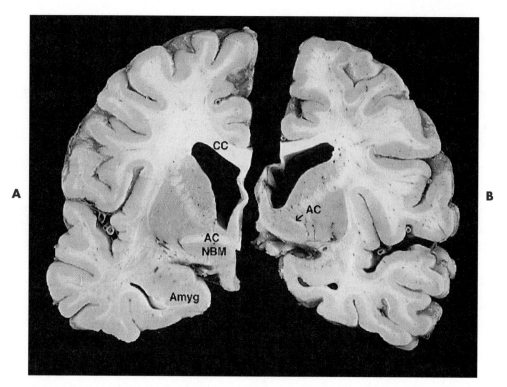

figure 3.3   Appearance of a hemibrain section from a normal individual **(A)** compared with that of an individual with Alzheimer's disease **(B)**. The Alzheimer's brain is significantly smaller than the normal brain, and specific structures appear atrophic. The corpus callosum and anterior commissure are narrower in the Alzheimer's brain. The nucleus basalis of Meynert and amygdala are shrunken by neuronal loss. *AC,* Anterior commissure; *Amyg,* amygdala; *CC,* corpus callosum; *NBM,* nucleus basalis of Meynert. *(Courtesy Dr. Richard E. Powers, Director, University of Alabama at Birmingham Brain Resource Program.)*

nicotinic and muscarinic. The nicotinic receptors, which are thought to be excitatory, are found in the peripheral nervous system at the myoneural junction of skeletal muscles and in the parasympathetic system at the ganglionic receptor. They are rarely found in the CNS. Nicotinic receptors use the first messenger system. Muscarinic receptors are found in the CNS and on the parasympathetic postganglionic receptors, including some of the cranial nerves. Muscarinic receptors use the second messenger system, causing both depolarization and hyperpolarization.

Chemicals that inhibit acetylcholinesterase, such as tacrine (Cognex), physostigmine, and donepezil (Aricept), and drugs that are chemically related to acetylcholine are referred to as cholinergics. Chemicals that block nicotinic receptors at the myoneural junction produce paralysis, whereas chemicals that block muscarinic receptors affect CNS functions (e.g., diminished acetylcholine can cause memory loss and confusion) and autonomic function. For example, antagonism of cranial nerves III, VII and IX, and X causes mydriasis, decreased salivation, and increased heart rate, respectively. Knowledge of the cholinergic system has implications for understanding and treating dementias (see Chapters 9 to 11), delirium (Chapter 12), and movement disorders (Chapter 13).

Amino Acids and Neuropeptides

Several amino acids meet the criteria for neurotransmitters. The most important of these are

Glutamate synthesis:

α-Ketoglutarate————————————————————→Glutamate

          α-Ketoglutarate aminotransferase

Glutamate metabolism:

Glutamate————————————————→GABA

          Glutamic acid decarboxylase

GABA (inhibitory) and glutamate (excitatory). Two other amino acids, glycine (powerful inhibitory influence) and aspartate (excitatory) are also significant neurotransmitters. Except for GABA, these amino acids are found in cells throughout the body. GABA is most highly concentrated in the CNS and spinal cord. All of these amino acids are products of the citric acid cycle.

Neuroactive neuropeptides fall into three categories: posterior pituitary neuropeptides, anterior pituitary neuropeptides, and neurotransmitter neuropeptides. Neuropeptide neurotransmitters such as the enkephalins and substance P are small chains of amino acids that modulate pain perception and emotional experiences. There are more than 50 known neuropeptides, and their dissimilarity from small molecule transmitters is a function of size and the site of synthesis (in the cell body). These large chains of amino acids are formed from the interaction between messenger ribonucleic acid (mRNA) and polyribosomes on the endoplasmic reticulum.[5,11] Most neurons containing neuropeptides also contain a small molecule neurotransmitter. In Chapter 13, it is noted that direct and indirect basal ganglia pathways differ. The direct pathway uses GABA and substance P, whereas the indirect pathway uses GABA and enkephalin.

Glutamate

Glutamate is an excitatory neurotransmitter and is found in the cortex, striatum, hippocampus, cerebellum, motor neurons, and spinal cord. Glutamate is the primary neurotransmitter for interneuronal excitatory synaptic discharges in the CNS.[8] Two receptors have been classified: N-methyl-D-aspartate (NMDA) and non-NMDA. Both receptors use the first messenger system and cause cellular depolarization, or cell firing. Extended exposure to glutamate leads to glutamate excitotoxicity, an event that can destroy neurons. Movement disorders (e.g., Huntington's disease) and epilepsy are negative outcomes linked to glutamate overexposure (see Chapters 13 and 14). (See the box above.)

When glutamate loses an ammonium ion (NH_4^+), glutamine is formed. Measuring glutamine cerebrospinal levels affords a reliable estimate of brain ammonia levels.[11] High ammonia levels can lead to coma and death.[7]

Gamma-Aminobutyric Acid

GABA is an inhibitory neurotransmitter and is said to have a ubiquitous CNS distribution. There are two types of GABA receptors: type A (first messenger) and type B (second messenger).[12] When these receptors are activated, chloride enters the cell, which leads to either hyperpolarization or inhibition. GABAB receptors are less numerous and render a relatively inferior role compared with GABAA receptors. The GABAA receptor is most accurately conceptualized as a GABA receptor complex and is the site of action of several CNS depressants, including barbiturates, alcohol, and benzodiazepines. These agents cause CNS depression by prolonging the time that chloride channels are open. However, the benzodiazepines attach to receptor sites that are different from the other depressants, which leads to the recognition of a benzodiazepine-specific site on the GABAA receptor complex.[14] The benzodiazepine receptor type is further differentiated as

GABA synthesis:

Glutamate————————————→**GABA**

   Glutamic acid decarboxylase

GABA metabolism:

GABA————————————→Succinic semialdehyde

   GABA aminotransferase

type I and type II.[12] Benzodiazepines are known to provide both sedative and anxiolytic effects. Interestingly, type I benzodiazepine receptors may be associated with sedation, and type II receptors may be associated with anxiolytic action.[14] This distinction intensifies the search for receptor-specific psychotropic agents (i.e., drugs that are anxiolytic and not sedating). (See the box above.)

The treatment of anxiety, as can be surmised, involves GABA neurotransmission (see Chapter 7). Furthermore, GABA inhibition plays a central role in maintaining the basal ganglia chemical balance required for smooth movement (see Chapter 13). An appreciation of GABA-mediated cell inhibition has been instrumental to the understanding and treatment of epilepsy (see Chapter 14).

Glycine and Aspartate

Glycine is a product of glycolysis and the citric acid cycle, and it is thought to be synthesized from serine. Glycine is found in the cortex, hippocampus, cerebellum, and spinal cord. It is inhibitory and uses the first messenger system. Aspartate is also a product of glycolysis and the citric acid cycle and is excitatory. Aspartate is found in the hippocampus and the dorsal root ganglion.

Substance P and Enkephalin

Substance P is a neuropeptide composed of a chain of 11 amino acids. It was isolated approximately 60 years ago in the gut and is classified as a gastrointestinal neuropeptide. It acts on smooth muscles and glands. In more recent times substance P has been found in the brainstem, pituitary gland, hypothalamus, and the ventral horn

of the spinal cord. It is also located in the striatum, where it combines with GABA in the direct pathway of the basal ganglia. Enkephalins are broadly dispersed in the CNS. In the mid-1970s enkephalins were found to bind to opioid receptors and reproduce the action of morphine. The indirect pathway of the basal ganglia uses GABA and enkephalin. When this pathway is altered, the overall inhibitory effect of the indirect pathway is compromised, which leads to movement disorders (see Chapter 13).

Blood-Brain Barrier

Life depends on isolating the brain from the normal physiological variability that is found in the periphery.[2] Whereas other body components may undergo shifts in body chemistry, even small flucuations in the brain may produce serious consequences. Hence, the physiological milieu of the brain is homeostatic. This segregation of body physiology from brain physiology is established by the blood-brain barrier. The blood-brain barrier governs the quantity of and rapidity with which substances in the blood penetrate the brain. Water, carbon dioxide, and oxygen readily cross the barrier; other substances are excluded from the brain. The blood-brain barrier can be compromised by disease or other factors. CNS infection and inflammation are the most common causes of barrier collapse.[10]

The blood-brain barrier has several dimensions: an anatomical barrier, a physiological barrier, and a metabolic barrier. The anatomical barrier is created by several features unique to brain capillaries.

First, the structure of the capillaries that supply blood to the brain differs from capillary structure in other parts of the body. The endothelial cells forming the tube of a brain capillary are joined by continuous tight junctions. These cells are physically joined together in contradistinction to peripheral capillaries, where molecules from the blood can slip between cells. Furthermore, channels running from the luminal to antiluminal border are not typically found in brain capillaries but are present in peripheral capillary membranes. Finally, brain capillaries are almost completely embraced by astrocyte foot processes that envelop the vessel. Together these distinctive anatomical features prevent many molecules from passing through the barrier, thus maintaining brain homeostasis.

The physiological barrier allows certain substances to enter the brain while preventing other blood constituents from doing so. A major determinant is lipid solubility. Highly lipid-soluble substances easily pass the blood-brain barrier, whereas highly water-soluble substances cross the barrier very slowly and in insignificant amounts. Lipid-soluble matter diffuses through the endothelial cells because the leaflets of the cells are composed of lipid molecules.[2] Nicotine, ethanol, heroin, caffeine, and diazepam (Valium) are examples of highly lipid-soluble substances that easily penetrate the blood-brain barrier. These molecules have a certain addictive quality that can be partially explained by the ease in which they penetrate the brain. On the other hand, penicillin, glycine, dopamine, epinephrine, albumin, sodium, and potassium are more water soluble and do not penetrate the blood-brain barrier well. Clinically this becomes significant because only drugs that are capable of crossing this barrier in significant amounts are effective in treating psychiatric or medical disorders of the brain. A good example of this assertion is dopamine. Parkinson's disease is related to decreased levels of dopamine (see Chapter 13). However, because dopamine crosses the blood-brain barrier only in miniscule amounts, it cannot be given to patients for CNS disorders. Researchers have discovered a precursor to dopamine that *does* cross the blood-brain barrier—levodopa. Levodopa was a major breakthrough for sufferers of Parkinson's disease, and the science behind its discovery became a prototype for other psychopharmacological research.

The metabolic barrier is the third restrictive wall that prevents molecules from entering the brain. Some molecules can cross the blood-brain barrier but are enzymatically reduced in the endothelial cell to a molecule that cannot pass the barrier. For example, the greater percentage of levodopa is converted to dopamine before it can enter the brain.

Continuous tight junctions, lipid solubility, and endothelial metabolism are key concepts in understanding the blood-brain barrier, but they do not explain how certain indispensable, non–lipid-soluble substances penetrate the barrier. For example, the brain would die if substances such as glucose, the brain's primary energy source, and essential amino acids could not enter. These substances are required for normal brain function. These vital components of brain function are escorted through the barrier by specific transport systems.[8] As previously stated, levodopa is noted to cross the blood-brain barrier much more readily than dopamine. However, levodopa's greater lipid solubility provides only a portion of the explanation; a specific transport system carries levodopa into the brain more rapidly than its lipid solubility alone can explain.

The blood-brain barrier isolates the brain from the rest of the body and in doing so preserves life. Drugs that would have an adverse effect on the CNS can be administered with little worry that they will enter the brain. However, the blood-brain barrier also makes the treatment of CNS infections more complex because many antibiotics do not pierce the barrier easily. For example, penicillin, at one time the only antibiotic available, crosses the barrier very poorly. In the past clinicians were able to successfully treat CNS infections only by the use of massive doses.

The blood-brain barrier is not complete. Certain brain sites that are in contact with ventricular walls are able to sample blood in the systemic circulation. These organs are referred to as *circumventricular organs* and include the pineal gland,

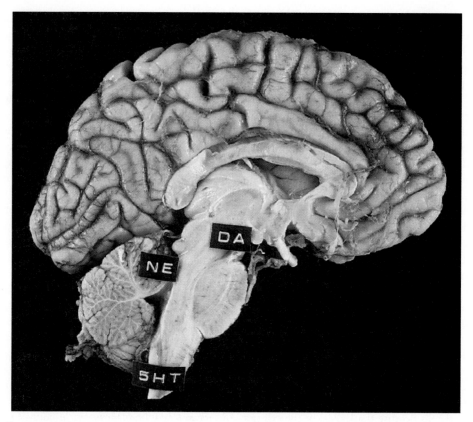

figure 3.4   Sagittal view of the brain, allowing visualization of major neurotransmitter synthesizing sites. *DA,* Dopamine; *NE,* norepinephrine; *5HT,* serotonin. *(Courtesy Dr. Richard E. Powers, Director, University of Alabama at Birmingham Brain Resource Program.)*

portions of the hypothalamus, and the pituitary gland.[8] These "holes" in the blood-brain barrier allow hormones in the systemic blood circulation to reach secretory neurons in the brain and complete the various psychoendocrine feedback systems. Chapter 6 provides a further discussion of these systems.

Summary

Effective psychopharmacological treatment of psychobiological disorders is achieved by manipulating neurotransmitter systems (Figure 3.4). System manipulation exploits key facts known about neurotransmitter synthesis and neurotransmission. For example, researchers have exploited their understanding of dopamine synthesis to boost systemic dopamine levels; a precursor to dopamine (levodopa) has been given to patients with remarkable initial results. Other psychotropic drugs mimic neurotransmitters. These agonists are "recognized" by a specific receptor and trigger responses like those caused by the endogenous chemical. Bromocriptine, a dopamine agonist used in the treatment of Parkinson's disease, elicits the same response as dopamine.

Using yet a different neurochemical strategy, some agents antagonize receptors. For example, neuroleptics block certain dopamine receptors, which accounts for both antipsychotic and extrapyramidal effects. Other psychotropics act by preventing the reuptake of chemicals into the presynaptic terminal. Both tricyclic antidepressants and serotonin reuptake inhibitors block reuptake, which precipitates prolonged receptor exposure to monoamines.

Finally, some agents block the enzymatic reduction of neurotransmitters. For example, tacrine inhibits acetylcholinesterase from degrading acetylcholine. Attempts to augment acetylcholine levels are consistent with knowledge about the role of the cholinergic system in dementia. As the understanding of chemical neuroanatomy continues to evolve, neurotransmitter systems will no doubt be more precisely manipulated to yield greater clinical efficacy.

REFERENCES

1. Axelrod J: Neurotransmitters, *Scientific American* 230(6):59-71, 1974.
2. Goldstein GW, Betz AL: The blood-brain barrier, *Scientific American* 255:74-83, 1986.
3. Graybeil AM: The basal ganglia, *Trends Neurosci* 18:60-62, 1995.
4. Hyman SE: What are second messengers? *The Harvard Medical Letter* 4:8, 1995.
5. Kandel ER, Schwartz JH, Jessell TM: *Priniciples of neural science*, ed 3, Norwalk, Conn, 1991, Appleton & Lange.
6. Mathews CK, Van Holde KE: *Biochemistry*, Redwood City, Calif, 1990, Benjamin-Cummings.
7. McGeer PL, McGeer EG: Amino acid neurotransmitters. In Siegal GJ et al, editors: *Basic neurochemistry*, New York, 1989, Raven Press.
8. Nolte J: *The human brain,* ed 3, St Louis, 1993, Mosby.
9. Patton HD: The autonomic nervous system. In Patton HD et al, editors: *Textbook of physiology,* vol 1, Philadelphia, 1989, WB Saunders.
10. Shlafer M: *The nurse, pharmacology, and drug therapy,* Redwood City, Calif, 1993, Addison-Wesley.
11. Sugerman R: Neuropharmacology. In Keltner NL, Folks DG: *Psychotropic drugs,* ed 2, St Louis, 1997, Mosby.
12. Suzdak PD, Jansen JA: A review of the preclinical pharmacology of tiagabine: a potent and selective anticonvulsant GABA uptake inhibitor, *Epilepsia* 36(6):612-626, 1995.
13. Weiner N, Molinoff PB: Catecholamines. In Siegal GJ et al, editors: *Basic neurochemistry,* New York, 1989, Raven Press.
14. Zorumski CF, Isenberg KE: Insights into the structure and function of GABA-benzodiazepine receptors: ion channels and psychiatry, *Am J Psychiatr* 148(2):162-173, 1991.

BIBLIOGRAPHY

1. Boss BJ, Stowe AC: Neuroanatomy, *J Neurosci Nurs* 18(4):214-228, 1986.
2. Kandel ER, Schwartz JH, Jessell TM: *Priniciples of neural science,* ed 3, Norwalk, Conn, 1991, Appleton & Lange.
3. McCance KL, Huether SE: *Pathophysiology: the biological basis for disease in adults and children,* ed 2, St Louis, 1994, Mosby.
4. Nolte J: *The human brain,* ed 3, St Louis, 1993, Mosby.
5. Ross G: *Essentials of human physiology,* ed 2, Chicago, 1982, Year Book Medical Publishers.
6. Sugerman R: Neuropharmacology. In Keltner NL, Folks DG, editors: *Psychotropic drugs,* ed 2, St Louis, 1997, Mosby.

chapter four

Brain Imaging

Neuroradiology is an expansive section of the neurosciences that has been growing extremely rapidly as a result of ongoing technological developments. Numerous textbooks of excellent quality have been written about various subdivisions of neuroradiology; the purpose of this chapter is to provide a brief introduction to the capabilities of neuroradiographic techniques in the diagnosis of patients with neuropsychiatric illnesses. In instances of coma or dementing illness, little other diagnostic information may be available, and imaging studies can be invaluable in determining localization of lesions.

Various planes are used in brain imaging. Whereas older radiographic techniques were able to provide views of only the anterior to posterior (AP) and lateral planes, the new systems enable photographs to be taken in the sagittal, coronal, and axial (or horizontal) planes (Figure 4.1).

Radiographs

Although of little general use today, plain x-ray films of the bones of the nervous system do have a few uses. They are beneficial in the evaluation of both skull fractures and compression or misalignment of the spinal axis, especially in circumstances of trauma.

Angiography

Angiography (or arteriography) is a neuroradiological procedure that uses intravenous or intraarterial dyes to identify abnormalities of the vascular system. It is used to search for aneurysms and arteriovenous malformations, as well as to as-

sess the extent of atherosclerosis. When used as part of the evaluation of brain tumors, angiography can determine the vascularity of a tumor (Figure 4.2), thereby indicating whether treatment is necessary to diminish the blood flow before a surgical procedure.

Ultrasonography

Unlike conventional radiographic procedures, the application of **ultrasonography** does not expose the patient to ionizing radiation. Mechanical waves are introduced over the surface of the body with a video probe to provide information concerning the structures below. Of much less clinical utility when the skull bone is intact, ultrasonography is clinically useful with children whose cranial sutures have not yet fused, and also intraoperatively, if a portion of the skull has been removed. It is also quite useful as a noninvasive procedure to determine the degree of atherosclerosis in the carotid arteries to assess the need for angiography.

Computed (Axial) Tomography

The development of computed tomography ([CT], or computed axial tomography [CAT]) scans was the beginning of the neuroradiological revolution in the late 1960s and early 1970s. This technology introduced views of the brain itself in cross section, thereby providing capabilities for diagnostic accuracy not previously available.

CT scanning is fairly noninvasive and is also rapid and safe. Although CT scans provide more detail than traditional procedures, they are not as sensitive as some of the newer techniques (Figure

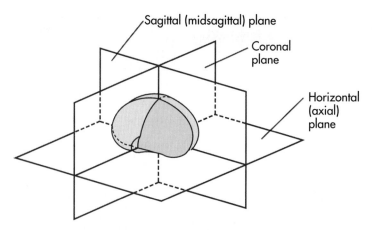

figure 4.1   Diagram of various planes used in brain imaging techniques. *(From Waxman SG: Correlative neuroanatomy, ed 23, Stanford, Conn, 1991, Appleton & Lange.)*

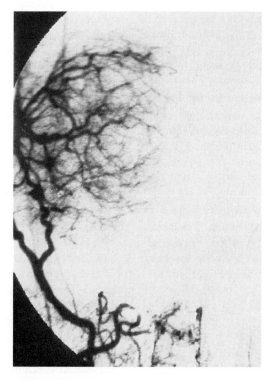

figure 4.2   This "tumor blush" is the result of an intraarterial dye injection in a patient with a vascular meningioma, a brain tumor of the meninges. *(Courtesy Dr. Cheryl A. Palmer, Division of Neuropathology, University of Alabama at Birmingham.)*

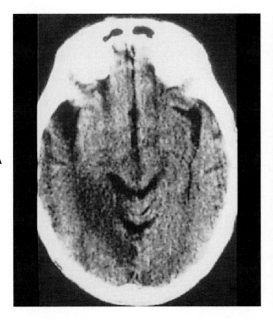

A

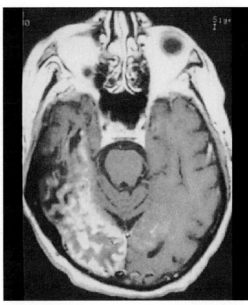

B

figure 4.3   **A,** In this CT scan without contrast dye, note that the central *black* region is part of the ventricular system, whereas the *white* on the outside is the skull. This scan depicts a right (*left* side of photograph) posterior cerebral artery infarction. **B,** The MRI of the same patient (T2-weighted image) reveals far greater detail than the CT scan. *(Courtesy Dr. Van B. Wadlington, Department of Radiology, University of Alabama at Birmingham.)*

4.3, *B*). CT, which provides axial images readily but requires computer reformatting for other planes, still remains the test of choice in the evaluation of calcification or bones, and it is much simpler to use in the case of emergency than other more laborious methods. In the image in Figure 4.3, *A, black* represents structures of low density (e.g., the cerebrospinal fluid [CSF] in the ventricular system, cysts) and *white* represents structures of higher density (e.g., bone, hemorrhage). CT scans of abnormalities in the posterior fossa are usually less than ideal because of the artifact induced by the dense bone in many planes in that region.

CT scans are often performed without contrast agents (intravenous dyes) and then duplicated with the use of contrast agents. Collections of contrast extravasation generally represent breakdown of the blood-brain barrier by infarctions or neoplastic or infectious processes.

Magnetic Resonance Imaging

Nuclear magnetic resonance (NMR) has been used in physical chemical laboratories since the 1950s. The radiographic technique of magnetic resonance imaging (MRI) was later developed for use in medicine from these earlier NMR techniques.

MRI images have the advantage that any plane can be obtained directly, and no computer reformatting is required. In addition to the usefulness of viewing differing planes in the brain, sagittal imaging of the spinal canal and spinal cord are valuable in evaluation of spinal anatomy and pathology. Two basic time sequences are used in MRI scanning: a short time sequence, which produces an image called a T1 and better defines brain and cord anatomy; and a longer time sequence, which produces a T2 image and excels in defining edema and subtle signal changes in the white matter (Figure 4.4).

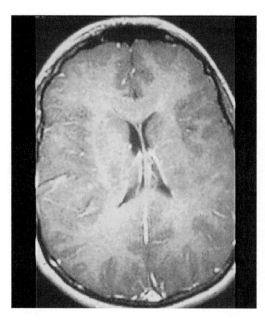
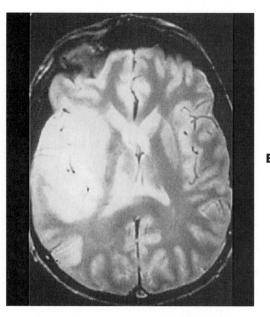

A

B

figure 4.4   The right hemisphere (*left* side of the photograph) in this T1-weighted image looks fuller than the opposite side (**A**), but the accompanying T2-weighted image actually reveals the extent of this glial tumor in the patient (**B**). *(Courtesy Dr. Van B. Wadlington, Department of Radiology, University of Alabama at Birmingham.)*

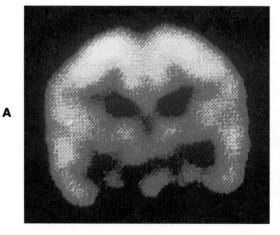
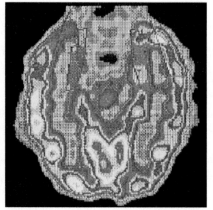

A

B

figure 4.5   **A,** An ictal (during a seizure) SPECT scan from a patient with frontal lobe epilepsy. Note the bright yellow spot in the left side of the photograph. **B,** A PET scan from a patient with temporal lobe epilepsy. The various regions are color-coded according to their metabolic activity. Less activity is occurring in this left temporal lobe. *(A, Courtesy Dr. Frank G. Gilliam, Department of Neurology, University of Alabama at Birmingham; B, Courtesy Dr. Ruben I. Kuzniecky, Department of Neurology, University of Alabama at Birmingham.)*

MRI scanning is rather slow and requires patient cooperation in altering the breathing cycle:
scans cannot be performed on patients who are
restless and unable to relax. Patients with ferro-
magnetic equipment such as pacemakers or steel
pins in bones cannot enter MRI units; neither can
patients who require artificial ventilation because
there is abundant metal in the respirators.

Single Photon Emission Computed Tomography

Unlike any of the previously discussed neuroradiographic techniques, which employ anatomical
information for diagnostic purposes, single photon emission computed tomography (SPECT)
scans use a functional imaging basis. The most
commonly used radiopharmaceutical in this procedure is Tc-99m-HMPAO, which can cross the
blood-brain barrier and diffuse into nerve cells
with the blood flow. This chemical remains distributed long enough for assessment of the relative
distribution of blood in the brain in thin slices.
Although these images do not have the anatomical precision of CT and MRI (Figure 4.5, *A*), they
are valuable in the study of epileptogenic foci (see
Chapter 14) and dementing illnesses, as well as in
determining the amount of brain tissue damage in
infarctions.

Positron Emission Tomography

Not available widely as a result of equipment
expense, positron emission tomography (PET)
scans have become a research tool in the field of
functional imaging. Most useful in the evaluation
of cerebral blood flow and brain metabolism, they
can generally determine hyperactive brain tissue
(e.g., tumor) versus necrotic, nonactive brain tissue (Figure 4.5, *B*). The isotopes used in this procedure decay quite quickly, which produces a
problem in their manufacture. In addition,
anatomical detail is far less than precise.

BIBLIOGRAPHY

1. deGroot J: *Correlative neuroanatomy*, ed 21, San
    Mateo, Calif, 1991, Appleton & Lange.
2. Osborn AG: *Diagnostic neuroradiology: a text/atlas*,
    St Louis, 1994, Mosby.

Biogenesis and Clinical Management of Mental Disorders

Schizophrenia and Psychosis

"To have forgotten that schizophrenia is a brain disease will go down as one of the great aberrations of twentieth century medicine"

(Ron, Harvey, 1990, p. 725).

Psychosis is a disruption of an individual's reality testing in which the person cannot distinguish internally generated sensory perceptions or ideas from external realities. Common symptoms of psychosis include hallucinations, delusions, and difficulty organizing thoughts. Psychosis is a nonspecific condition that can be present in schizophrenia, acute mania, depression, drug intoxication, dementia, delirium, and multiple other clinical conditions. The symptoms of psychosis do not identify the cause of brain malfunction.

Schizophrenia is one of the most common causes of psychosis. It is a biological brain disorder with symptoms that usually appear in late adolescence or early adulthood. Patients manifest disturbances in thought and sensory perceptions (e.g., hallucinations, delusions), thought disorders, and a deterioration of psychosocial function. A typical patient is a 21-year-old college student who withdraws socially and drops out of the university after experiencing auditory hallucinations and paranoid delusions. Five years later, this person holds a low-paying job and lives with his or her parents.

The term *schizophrenia* comes from the Greek terms *schizo* (to split) and *phrenia* (thought) and denotes the disconnection between thought and emotion. Classic psychodynamic explanations for schizophrenia included suggestions that poor parenting and family stress caused the disease. The absence of physical or neurological findings coupled with an intact intellect led clinicians to believe that schizophrenia was a functional rather than a biological disease.

Schizophrenia is characterized by a severe disturbance in personality and disruptions in thinking. Symptoms associated with schizophrenia can be roughly classified as positive (delusions, hallucinations, conceptual disorganization, grandiosity, hostility, persecution, suspiciousness, excitement) and negative (blunted affect, withdrawal, poor rapport, passive social withdrawal, difficulty in abstract thinking, difficulties in communication).[3]

Epidemiology and Demographics

Epidemiological and demographical statistics for schizophrenia have remained relatively constant since 1978, when sophisticated measurements were initiated by The President's Commission on Mental Health.[52] Approximately 1% of the U.S. population has been diagnosed with schizophrenia. Regier et al[54] found that in any given year 1.1% of adults over 17 years of age were diagnosed with schizophrenia. They illustrate the chronicity of the condition by noting that twice as many individuals had the disorder at the beginning of the year (0.7%) as developed the disorder or relapsed during the year (0.3%). Regier et al have estimated that 1.7 million adults are afflicted with schizophrenia. Approximately 1 million of these patients are treated on an outpatient basis, which accounts for 16.7 million visits, or approximately 16 visits per patient per year.[46] Another 295,000 patients receive inpatient treatment for schizophrenia.[46] Although no study of mental health treatment comprehensively addresses the extent of that treatment, it is estimated that 90% of individuals with severe mental illness (including schizophrenia) receive professional help in a given year.

Kraepelin[35] described schizophrenia, which he termed *dementia praecox*, as a disorder of young men. However, current demographic studies do not fully support Kraepelin's view. Women have a higher incidence of schizophrenia than men; however, the ratios are not nearly so strikingly different as the gender differences found in affective and anxiety disorders. Kraepelin's observation that schizophrenia is a disorder of youth has been supported; that is, schizophrenia is a disorder that emerges in late adolescence or early adulthood.[71] Approximately 2.5% of men and 3.3% of women between the ages of 18 and 24 suffer from schizophrenia. By the time men and women reach the ages of 55 to 64, only 0.5% and 0.6%, respectively, are afflicted with schizophrenia.[26,47] Overall, Kessler et al[32] found a 12-month prevalence rate of 0.5% for men and 0.6% for women. Lifetime prevalence rates are 0.6% and 0.8%, respectively.

Socioeconomically, schizophrenia is eight times more likely to occur in those who are poor. Whether poverty is a consequence or cause of schizophrenia is eloquently debated in other texts. When socioeconomic variables are controlled for, schizophrenia is found in similar numbers across ethnic and racial groups.[48] Kessler et al[32] found regional differences in prevalence rates for all mental disorders. Individuals living in the southern United States demonstrated significantly lower rates of mental illness. It is not known whether these findings reflect real geographical differences or merely cultural differences reflected through treatment-seeking behaviors or a reluctance to discuss personal health concerns.

Other epidemiological and treatment issues include the high incidence of comorbidity present in persons with schizophrenia. A high percentage of individuals with chronic mental illness also abuse alcohol and/or drugs. Among those who are homeless and mentally ill, more than 50% are thought to abuse such substances.[22] Furthermore, depression is common among persons with schizophrenia and is often associated with poor outcome and relapse.[7,41,44]

Psychobiological Considerations
Macroscopic Brain Alterations

Modern schizophrenia research began with the work of Johnstone et al[31] in 1976 when they published their findings of enlarged ventricles among some individuals with schizophrenia.[45] Evidence continues to accumulate to support the idea that schizophrenia is related to physiological and anatomical disorders in the brain.[4,5,18] Although negative schizophrenia and positive schizophrenia have different neurophysiological profiles,[25] it seems that physiological changes are more closely associated with positive symptoms, whereas anatomical changes are more closely linked to negative symptoms.

Although many of the anatomical changes that occur in schizophrenia are microscopic, several important anomalies are macroscopic and have attracted serious research investigations. These alterations include ventricular enlargement and other anatomical abnormalities that together can manifest in such proportion as to be visible to the unaided eye. A majority of studies find that, as a group, patients with schizophrenia have significantly smaller limbic structures than do normal controls.[38] Volume reductions are found in the temporal lobe grey matter, hippocampus (up to 20% neuronal loss histologically), entorhinal cortex (up to 20% neuronal loss), and cortex grey matter. Collectively these "smaller" structures can contribute to an overall reduction in brain weight (up to 5%) and length.[15,38,55,77]

Ventricular Enlargement (Ventriculomegaly)

Although not peculiar to schizophrenia, enlarged third and lateral ventricles or increased ven-

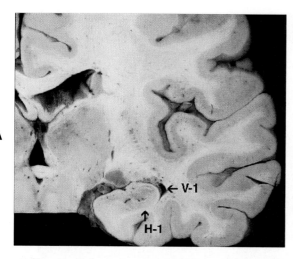 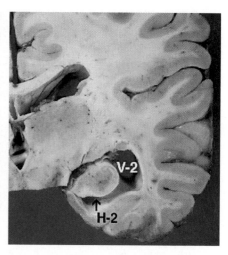

figure 5.1 Comparison of the temporal lobe of a normal individual (**A**) to that of a patient with schizophrenia (**B**). The inferior horn of the lateral ventricle (V-1) in the normal individual is conspicuously smaller than the ventricle of the patient with schizophrenia (V-2). In contrast, the hippocampus of the patient with schizophrenia (H-2) is smaller than that of the normal subject (H-1). *(Courtesy Dr. Richard E. Powers, Director, University of Alabama at Birmingham Brain Resource Program.)*

tricular brain ratios (VBRs) are found in patients with this chronic disease.* This observation originated in postmortem findings, which suggested a significant increase in ventricular size among patients with schizophrenia. Computed tomography (CT) and magnetic resonance imaging (MRI) studies confirm these earlier reports. Ventricular enlargement has two etiologies: (1) ventricles can expand like a balloon because of increased amounts of cerebrospinal fluid (CSF), and (2) ventricles may fill a "vacuum" when cortical or subcortical tissue either dies and atrophies or does not fully develop.

Ventricular expansion resulting from increased pressure. When ventricles expand because of increased volumes of CSF, a condition known as *hydrocephalus* occurs. There is no established link between hydrocephalus and schizophrenia. Depending on the etiology, hydrocephalus is usually described as communicating or noncommunicating. **Communicating** hydrocephalus is related to inadequate CSF resorption into venous sinuses.

This phenomenon is often a result of injury to the arachnoid villi by an inflammatory process or trauma. **Noncommunicating** hydrocephalus is caused by a blockage of the ventricular system. The accumulation of CSF causes expansion of the ventricles. Hydrocephalus can be successfully treated with surgery, typically by implanting a catheter in the anterior horn of the lateral ventricle, with drainage into the peritoneal cavity (VP shunt).

Ventricular expansion resulting from cell death. Ventricular enlargement related to cell death or atrophy (ex-vacuo) is *not* treatable and is prominent in Alzheimer's disease and other conditions. Ventricular enlargement associated with schizophrenia may be a result of a developmental lag. It is important to note that, unlike with Alzheimer's disease, the ventricular enlargement found in patients with schizophrenia is not thought to be associated with neurodegeneration.[12,16,38,55,64]

Figure 5.1 contrasts the ventricles of a "normal" brain with the brain of a person with schizophrenia. In this figure the difference in ventricular size is readily apparent, but not all cases are so com-

*References 4, 23, 26, 36, 53, 69, 70.

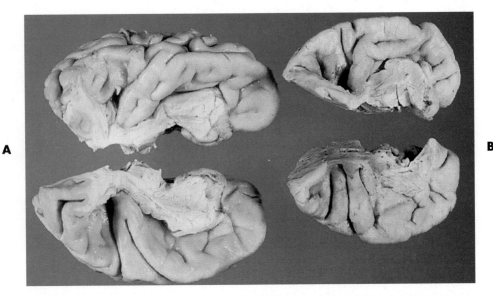

figure 5.2   The temporal lobes of a patient with schizophrenia **(B)** are significantly smaller than the temporal lobes of an age- and gender-matched normal subject **(A)**. Abnormalities of the superior temporal gyrus are related to the severity of auditory hallucinations. *(Courtesy Dr. Richard E. Powers, Director, University of Alabama at Birmingham Brain Resource Program.)*

pelling. Approximately 50% of patients with schizophrenia fall within the range of control or "normal" subjects.[15] The search for a grossly apparent anatomical marker of schizophrenia is further complicated by ventricular variability; that is, ventricle size varies among persons who do not have schizophrenia. Historically, defining acceptable control comparisons has been a major challenge to schizophrenia researchers.

The search for an adequate comparison population has led researchers to what might be the perfect control; a monozygotic, unaffected twin of a patient with schizophrenia. As a group, first-degree relatives have a high (70% to 100%) sensitivity ratio for ventricular enlargement,[15] and it is consistent with genetic theory to assume that monozygotic twins occupy the higher end of this range. However, without the "perfect" control, a twin with schizophrenia may not have a discernably larger ventricle. These findings suggest a continuum of disease among individuals with schizophrenia—from seemingly slight to gross pathoanatomical changes. Hence, even small vol-

umetric losses of brain tissue can have a profound impact on mental function.

Genetic considerations. A peripheral yet significant issue raised by twin studies is that of genetic influences. Monozygotic twins share identical genes; therefore discordancy for schizophrenia among this select population underscores the role of environment (common sense would suggest prenatally) as a causative factor. In other words, a strictly genetic model for schizophrenia could not account for ventricular variability.

Temporal Lobe Reduction

Evidence suggests that a reduction in temporal lobe grey matter is also a pathoanatomical phenomenon that occurs in schizophrenia (Figure 5.2).[23,29,51,70,74] A reversal of normal temporal lobe asymmetry (the left is "normally" slightly larger than the right) was noted in two studies.[51,70] Of particular interest has been the planum temporale, which lies on the superior aspect of the temporal lobe and is involved in the generation and under-

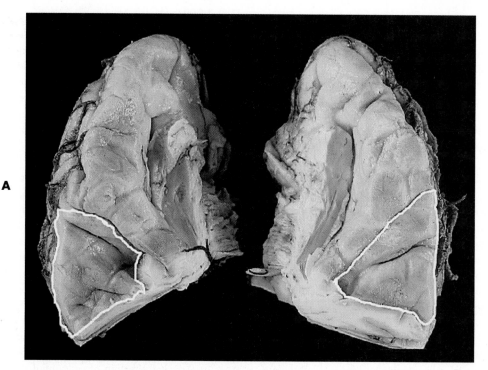

figure 5.3   The left (**A**) and right (**B**) temporal lobes from a patient with schizophrenia demonstrate the reversal of normal asymmetry of the planum temporale. In normal subjects the left planum temporale is larger than the right, but the opposite can be true in those with schizophrenia. Abnormalities of the planum temporale are related to the severity of thought disorder. *(Courtesy Dr. Richard E. Powers, Director, University of Alabama at Birmingham Brain Resource Program.)*

standing of language.[51] The planum temporale suffers cell loss, and this reduction could explain the language difficulties commonly associated with schizophrenia (Figure 5.3).

Association Cortex Changes and Hallucinations

Hallucinations are experienced in all sensory modalities; these occurrences may result from electrophysiological malfunction in the respective cortices. Sensory cortices are divided into three general regions: (1) primary sensory receptive cortex, (2) unimodal association cortex, and (3) multimodal or heteromodal association cortex. Each of the five sensory modalities has association cortices that integrate specific sensory information. Adjacent multimodal association cortices integrate the sensory message into the environmental context. Auditory, visual, olfactory, and kines-

thetic hallucinations occur with schizophrenia and other neurological disorders (e.g., temporal lobe epilepsy, Alzheimer's disease). These symptoms are specific to the brain region—not the disease.

The auditory cortex is a good example of a brain region in which complex sensory information is interpreted and integrated. Auditory input is processed from the cranial nerve VIII via the medial geniculate nucleus in the transverse temporal gyrus. Auditory input is interpreted in the superior temporal gyri and in the inferior parietal lobule and other temporal areas. Very sophisticated interpretation occurs in the cortex immediately posterior to the superior temporal gyrus, which is often referred to as the planum temporale. Multimodal associations probably occur in the temporal pole and in other areas.

Accurate interpretation of spoken communication involves (1) understanding the language, (2) interpreting the tone and emotional quality of the speaker's voice, and (3) integrating the information into the context of the total environment. The emotional tone and intellectual content of language can be disconnected by brain damage; patients with such damage may speak with a loud angry voice when they are actually experiencing calm, happy emotions. The musical, rhythmic, and emotional quality of language is called *prosody*. For example, the words "aren't you smart" have a different meaning if spoken with a friendly, calm, warm voice versus a loud angry voice. The words "are you feeling lucky" have two different meanings when spoken by your friends on a tennis court or by three large, threatening individuals following you down a dark, lonely street. Although the script of these words is exactly the same, the prosody and context of the message carries great weight for the meaning. The multimodal association cortex may help distinguish between a friendly greeting and impending threats.

Damage to the auditory association cortex can cause receptive aphasia (an inability to interpret spoken words) or auditory hallucinations. Alzheimer's disease also destroys association cortex and causes receptive aphasia. Electrical stimulation of the superior temporal gyrus causes auditory hallucinations similar to those experienced by patients with schizophrenia. Neurosurgical patients report hearing voices, sounds, and music when their temporal lobe is electrically stimulated in the wake state during operations. Abnormalities of the planum temporale may relate to thought disorder (the inability to organize internal, verbal thoughts) or dyslexia (difficulty assembling or interpreting written language).

Hippocampal Reductions

The most prominent functions of the hippocampus are learning and memory. Although hippocampal reductions are not found consistently in the schizophrenia literature, a growing body of evidence does suggest hippocampal involvement in schizophrenia. These anatomical changes are by definition quite subtle; only as

imaging technology has advanced has the ability to capture these minor variations improved. The number of positive findings has increased significantly in the past few years, and a reduction in hippocampal volume has been reported by several researchers.* Other studies suggest that certain cellular level abnormalities may eventually culminate into macroscopic changes (e.g., decrease in hippocampal synaptic density and activity,[19] hypofunction of hippocampal glutaminergic neurons,[68] decreased numbers of nicotinic receptors,[24] and smaller neuron size[6]). Roberts, Leigh, and Weinberger[55] and Bogerts et al[11] indicate that hippocampal neuron loss may reach 20%. Reduced volume in the hippocampus and associated structures appears to be linked to an increased severity of schizophrenic symptoms.[12]

One of the more interesting hypotheses concerning hippocampal involvement in schizophrenia has been advanced by Torrey.[67] He believes that hippocampal damage is a major cause of schizophrenia and that this damage probably arises from a viral infection of early infancy. This hypothesis is bolstered by observations that birth dates in the winter (when viral infections are more prevalent) are overrepresented among individuals with schizophrenia.

Entorhinal Cortex Reductions

The entorhinal cortex, a subdivision of the parahippocampal gyrus, plays a major role in learning, memory, and social behavior. It links the limbic system to the neocortex and is continuous with the hippocampal formation, lying just below that area. It has also been implicated in schizophrenia.[1,16] Arnold et al[6] found reductions in neuron size and volume in the entorhinal cortex of persons with schizophrenia as compared with unaffected individuals. Because the entorhinal cortex and surrounding hippocampal structures maintain efferent and afferent connections to many cortical and subcortical sites (e.g., entorhino-hippocampal loop, entorhinal-insula and entorhino-orbitofrontal reciprocal connections), reductions may well re-

---

*References 8, 11, 13, 38, 57, 63, 65, 72.

flect impairment and be related to consequential dysfunctional behaviors.[30]

Cortical Atrophy

More than 100 years ago Alzheimer described a loss of cells in the cortices of patients with schizophrenia. Modern day researchers have reinforced these findings.[10] Pathological changes in the frontal lobe may indeed account for many of the negative symptoms associated with schizophrenia (e.g., cognitive deficits, alogia, avolition, anergia, apathy, withdrawal, and inappropriate affect).[10] (Figure 5.4 exhibits the loss of cells from an accident.)

Microscopic Brain Alterations

Persons with schizophrenia also display changes at the cellular level of the brain. Pathological evidence indicates that the brain of a person with schizophrenia is slightly reduced in weight[50] and length.[14] As noted in Chapter 2, the neocortex is composed of six layers of neurons. Cellular changes may occur in a few specific layers or may have a broader distribution. Cellular changes found in schizophrenia include decreased volume, a change in shape, and a change in neuronal cytoarchitecture (cell pattern), including migrational deficits.

Decreased Cellular Volume

Selemon, Rajkowska, and Goldman-Rakic[61] state that neuronal atrophy is the (possible) anatomical substrate for "deficient information processing in schizophrenia." They note a reduction in dendritic trees, synapses, and axonal projections from these neurons, but not necessarily a loss of neurons. They suggest that the cortical thinning found among persons with schizophrenia may be related to an overall atrophic process that results in a 7% reduction in cortical thickness.[61]

Neuronal cell count reductions of up to 20% have been described in the anterior hippocampus and in layer 2 of the entorhinal cortex.[10,55] Smaller reductions have been found in layer 5 of the cingulate and layer 6 of the prefrontal cortex. Other

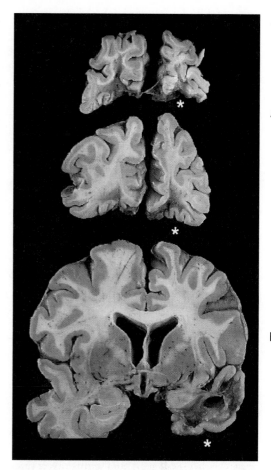

A

B

figure 5.4   This 28-year-old individual developed psychosis and explosive speech following a severe motor vehicle accident. The frontal lobes **(A)** sustained severe contusions *(asterisks)* in the orbital frontal region, and the temporal lobe **(B)** sustained extensive damage. The frontal lobe damage produced irritable, hostile behavior, and the temporal lobe damage caused auditory hallucinations and aprosodic speech. *(Courtesy Dr. Richard E. Powers, Director, University of Alabama at Birmingham Brain Resource Program.)*

studies have found a significant reduction in neuronal count in the amygdala, stria terminalis, and caudate nucleus.[10,13]

Changes in Cell Shape

Persons with schizophrenia may have smaller neurons in some cortical areas. A great deal of at-

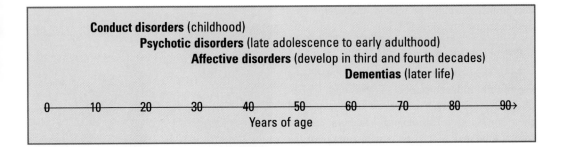

tention has focused on layer 2 of the entorhinal cortex, but other regions can be found to demonstrate smaller cell size.[6,30]

Changes in Cytoarchitecture and Migrational Defects

Cytoarchitectural disturbances and neuron misarrangement are difficult to quantify, but available evidence suggests that migrational defects play a significant role in schizophrenia.[55] Jakob and Beckmann[30] speculate that these migrational problems begin during pregnancy. Potential consequences include "downstream" synaptic disruptions and distortion of sensory input and post-synaptic integration.[55] Weinberger[71] provides an excellent example by describing a child with perinatal hypoxic encephalopathy. He explains that the child may have spastic diplegia or hemiparesis at age 2, athetosis at age 4, and seizures a few years later. The lesion does not change, but the *effects* of the lesion change as the nervous system develops. Weinberger suggests a similar model for schizophrenia. A prenatal insult may remain silent and emerge as schizophrenia only when the developmental timetable is disrupted at some later date; this model leads to Weinberger's explanation for the onset of schizophrenia in late adolescence (see the box above). Evidence exists to suggest that the final synaptic connections in schizophrenia occur in the dorsolateral prefrontal cortex during late adolescence or early adulthood.

Neurophysiological Brain Alterations
The Role of Neurotransmitters in Schizophrenia

Dopamine. The most common neurochemical explanation for schizophrenia is what is referred to as the dopamine hypothesis. Matthysee[40] described

dopamine as a contributing if not causative factor in schizophrenia. It had been observed that L-dopa, an early 1950s scientific breakthrough for patients with Parkinson's disease, worsened schizophrenia and often caused psychotic symptoms in these patients.[76] Because the chief effect of L-dopa is dopaminergic and because chlorpromazine antagonizes dopamine, Matthysee concluded that excessive dopamine bioavailability was instrumental in the development and expression of schizophrenia.[40]

The role of dopamine in schizophrenia is well studied, and this hypothesis continues to provide the most compelling explanation for the disease. Evolving research reveals a number of dopamine receptor subtypes. Seeman and Van Tol[60] categorized dopamine receptors as D1-like (D1 and D5 receptors) and D2-like (D2, D3, and D4) (Box 5.1). They reported that D2 and D3 receptor density increased 10% in schizophrenia, whereas the number of D4 receptors increased 600%.[60] Most antipsychotic drugs block D2 receptors, and potency estimations are based on the antagonism of this receptor. Clozapine primarily antagonizes D4 receptors, which partially explains its efficacy in the treatment of refractory schizophrenia. Many future antipsychotic drug research projects will no doubt focus on D4 receptors and their role in schizophrenia and schizophrenia treatment.

Figure 5.5 outlines three major dopaminergic tracts in the brain with their proposed role in schizophrenia: the nigrostriatal (from the substantia nigra to the striatum), mesolimbic (from the ventral tegmental area [VTA] to the mesial limbic area), and mesocortical (from the VTA to the mesial cortex) tracts. Not included in this figure is

Dopamine Receptors and Their Subtypes

There are basically two categories of dopamine receptors: D_1-like, which includes D_1 and D_5 receptors, and D_2-like, which includes D_2, D_3, and D_4 receptors.

1. **D_1-like receptors:** D_1, D_5, $D_{5\text{ pseudo-1}}$, $D_{5\text{ pseudo-2}}$
2. **D_2-like receptors:** D_{2L}, D_{2S}, $D_{2\text{Ala96}}$, $D_{2\text{ Ser310}}$, $D_{2\text{ Cys311}}$, D_3, $D_{3\text{ Gly9}}$, $D_{3\text{ nf}}$, $D_{3\text{ TM4 d}}$, $D_{3\text{ TM3 d}}$, $D_{4.0}$, $D_{4.1}$, $D_{4.2}$, $D_{4.3}$, $D_{4.4}$, $D_{4.5}$, $D_{4.6}$, $D_{4.7}$, $D_{4.8}$, $D_{4.9}$, $D_{4.10}$, $D_{4\text{ d}}$

Modified from Seeman P, Van Tol HM: Dopamine receptor pharmacology, *Trends Pharmacol Sci* 15(7):264-270, 1994.

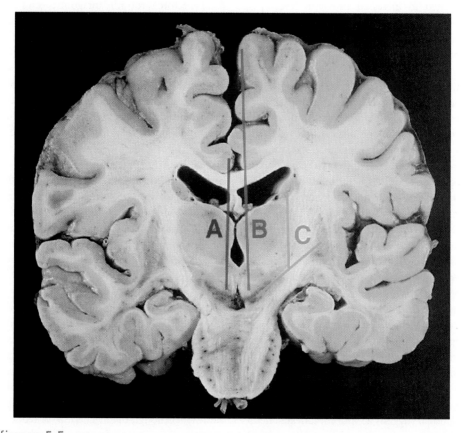

figure 5.5   Three major dopaminergic tracts arising from the brainstem. Tract A *(blue)* represents the mesolimbic tract; hypersecretion of dopamine in this tract leads to positive symptoms of schizophrenia. Tract B *(red)* is the mesocortical tract; hyposecretion of dopamine in this tract may lead to negative symptoms. Tract C *(green)* is the nigrostriatal tract; dopaminergic antagonism in this tract by antipsychotic drugs causes extrapyramidal side effects. *(Courtesy Dr. Richard E. Powers, Director, University of Alabama at Birmingham Brain Resource Program.)*

the tuberoinfundibular tract. According to current thinking, traditional neuroleptics (those that chiefly block D2 receptors) have antipsychotic effects because of their antagonistic actions in the mesolimbic area. Unfortunately, in achieving sufficient antagonism of this tract, the nigrostriatal tract is also affected. Extrapyramidal side effects (EPSEs) occur when receptor occupancy of the nigrostriatal tract reaches a certain threshold (75% to 90%). Furthermore, because dopamine inhibits prolactin levels, dopamine receptor antagonism causes a disinhibition of prolactin. Therefore some patients occasionally experience side effects related to increased prolactin levels (e.g., galactorrhea and gynecomastia); these effects directly result from antagonism of the tuberoinfundibular tract. Finally, traditional antipsychotics may actually worsen negative symptoms by antagonism of the mesocortical tract. Because negative symptomatology may be a *hypo*dopaminergic phenomenon, dopamine blockade could theoretically compound the pathological condition.

Although researchers continue to study the roles of other neurotransmitters in schizophrenia, the dopamine hypothesis continues to have great heuristic value. Supporting evidence includes the following findings: [21,65]

1. Dopaminergic drugs (e.g., L-dopa, amphetamines) can cause psychotic symptoms.
2. Clinically effective antipsychotic drugs occupy approximately 70% to 80% of D2 receptors.
3. Postmortem studies of persons with schizophrenia reveal elevated levels of dopamine receptors.

Critics of the dopamine hypothesis point out the time lag between dopamine receptor blockade, which occurs rapidly, and therapeutic effects, which require weeks to months. At a minimum, this argument suggests a more complicated neurophysiological process than that proposed by the dopamine hypothesis.

Serotonin. As early as 1954, Woolley and Shaw[75] proposed a role for serotonin in schizophrenia. Serotonin inhibits dopamine synthesis; therefore agents that occupy serotonin receptors may in-

crease dopamine levels and be therapeutic in patients with negative symptoms. This argument can be outlined as follows:

1. The negative symptoms of schizophrenia are thought to be related to a hypodopaminergic phenomenon in the frontal cortex.
2. Serotonergic receptors are evenly distributed throughout the six neuronal layers of frontal cortex.
3. Serotonin inhibits dopamine.
4. Serotonin antagonists block the inhibition of dopamine, resulting in increased dopamine in the frontal cortex.
5. Therefore serotonin antagonists can be therapeutic in the treatment of negative schizophrenia symptoms (alogia, flattened affect, avolition, anergia).

The new atypical antipsychotic drugs such as clozapine (Clozaril), risperidone (Risperdal), and olanzapine (Zyprexa) are marketed as serotonin/dopamine antagonists (SDAs) and have proven effectiveness in the treatment of the negative symptoms of schizophrenia. Similar agents soon to be available include sertindole, quetiapine (Seroquel), and ziprasidone. Furthermore, because serotonin neurons project to the substantia nigra, the serotonergic inhibitory influence of these atypical agents may account for the decreased incidence of EPSEs associated with their use.[48a] In other words, they increase dopamine activity in the nigrostriatal pathway.

Glutamate and glycine. Glutamate is a product of the Krebs' cycle, whereas glycine is synthesized directly from serine, which is derived from glycolysis.[42] Glutamate is excitatory, and glycine is inhibitory. Kim et al[33] were the first to suggest a role for decreased glutamate levels in schizophrenia. Other researchers have supported this speculation.[62,68] Although the mechanism of reduced glutamate activity is not clear, studies indicate that a hypoglutaminergic process occurs in schizophrenia that can account for both positive and negative symptoms. Both glutamate and glycine contribute to the regulation of *N*-methyl-D-aspartate (NMDA) receptors. It is suspected that endogenous disruption of this system is related to schizophrenia because NMDA receptors are instrumental to cognitive processes. Several attempts have been made to enhance glutaminergic modulation of NMDA receptors by administering glycine. Moderate therapeutic success can be explained in part by the poor penetration of glycine through the blood-brain barrier.

Functional Changes in Schizophrenia

Numerous studies have substantiated decreased regional cerebral flood flow (rCBF) to areas of the brain in persons with schizophrenia. The prefrontal cortex (specifically, the dorsolateral prefrontal cortex [DLPC]) is the site of cognitive and inhibition processes, goal setting, abstraction, spontaneity, and recent memory. In schizophrenia, this area shows decreased activity in brain function tests—a phenomenon referred to as *hypofrontality*.

Brain Imaging Techniques, Findings, and Research

Brain imaging techniques are perhaps the most active areas of current schizophrenia research. These techniques have provided rich evidence that schizophrenia is associated with structural brain abnormalities.[49] As noted in Chapter 4, a variety of new techniques are available and allow for study of the human brain in vivo. CT and MRI imaging have demonstrated the neuroanatomical changes previously discussed in this chapter, including increased ventricle-brain ratios, temporal lobe reductions, hippocampal reductions, and cortical atrophy. On the other hand, positron emission tomography (PET) and single photon emission computed tomography (SPECT) studies have enabled scientists to study the actual function of the brain. Decreased cerebral brain flow and hypometabolism have been demonstrated consistently in persons with schizophrenia. A mental performance assignment such as the Wisconsin Card Sorting Task is often given to a subject while glucose use (a marker of brain activity) is monitored by PET technology. Repeated studies have confirmed a lower level of brain activity in patients with schizophrenia versus control groups.

Clinical Applications

Clinical Findings and Course

As previously noted, schizophrenia can be roughly divided into two groups of patients: those with positive symptoms and those with negative symptoms (Table 5.1).

The course of schizophrenia has not been satisfactorily studied. Roberts, Leigh, and Weinberger[55] postulate the following in regard to persons with schizophrenia:

- One fifth recover to a premorbid state after a bout with one or several psychotic episodes.
- Another one fifth experience a devastating course that is deteriorating in nature and overwhelming in consequence.
- The middle three fifths have an up-and-down course and may experience exacerbation and remission over a lifetime.

Both Murray[45] and Kopelowicz and Bidder[34] endorse Kraepelin's diagnostic term *dementia praecox,* which suggests that it continues to have meaningful application today. They reserve this diagnosis for those who experience a progressive, deteriorating course (10% according to Kopelowicz and Bidder, and 20% according to Murray).[34,45]

For persons with schizophrenia, positive symptoms tend to dominate the early clinical picture; negative symptoms eventually become more significant.[43] However, this clear dichotomy is elusive in clinical practice. Few patients exhibit purely positive or negative symptoms over time. Approximately one half to two thirds of older patients with schizophrenia (>55 years of age) recover or enjoy significant improvement.[17] These and other findings indicate that multiple outcomes occur, some of which are devastating to the individuals, their families, and society.

Clinical Consequences

As noted by Weinberger,[71] schizophrenia typically emerges in late adolescence or early adulthood. Schizophrenia may either have a rapid onset or develop over several years. A rapid onset is more closely associated with positive schizophrenia, whereas a slower development is associated

table 5.1 ▮▮▮▮▮▮▮▮
Positive and Negative Symptoms of Schizophrenia

SYMPTOM CATEGORY	SYMPTOMS
Positive (Type I)	
Prognosis: good	Abnormal thought form
Precipitating factors: yes	Agitation, tension
Onset: acute	Associational disturbances
Sensorium: dreamlike quality	Bizarre behavior
Intellectual impairment: none	Conceptual disorganization
Pathophysiology: D_2 hyperactivity	Delusions
Pathoanatomy: VBRs usually normal	Excitement
Response to typical neuroleptics: good	Feelings of persecution
Effect of levodopa: increases symptoms	Grandiosity
	Hallucinations
	Hostility
	Ideas of reference
	Illusions
	Insomnia
	Suspiciousness
Negative (Type II)	
Prognosis: poor	Alogia
Onset: chronic	Anergia
Family history: more than type I	Anhedonia
Sensorium: clear	Asocial behavior
Intellectual impairment: yes	Attention deficits
Pathophysiology: possibly hypodopaminergic, decreased CBFs	Avolition
Pathoanatomy: increased VBRs, other changes (see text)	Blunted affect
Response to typical neuroleptics: varies	Communication difficulties
Response to atypical neuroleptics: fair to good	Difficulty with abstractions
Effect of levodopa: minimal	Passive social withdrawal
	Poor grooming and hygiene
	Poor rapport
	Poverty of speech

with negative schizophrenia. A favorable outcome is associated with a later age of onset, higher premorbid social functioning, female gender, positive symptoms, and an acute onset.[17]

Age of Onset

Typically, the earlier the age at onset, the poorer the long-term prognosis.[2,27,28,59,66]

Premorbid Social Adjustment

An improved prognosis is also associated with higher premorbid social functioning.[17,28,45] That

is, individuals who have experienced successful negotiation of their social world are more likely to function better than those who have not.

Female Gender

Women with schizophrenia have a better long-term prognosis than do men.[17,26,28,45,66] This greater resilience has been linked to two factors: (1) women develop schizophrenia later in life than do men (mean = 5 years), which provides a longer period of premorbid social skill development, and (2) women are partially protected from the development of schizophrenia during their reproductive years because of estrogen, which is thought to have antidopaminergic properties.

Positive versus Negative Symptoms

Individuals with positive symptoms tend to have a better prognosis than individuals with negative symptoms.[27,34,45,55] This observation is somewhat muted by more recent studies that indicate a merging of positive and negative symptoms over time.[20,37] In other words, positive symptoms evolve to or merge with negative symptoms as the disorder persists, leaving a minority of patients (25%) on a "monomorphous course."[37]

Acute versus Insidious Onset

The more acute the onset of schizophrenia, the greater the likelihood of a favorable outcome.[17,34,55] An acute onset is typically characterized by positive symptoms (e.g., frank delusions and hallucinations). An insidious onset displays an evolving quality to the development of schizophrenia. Families often report a childhood marked by behavior problems, neuromotor disabilities, and the beginnings of asociality (shyness, few friendships, loner behavior).

Clinical Management Implications

The psychosocial/behavioral, psychopharmacological, and environmental implications of working with patients with schizophrenia are briefly addressed in the following sections, specifically as they relate to the biological variables previously discussed. More complete works address the issue of psychotherapeutic interventions with this population.

Perhaps one of the more compelling issues raised by the biological framework is the sense of "inevitability." In other words, if a patient's disorder is biological, there may be clinicians and patients who dismiss nonpharmacological treatment as a waste of time; furthermore, they may invest little hope in preventive measures. Rubenstein has said that the biological approach "even suggests, quite misleadingly, that the only reality is biochemical."[58] Such a view minimizes the personhood of the patient with schizophrenia.

Psychosocial/Behavioral Implications

A biological understanding of schizophrenia enables the clinician to differentiate between behaviors not immediately controllable by the patient and behaviors that may be. For example, many behaviors associated with both positive and negative schizophrenia (see Table 5.1) are not amenable to suggestion, will power, or "insight." Apathy, anergia, and other symptoms associated with negative schizophrenia can be recognized as part of the disorder rather than as intentional obstructionism or defiance. Second, adverse responses to antipsychotic agents commonly occur and can be confused with negative symptoms; an understanding of the biology of schizophrenia and the effect of antipsychotic drugs on the body can facilitate the correct interpretation of behavior.

Other significant psychosocial/behavioral interventions include the following:

- *Minimize stressful interactions.* Stress exacerbates or intensifies symptoms. Stressors include loneliness, doubts about the future, excessive free time, crime, regrets, and fear of rejection. Intervention is aimed at reducing stress and/or improving coping skills.

- *Treat depression.* Approximately 25% of patients with schizophrenia experience depression as their psychosis lifts,[73] and 10% of these people commit suicide.[9] Treatment with antidepressants helps these individuals.[39]

- *Work with the family.* One of the most significant accomplishments of the biological framework has been the alliance with the family. Former models that were purely psychodynamic seemed to blame the family and alienated family members from the treatment process.

- *Avoid lengthy, intense verbal interactions.* Historically, many mental health workers have attempted to use "insight" therapy with patients with schizophrenia. Such intrusive approaches have often proven counterproductive.

- *Treat substance abuse.* More than half of the patients with schizophrenia abuse drugs and/or alcohol. This abuse inhibits treatment and confounds existing poor judgment.

table 5.2 ▮▮▮▮▮▮▮▮▮▮▮▮▮▮▮▮▮▮▮▮▮
Selected Antipsychotics Categorized by Potency and Atypicality

NEUROLEPTIC	GENERAL DOSAGE RANGE	MOST COMMON SIDE EFFECT
High-Potency Agents		
Fluphenazine (Prolixin)	Daily adult dosages range from	EPSEs are the most common
Haloperidol (Haldol)	1-30 mg/day, with trifluoper-	side effects
Thiothixene (Navane)	azine slightly above and	
Trifluoperazine (Stelazine)	haloperidol slightly below this	
	range	
Moderate-Potency Agents		
Loxapine (Loxitane)	Daily adult dosages range from	EPSEs
Molindone (Moban)	15-250 mg/day	
Low-Potency Agents		
Chlorpromazine (Thorazine)	Daily adult dosages range from	Orthostatic hypotension and an-
Thioridazine (Mellaril)	30-800 mg/day	ticholinergic side effects are
		most common
Atypical Neuroleptic		
Clozapine (Clozaril)	Clozapine 300-900 mg/day	Basically a good side effect pro-
Olanzapine (Zyprexa)	Olanzapine 10 mg/day	file; orthostatic hypotension is
Risperidone (Risperdal)	Risperidone 4-6 mg/day	more common with clozapine
		and risperidone

Psychopharmacology

Psychopharmacological intervention is discussed in this section to provide basic information about this important treatment strategy. For a more definitive review of psychopharmacology, refer to the companion text, *Psychotropic Drugs,* second edition.[31a]

As previously noted, the dopamine hypothesis suggests that a hyperdopaminergic state is pathognomonic of schizophrenia. Antipsychotic agents antagonize dopamine. Table 5.2 lists the most commonly used antipsychotic agents. This relatively long list of drugs can be categorized in three ways: chemical structure, potency, or typicality. The major advantage of categorizing by chemical structure is that the clinician is directed to a new chemical class when a particular drug is ineffective. For instance, if a patient does not respond to trifluoperazine (Stelazine), the clinician would in most cases select a drug from a different chemical class (e.g., haloperidol [Haldol])—not another phenothiazine (e.g., fluphenazine [Prolixin]).

A more useful distinction between antipsychotic drugs is based on potency. Table 5.2 categorizes antipsychotics by potency. Because all of the traditional or typical antipsychotic drugs are equieffective, drug selection is often based on the side effect profiles of a given drug. High-potency agents tend to cause a higher frequency of EPSEs, whereas lower potency drugs are prone to cause orthostasis and anticholinergic effects.

The final category—typicality—contrasts the older or traditional drugs with the newer or atypical antipsychotics clozapine, risperidone, olanzapine, quetiapine, sertindole, and ziprasidone. These newer agents are also described as SDAs because their effectiveness is thought to result in part from their ability to block serotonin receptors. The nontraditional antipsychotics have proven to be effective for patients refractory to traditional drug treatment.

Environmental Implications

The patient's environment affects him or her and may contribute to recovery from or aggravation of the disorder. Significant environmental barriers to optimum functioning are an inability to cope with the activities of daily living or to find, secure, and maintain work; inadequate or no housing; substance abuse; severance of longstanding relationships and poor, few, or no current relationships; and poor wellness activities. Environmental interventions that can diminish or perhaps neutralize these concerns include but are not limited to the following:

- *Monitor for substance abuse.* Alcohol and drug abuse is common among patients with schizophrenia. It compromises treatment and is a contributor to homelessness and noncompliance. Although motivations for substance abuse are multifaceted, self-medication ranks high among those identified by clinicians.
- *Find adequate housing.* Without adequate housing, other interventions are not very meaningful.
- *Ensure compliance with medications.* A high percentage of patients with schizophrenia are noncompliant with antipsychotic therapy, and decompensation results. Injectable depot forms of haloperidol and fluphenazine are valuable approaches to fighting this problem. Furthermore, because disturbing side effects and multiple daily dosing contribute to noncompliance, atypical agents that have a good side effect profile and once-a-day dosing (e.g., olanzapine) can increase compliance.[48a]
- *Reduce stress.* As stated earlier, stress is a fundamental element in the development of schizophrenia. As the environment is manipulated to make it less stressful (e.g., moving from a crime-ridden neighborhood), the patient is positioned to improve.

Summary

Schizophrenia is not a neurodegenerative process. Positive symptoms of schizophrenia are typically associated with physiological alterations in the brain (e.g., a hyperdopaminergic process in mesolimbic areas). Negative symptoms of schizophrenia are typically associated with a hypodopaminergic process and anatomical alterations in the brain. However, it should be noted that reductions in amine activity are related to structural changes.

Increased ventricular-brain ratios; reductions in limbic, temporal lobe, hippocampal, and entorhinal cortex mass; and cytoarchitectural disturbances (cell disorganization and neuronal loss) are associated with schizophrenia.

REFERENCES

1. Akil M, Lewis DA: The distribution of tyrosine hydroxylase–immunoreactive fibers in the human entorhinal cortex, *Neurosci* 60(4):857-874, 1994.
2. Alaghband-Rad J, McKenna K, Gordon CT et al: Childhood-onset schizophrenia: the severity of premorbid course, *J Am Acad Child Adolesc Psychiatry* 34(10):1273-1283, 1995.
3. American Psychiatric Association: *Diagnostic and statistical manual IV,* Washington, DC, 1994, American Psychiatric Association.
4. Andreasen NC: Positive vs negative schizophrenia: a critical evaluation, *Schizophr Bull* 11:380-389, 1985.
5. Andreasen NC, Flaum M, Swayze VW et al: Positive and negative symptoms in schizophrenia, *Arch Gen Psychiatry* 47(7):615-621, 1990.
6. Arnold SE, Franz BR, Gur RC et al: Smaller neuron size in schizophrenia in hippocampal subfields that mediate cortical-hippocampal interactions, *Am J Psychiatry* 152(5):738-748, 1995.
7. Azorin JM: Long-term treatment of mood disorders in schizophrenia, *Acta Psychiatr Scand Suppl* 388:20-23, 1995.
8. Bartzokis G, Mintz J, Marx P et al: Reliability of in vivo volume measures of hippocampus and other brain structures using MRI, *Magn Reson Imaging* 11(7):993-1006, 1993.
9. Becker RE: Depression in schizophrenia, *Hosp Commun Psychiatry* 39:1269, 1988.
10. Bogerts B: Recent advances in the neuropathology of schizophrenia, *Schizophr Bull* 19(2):431-435, 1993.
11. Bogerts B, Falki P, Haupts M et al: Post-mortem volume measuremens of limbic and basal ganglia structures in chronic schizophrenia, *Schizophr Res* 3(5-6):295-301, 1990.

12. Bogerts B, Lieberman JA, Ashtari M et al: Hippoccampus-amygdala volume and psychopathology in chronic schizophrenia, *Biol Psychiatry* 33(4):236-246, 1993.

13. Breier A, Buchanan RW, Elhasfef A et al: Brain morphology and schizophrenia: a magnetic resonance imaging study of limbic, prefrontal cortex, and caudate structures, *Arch Gen Psychiatry* 49(12):921-926, 1992.

14. Bruton CJ, Crow TJ, Frith CD et al: Schizophrenia and the brain: a prospective cliniconeuropathological study, *Psychol Med* 20:285-304, 1990.

15. Cannon TD, Marco E: Structural brain abnormalities as indicators of vulnerability to schizophrenia, *Schizophr Bull* 20(1):89-102, 1994.

16. Casanova MF, Carosella NW, Gold JM et al: A topographical study of senile plaques and neurofibrillary tangles in the hippocampi of patients with Alzheimer's disease and cognitively impaired patients with schizophrenia, *Psychiatry Res* 49(1): 41-62, 1993.

17. Cohen CI: Studies of the course of outcome of schizophrenia in later life, *Psychiatr Serv* 46(9): 877-879, 889, 1995.

18. Crow TJ: Molecular pathology of schizophrenia: more than one disease process? *Br Med J* 280:66-68, 1980.

19. Eastwood SL, Burnet PW, Harrison PJ: Altered synaptophysin expression as a marker of synaptic pathology in schizophrenia, *Neurosci* 66(2):309-319, 1995.

20. Eaton WW et al: Structure and course of positive and negative symptoms in schizophrenia, *Arch Gen Psychiatry* 52(2):127-134, 1995.

21. Ereshefsky L, Tran-Johnson TK, Watanabe MD: Pathophysiologic basis for schizophrenia and the efficacy of antipsychotics, *Clin Pharm* 9(11):682-707, 1990.

22. Federal Task Force on Homelessness and Severe Mental Illness: *Outcasts on main street,* Washington, DC, 1992, National Institute of Mental Health.

23. Flaum M, Swayze VW, O'Leary DS et al: Effects of diagnosis, laterality, and gender on brain morphology in schizophrenia, *Am J Psychiatry* 152(5): 704-714, 1995.

24. Freedman R, Hall M, Adler LE et al: Evidence in postmortem brain tissue for decreased numbers of hippocampal nicotinic receptors in schizophrenia, *Biol Psychiatry* 38(1):22-23, 1995.

25. Gerez M, Tello A: Selected quantitative EEG (QEEG) and event-related potential (ERP) variables as discriminators for positive and negative schizophrenia, *Biol Psychiatry* 38(1):34-49, 1995.

26. Goldstein JM, Tsuang MT: Gender and schizophrenia: an introduction and synthesis of findings, *Schizophr Bull* 16(2):179-183, 1990.

27. Gupta S, Rajaprabjalaran R, Arndt S et al: Premorbid adjustment as a predictor of phenomenological and neurobiological indices in schizophrenia, *Schizophr Res* 16(3):189-197, 1995.

28. Hafner H, Nowotny B: Epidemiology of early-onset schizophrenia, *Eur Arch Psychiatry Clin Neurosci* 245(2):80-92, 1995.

29. Howard R, Mellers J, Petty R et al: Magnetic resonance imaging volumetric measurements of the superior temporal gyrus, hippocampus, parahippocampal gyrus, frontal and temporal lobes in late paraphrenia, *Psychol Med* 25(3):495-503, 1995.

30. Jakob H, Beckmann H: Circumscribed malformation and nerve cell alterations in the entorhinal cortex of schizophrenics: pathogenetic and clinical aspects, *J Neural Transm* 98(2):83-106, 1994.

31. Johnstone EC, Crow TC, Frith CD et al: Cerebral ventricular size and cognitive impairment in chronic schizophrenia, *Lancet* 2(7992):924-926, 1976.

31a. Keltner N, Folks DG: *Psychotropic drugs,* St Louis, ed 2, 1997, Mosby.

32. Kessler RC, McGonagle KA, Zhao S et al: Lifetime and 12-month prevalence of DSM-III-R psychiatric disorders in the United States, *Arch Gen Psychiatry* 51(1):8-19, 1994.

33. Kim JS, Kornhuber HH, Schmid-Burgk W et al: Low cerebrospinal fluid glutamate in schizophrenic patients and a new hypothesis on schizophrenia, *Neurosci Lett* 20:379-382, 1980.

34. Kopelowicz A, Bidder GT: Dementia praecox: inescapable fate or psychiatric oversight? *Hosp Commun Psychiatry* 43(9):940-941, 1992.

35. Kraepelin E: *Dementia praecox and paraphrenia,* 1919 (Translated by Barclay RM New York, 1971, RE Krieger).

36. Lewine RR, Hudgins P, Brown F et al: Differences in qualitative brain morphology findings in schizophrenia, major depression, bipolar disorder, and normal volunteers, *Schizophr Bull* 15(3):253-259, 1995.

37. Marneros A, Rohde A, Deister A: Validity of the negative/positive dichotomy of schizophrenic disorders under long-term conditions, *Psychopathology* 28(1):32-37, 1995.

38. Marsh L, Suddath RL, Higgins N et al: Medial temporal lobe structure in schizophrenia: relationship of size to duration of illness, *Schizophr Bull* 11(3):225-238, 1994.

39. Mason SE, Gingerich S, Siris SG: Patient's and caregiver's adaptation to improvement in schizophrenia, *Hosp Commun Psychiatry* 41:541, 1990.

40. Matthysee S: The role of dopamine in schizophrenia. In Usdin E, Hamburg D, Barchas J, editors: *Neuroregulators and psychiatric disorders,* New York, 1977, Oxford University Press.

41. Mauri MC, Bravin S, Mantero M et al: Depression in schizophrenia: clinical and pharmacological variables, *Schizophr Bull* 14(3):261-262, 1995.

42. McGeer PL, McGeer EG: Amino acid neurotransmitters. In Siegal GJ et al, editors: *Basic neurochemistry*, New York, 1989, Raven Press.

43. McGlashen TH, Fenton WS: The positive-negative distinction in schizophrenia: review of natural history validators, *Arch Gen Psychiatry* 49:63-72, 1992.

44. Moller HJ: The negative component of schizophrenia, *Acta Psychiatr Scand Suppl* 388:11-14, 1995.

45. Murray RM: Neurodevelopmental schizophrenia: the rediscovery of dementia praecox, *Br J Psychiatry Suppl* 25:6-12, 1994.

46. Narrow WE, Regier DA, Rae DS et al: Use of services by persons with mental and addictive disorders: findings from the National Institute of Mental Health Epidemiologic Catchment Area Program, *Arch Gen Psychiatry* 50(2):95-107, 1993.

47. National Foundation for Brain Research: *The cost of disorders of the brain,* Washington, DC, 1992, National Foundation for Brain Research.

48. National Institute of Mental Health: *Caring for people with severe mental disorders: a national plan of research to improve services,* DHHS Pub No (ADM)91-1762, Washington, DC, 1991, US Government Printing Office.

48a. Nihart MA: Atypical antipsychotics and the pharmacology of olanzapine, *J Am Psych Nurs Assoc* 3(1):S2-S7, 1997.

49. Nopoulos P, Torres I, Flaum M et al: Brain morphology in first-episode schizophrenia, *Am J Psychiatry* 152(12):1721-1723, 1995.

50. Pakkenberg B: Post-mortem study of chronic schizophrenic brains, *Br J Psychiatry* 151:744-752, 1987.

51. Petty RG, Barta PE, Pearlson GD et al: Reversal of asymmetry of the planum temporale in schizophrenia, *Am J Psychiatry* 152(5):715-721, 1995.

52. The President's Commission on Mental Health: *Report to the President from the President's Commission on Mental Health,* Washington, DC, 1978, President's Commission on Mental Health.

53. Rao ML, Moller HJ: Biochemical findings of negative symptoms in schizophrenia and their putative relevance to pharmacologic treatment: a review, *Neuropsychobiology* 30(4):160-172, 1994.

54. Regier DA, Narrow WE, Rae DS et al: The de facto US mental and addictive disorders service system: epidemiologic catchment area prospective 1-year prevalence rates of disorders and services, *Arch Gen Psychiatry* 50(2):85-94, 1993.

55. Roberts GW, Leigh PN, Weinberger DR: *Neuropsychiatric disorders,* London, 1993, Wolfe.

56. Ron MA, Harvey I: The brain in schizophrenia, *J Neurol Neurosurg Psychiatry* 53(9):725-726, 1990.

57. Rossi A, Stratta P, Mancini F et al: Magnetic resonance imaging findings of amygdala-anterior hippocampus shrinkage in male patients with schizophrenia, *Psychiatry Res* 52(1):43-53, 1994.

58. Rubenstein LS: Discrimination by any other name, *Psychiatr Serv* 47(6):557, 1996.

59. Schmidt M, Blanz B, Dippe A et al: Course of patients diagnosed as having schizophrenia during first episode occurring under age 18 years, *Eur Arch Psychiatry Clin Neurosci* 245(2):93-100, 1995.

60. Seeman P, Van Tol HM: Dopamine receptor pharmacology, *Trends Pharmacol Sci* 15(7):264-270, 1994.

61. Selemon LD, Rajkowska G, Goldman-Rakic PS: Abnormally high neuronal density in the schizophrenic cortex: a morphometric analysis of prefrontal area 9 and occipital area 17, *Arch Gen Psychiatry* 52:805-818, 1995.

62. Sherman AD, Davidson AT, Baruah S et al: Evidence of glutamatergic deficiency in schizophrenia, *Neurosci Lett* 121(1-2):77-80, 1991.

63. Slater E, Beard AW: The schizophrenia-like psychosis of epilepsy, *Proc R Soc Med* 55:1-7, 1962.

64. Sponheim SR, Iacono WG, Beiser M: Stability of ventricular size after the onset of psychosis in schizophrenia, *Psychiatry Res* 40(1):21-29, 1991.

65. Syvalahti EK: Biological factors in schizophrenia: structural and functional aspects, *Br J Psychiatry Suppl* (23):9-14, 1994.

66. Szymanski S, Lieberman JA, Alvir JM et al: Gender differences in onset of illness, treatment response, course, and biologic indexes in first-episode schizophrenia, *Am J Psychiatry* 152(5):698-703, 1995.

67. Torrey EF: A viral-anatomical explanation of schizophrenia, *Schizophr Bull* 17(1):15-18, 1991.

68. Tsai G, Passani LA, Slusher BS et al: Abnormal excitatory neurotransmitter metabolism in schizophrenic brains, *Arch Gen Psychiatry* 52(10):829-836, 1995.

69. Vita A, Dieci M, Giobbio GM et al: A reconsideration of the relationship between cerebral structural abnormalities and family history of schizophrenia, *Psychiatry Res* 53(1):41-55, 1994.

70. Vita A, Dieci M, Giobbio GM et al: Language and thought disorder in schizophrenia: brain morphological correlates, *Schizophr Res* 15(3):243-251, 1995.

71. Weinberger DR: Implications of normal brain development for the pathogenesis of schizophrenia, *Arch Gen Psychiatry* 44(7):660-668, 1987.

72. Weinberger DR, Berman KF, Suddath R et al: Evidence of dysfunction of a prefrontal-limbic network in schizophrenia: a magnetic resonance imaging and regional cerebral blood flow study of discordant monozygotic twins, *Am J Psychiatry* 149(7):890-897, 1992.

73. Weiss KJ, Valdiserri EV, Dubin WR: Understanding depression in schizophrenia, *Hosp Commun Psychiatry* 40:849, 1989.

74. Wibble CG, Shenton ME, Hokama H et al: Prefrontal cortex and schizophrenia: a quantitative magnetic resonance imaging study, *Arch Gen Psychiatry* 52(4):279-288, 1995.

75. Woolley DW, Shaw E: A biochemical and pharmacological suggestion about certain mental disorders, *Proc Natl Acad Sci U S A* 40:228-231, 1954.

76. Yaryura-Tobias Y, Diamond B, Merlis S: The actions of L-dopa on schizophrenic patients: a preliminary report, *Curr Ther Res* 12:528-531, 1970.

77. Zipursky RB, Marsh L, Lim KO et al: Volumetric MRI assessment of temporal lobe structures in schizophrenia, *Biol Psychiatry* 35(8):510-516, 1994.

Mood Disorders

The mood disorders are a spectrum of clinical conditions with varying degrees of depression, elation, or irritability. Signs and symptoms occur for a specified time, resulting in significant disability with social functioning and interpersonal relationships. The *Diagnostic and Statistical Manual of Mental Disorders*, fourth edition (DSM-IV)[2] provides the most widely used criteria for diagnosing mood disorders. This chapter focuses on major depressive disorder and bipolar I disorder. Subtypes of depressive disorders (dysthymic disorders, adjustment disorder with depressed mood, and depressive disorder not otherwise specified) and variants of bipolar disorder (bipolar II disorder, cyclothymic disorder, and bipolar disorder not otherwise specified) are discussed briefly. In general, mood disorders may result from a general systemic condition or may be induced by substances or prescribed medications.

Epidemiology and Demographics

Studies of major depressive disorder have reported a wide range of values for incidence and prevalence. According to DSM-IV,[2] major depressive disorder has a lifetime prevalence of approximately 15%, with prevalence rates as high as 25% for women. The incidence approaches 10% in a primary care setting and 15% in a medical inpatient setting. In the community, the lifetime risk of major depressive disorder is between 10% and 25% in women and between 5% and 12% in men. Some studies have estimated that between 13% and 20% of the population has some symptoms of clinical depression at any given time; approximately 2% to 3% of the population is hospi-

talized or seriously impaired because of major mood disorders.[20] The prevalence of major depressive disorder does not appear to be associated with education, income, marital status, or ethnic origin.[2]

For adolescents and adults, major depressive disorder occurs twice as often in women as in men. However, prepubertal boys and girls are equally affected. The 25- to 44-year-old age group has the highest rates of major depressive disorder for both men and women, whereas after age 65 years, rates are lower for men and women. This disorder is 1.5 to 3 times more common among first-degree biological relatives as compared with the general population. Culture may influence the experience in the communication of depressive symptoms. An increased risk of alcohol dependence exists in adult first-degree biological relatives, and an increased incidence of attention-deficit/hyperactivity disorder exists in the children of adults with major depressive disorder.[2]

Bipolar I disorder is less common than major depressive disorder; it has a lifetime prevalence of approximately 1%, which is similar to the figure for schizophrenia. The incidence of bipolar I disorder is approximately equal in men and women, and no studies indicate that this disorder is associated with race or ethnic origin. However, the *order* of appearance of manic and depressive episodes does appear to be related to gender. In men, the first episode is more likely to be a manic episode, whereas a major depressive episode is more likely to be the first episode in women. Women with bipolar I disorder have an increased risk for additional episodes immediately post partum. First-degree biological relatives have elevated rates of bipolar I disorder (4% to 24%); a genetic influence has been strongly supported by twin and adoption studies.[2]

Psychobiological Considerations

Biological research findings support the hypothesis that mood disorders involve dysfunction of the limbic system, basal ganglia, and hypothalamus. The limbic system and basal ganglia play a major role in the production of emotion. Therefore neurological disorders of the basal ganglia (e.g., Parkinson's disease) or limbic system (e.g., Alzheimer's disease) may present with depressive symptoms. Dysfunction of the hypothalamus in an individual with depressive symptoms is also suggested by alterations in sleep, appetite, and sexual behavior and by biological changes in endocrine, immunological, and chronobiological measures.

Macroscopic Brain Alterations

A survey of the literature suggests that only 30 neuropathological studies of mood disorders have been reported in the last 25 years. Of the studies published between 1970 and 1993, only three of six included nonschizophrenic control subjects.[9] These three studies examined the peripheral motor neuron branching patterns; cerebellar branching cells, multipolar cells, and dentate nucleus; and several regions in the basal ganglia and temporal lobe.[4] In a small study (N = 8), Beckmann and Jakob[3] found subtle migrational malformations in the entorhinal cortex and cell loss in the ventral insular cortex of patients with manic depression. Casanova et al[5] morphometrically compared five patients with mood disorder who had undergone previous lobotomies with five nonpsychiatric lobotomized control subjects; they also compared six leucotomized patients with schizophrenia with eight nonleucotomized control subjects with no history of neuropsychiatric impairment. They found marked neuronal reductions in the entorhinal cortex of patients with schizophrenia or mood disorder as compared with the nonpsychiatric control subjects.

On the basis of animal models, depressive symptoms and behavioral disturbances are commonly associated with hypothalamic and limbic system defects. Disturbed regulation of glucocorticoid secretion and abnormalities of circadian rhythms are thought to be caused by dysfunction in these structures. A number of postmortem studies of depression and suicide have detected abnormalities in monoamine concentration and metabolism. These findings indicate the need for neurohistological studies in brain regions where functions are believed to be disturbed in mania and depression. Areas of study would preferentially include the septum/hypothalamus region, where the neuronal generators of the more phylogenetically primitive drives and emotions are situated; the limbic structures of the temporal lobe and orbital cortex, which are structurally and functionally interposed between the neocortex and hypothalamus and regulate both neocortical and hypothalamic activities; and the monoaminergic and cholinergic brainstem systems, which are the main targets of antidepressant drugs and currently play a major role in the biological theories of mood disorders.[8]

Neurophysiological Brain Alterations

A large number of studies of depression have reported various abnormalities in biogenic amine metabolites (e.g., 5-hydroxyindoleacetic acid [5-HIAA], homovanillic acid [HVA], and 3-methoxy-4-hydroxyphenylglycol [MHPG]) in the blood, urine, and cerebrospinal fluid (CSF) of patients with mood disorders (Table 6.1). The data reported are most consistent with the hypothesis that mood disorders are associated with heterogenous dysregulations of the biogenic amines; *norepinephrine* and *serotonin* are the two neurotransmitters most often implicated in the pathophysiology of mood disorders. Evidence also points to dysregulation of dopamine and acetylcholine.

In animal models, virtually all effective somatic antidepressant treatments have been associated with a decrease in the sensitivity of the postsynaptic β-adrenergic and serotonin type 2 (5HT$_2$) re-

table 6.1

Commonly Reported Neurotransmitter and Metabolite Changes in Some Patients with Depression (Compared with Normal Controls)

	NE	MHPG	NM	VMA	Epi	MET	DA	HVA	5HT	5-HIAA	GABA	GAD	CRH	ENDOCRINE
CSF	nd	↓→	nd	nd	nd	nd	nd	→↓ ↑ psychotic depression	nd	↓↔	→	nd	↑	↑ mania ↔ depression
Plasma	nd	nd	nd	nd	nd	nd	nd	nd	→	nd	→	nd	nd	↑↔
Uptake into platelets	nd	nd	nd	nd	nd	nd	nd	nd	→	nd	nd	nd	nd	nd
Urine	↑↔	↓→	↑↔	↑↔	↑↔	↑↔	↑ mania	nd	nd	nd	nd	→↓	nd	nd
Brain tissue	nd	nd	nd	nd	nd	nd	nd	nd	→	→	nd	→↔	nd	nd

From Caldecott-Hazard S, Morgan DG, DeLeon-Jones F et al: Clinical and biochemical aspects of depressive disorders. II. Transmitter/receptor theories, *Synapse* 9:253, 1991. *nd*, No data in this review; ↑, increased levels as compared with controls; ↓, decreased levels as compared with controls; ↔, no change as compared with controls; *NE*, norepinephrine; *MHPG*, 3-methoxy-4-hydroxyphenylglycol; *NM*, normetanephrine; *VMA*, 3-methoxy-4-hydroxymandelic acid; *Epi*, epinephrine; *MET*, metanephrine; *DA*, dopamine; *HVA*, homovanillic acid; *5HT*, serotonin; *5-HIAA*, 5-hydroxyindoleacetic acid; *GABA*, γ-aminobutyric acid; *GAD*, glutamic acid decarboxylase; *CRH*, corticotropin-releasing hormone.

table 6.2

Antidepressant-Induced Changes in Neurotransmitters, Metabolites, and Their Receptors in Humans and Animals

WHAT WAS MEASURED	DRUGS					
	TRICYCLICS	MAOIs	SUBs	IPRINDOLE	Li	ECT
Concentrations in brain tissue						
MHPG	$\uparrow$	nd	nd	nd	nd	nd
Enkephalins	$\uparrow$	nd	nd	$\uparrow$	nd	$\uparrow$
Concentrations in CSF						
MHPG	$\downarrow$	$\downarrow$	$\downarrow$	nd	nd	nd
HVA	nd	$\downarrow$	nd	nd	nd	nd
5-HIAA	$\downarrow$	$\downarrow$	$\downarrow$	nd	nd	nd
β-Endorphin	nd	nd	nd	nd	nd	$\uparrow$
Concentrations in urine						
MHPG	$\downarrow \uparrow \leftrightarrow$	nd	nd	nd	nd	nd
Effects on uptake						
NE	$\downarrow$	nd	$\leftrightarrow$	$\leftrightarrow$	nd	nd
5HT	$\downarrow$	nd	$\downarrow$	$\leftrightarrow$	nd	nd
GABA	$\downarrow$	nd	nd	nd	nd	nd
Number of receptors						
Brain α_2	$\downarrow \leftrightarrow$	nd	nd	nd	nd	nd
Platelet α_2	nd	nd	nd	nd	$\downarrow$	nd
Brain α_2	$\uparrow \leftrightarrow$	nd	nd	nd	$\uparrow$	nd
Brain β	$\downarrow$	$\downarrow$	$\downarrow \leftrightarrow$	$\downarrow$	nd	$\downarrow$
Brain $5HT_2$	$\downarrow$	$\downarrow$	$\downarrow$	$\downarrow$	nd	$\uparrow$
Brain $5HT_1$	$\downarrow \uparrow \leftrightarrow$	$\downarrow$	$\downarrow \leftrightarrow$	nd	nd	nd
Brain mACh	$\uparrow$	nd	nd	nd	$\uparrow \leftrightarrow$	nd
Brain dopamine-1	$\downarrow$	nd	nd	nd	nd	$\downarrow$
Brain $GABA_B$	$\uparrow \leftrightarrow$	$\uparrow$	$\uparrow$	nd	nd	$\uparrow$
Brain μ and $\triangle$ opioid	nd	nd	nd	nd	nd	$\uparrow \downarrow$
Sensitivity of somatodendritic DA receptors	$\downarrow \leftrightarrow$	$\downarrow$	nd	nd	nd	$\downarrow$
Effect on stimulation of cAMP by NE	$\downarrow$	$\downarrow$	$\downarrow$	$\downarrow$	nd	$\downarrow$
Effect of stimulation of PI by muscarinic agonists	nd	nd	nd	nd	$\downarrow \leftrightarrow$	nd
Amount of glucocorticoid mRNA or receptor sites in brain	$\uparrow \downarrow$	nd	nd	nd	nd	nd

From Caldecott-Hazard S, Morgan DG, DeLeon-Jones F et al: Clinical and biochemical aspects of depressive disorders. II. Transmitter/receptor theories, *Synapse* 9:254, 1991.
nd, No data in this review; $\uparrow$, increased; $\downarrow$, decreased; $\leftrightarrow$, no change. Arrows represent the most commonly observed (not necessarily all) effects of the drugs in each group. *MAOI,* Monoamine oxidase inhibitor; *SUB,* serotonin uptake blocker; *Li,* lithium; *ECT,* electroconvulsive therapy; *CSF,* cerebrospinal fluid; *MHPG,* 3-methoxy-4-hydroxyphenylglycol; *HVA,* homovanillic acid; *5-HIAA,* 5-hydroxyindoleacetic acid; *5HT,* serotonin; *NE,* norepinephrine; *DA,* dopamine; *GABA,* γ-aminobutyric acid; *mACh,* muscarinic cholinergic; *cAMP,* cyclic adenosine monophosphate; *PI,* phosphoinositide; *mRNA,* messenger ribonucleic acid.

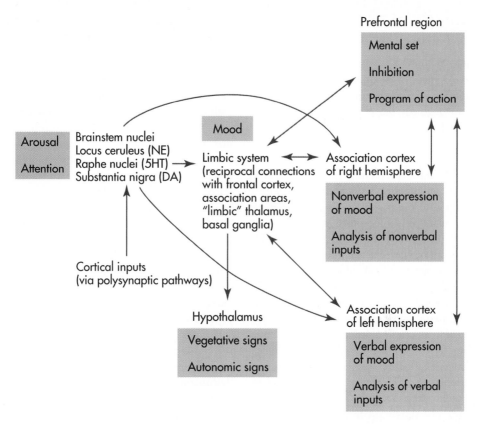

figure 6.1   Mood and its expression. *NE,* Norepinephrine; *5HT,* serotonin; *DA,* dopamine. *(From Yudofsky SC, Hales RE, editors:* The American Psychiatric Press textbook of neuropsychiatry, Washington, *DC, 1992, American Psychiatric Press.)*

ceptors after long-term treatment. Other various changes resulting from long-term treatment with antidepressants have also been reported (Table 6.2). The temporal response of receptor changes in animal models correlates with the 1- to 3-week delay in clinical improvement usually seen in patients treated with antidepressant medications.

Norepinephrine Alterations

Down-regulation of β-adrenergic receptors represents a homeostatic response to the acute actions of antidepressant drugs (Figure 6.1). Acute increased synaptic levels of norepinephrine ultimately result in a homeostatic drive to decrease β-adrenergic receptor levels and restore baseline noradrenergic signal transduction levels within the postsynaptic neuron. Other evidence has implicated the presynaptic α_2-adrenergic receptors in

depression because activation of those receptors results in a decrease in the amount of norepinephrine released. Presynaptic α_2-adrenergic receptors are also located on serotonergic neurons and regulate the amount of serotonin released. The existence of almost purely noradrenergic and clinically effective antidepressant drugs (e.g., desipramine) further supports the role of norepinephrine in the pathophysiology of at least the symptoms of depression. A potential problem with the β-adrenergic receptor hypothesis is the observation that a number of atypical antidepressants (e.g., bupropion) are clinically effective but do *not* down-regulate β-adrenergic receptors in the rat brain. Thyroid hormone has also been shown to be helpful as an adjunct in the therapy of depression despite the fact that it augments rather than diminishes β-adrenergic receptor function. Yohimbine, a compound that facilitates the development of β-adrenergic receptor down-regulation in response to tricyclic antidepressants, does not augment the clinical efficacy of these compounds.

Serotonergic Alterations

Chronic antidepressant treatment produces changes in serotonergic neurotransmission within the brain. Most types of antidepressant drugs down-regulate $5HT_2$ receptors as demonstrated by binding assays. Such down-regulation of $5HT_2$ receptors can be viewed as a homeostatic response to increased synaptic levels of serotonin—similar to the mechanisms implicated for down-regulation of the adrenergic receptors. Antidepressants have also been found to facilitate serotonergic synaptic transmission at certain cortical and hippocampal synapses as determined by electrophysiological recordings. The mechanisms underlying this augmentation of serotonergic neurotransmission remains unknown but may be mediated via $5HT_{1A}$ receptors. The significant impact of the selective serotonin reuptake inhibitors (SSRIs) on the serotonin biogenic amine neurotransmitter is now well established. The discovery of multiple 5HT receptor subtypes enables the development of even more specific treatments for depression and provides further evidence that serotonin is involved in the pathophysiology of depression.

The depletion of serotonin may precipitate depression. Some suicidal patients have shown low CSF concentrations of serotonin metabolites and low concentrations of serotonin uptake sites on platelets as measured by imipramine binding to platelets. Some patients with depression also have abnormal neuroendocrine responses, such as growth hormone, prolactin, and adrenocorticotropic hormone secretion in response to challenge with serotonergic agents. Although current serotonergic antidepressants act primarily through the blockade of serotonin reuptake, future generations of antidepressants have other serotonin system effects, including the antagonism of serotonin receptors (e.g., nefazodone [$5HT_2$]) and agonism of the serotonin receptor (e.g., buspirone [$5HT_{1A}$] and mirtazapine [$5HT_2$, $5HT_3$]).

Dopaminergic Alterations

Although norepinephrine and serotonin are the biogenic amines most often associated with the pathophysiology of depression, dopamine has also been theorized to play a role. Dopamine activity may be reduced in depression and increased in mania. The discovery of new subtypes of dopamine receptors and an increased understanding of the presynaptic and postsynaptic regulation of dopamine function have further enriched research into the relationship between dopamine and mood disorder. Depressive symptoms are associated with drugs that reduce dopamine concentration, such as reserpine, and with diseases that reduce dopamine concentration, such as Parkinson's disease. Drugs that increase dopamine concentration, such as bupropion, reduce the symptoms of depression. There are two recent theories regarding dopamine and mood disorder: (1) the mesolimbic dopamine pathway may be dysfunctional, and (2) the dopamine type 1 (D1) receptor may be hypoactive in depression and hyperactive in mania.

Cholinergic Alterations

Considerable evidence suggests that the cholinergic nervous system, acting either alone or together with other neurotransmitters, may play an important role in the regulation of mood. Pharmacologically induced changes in acetylcholine may cause perturbations in depression-relevant systems other than the cholinergic nervous system. Pharmacologically induced acetylcholine alterations could cause a "model depression" through governing neurotransmitters (e.g., γ-aminobutyric acid [GABA], serotonin, dopamine, norepinephrine) or through second-messenger systems in patients with affective disorders. The fundamental biochemical changes in depression could then result from relatively low-level norepinephrine or serotonin activity, which explains these hypothesized observations.

Cholinergic supersensitivity is observed in many patients with depression and may be a reflection of altered second messengers, including G proteins. Cholinomimetics could cause a "model depression," with elevated levels of adrenocorticotropic hormone (ACTH), cortisol, β-endorphin, and epinephrine; sleep architecture changes; and increased pulse rates and blood pressure. This presumed pharmacological phenomenon may ultimately offer greater comprehension of the pathophysiology of mood disorders, with subsequent treatment implications. Cholinomimetic experiments may further clarify the actual neurobiology of mood disorders. Alternatively, acetylcholine may prove to be involved directly in the etiology and expression of mood disorders, either alone or through other relevant neurotransmitters or second messengers.

Hypothalamic Alterations

The hypothalamus is central to the regulation of the neuroendocrine axes and receives many neuronal inputs that use biogenic amine neurotransmitters. A variety of neuroendocrine dysregulations have been reported in patients with mood disorders. The abnormal regulation of neuroendocrine axes may result from abnormal functioning of biogenic amine-containing neurons. For example, with the thyroid or adrenal axis, dysregulations may be reflections of a fundamental underlying brain disorder. Other neuroendocrine abnormalities described in patients with mood disorders include decreased nocturnal secretion of melatonin, decreased prolactin release to tryptophan administration, decreased basal levels of follicle-stimulating hormone (FSH) and luteinizing hormone (LH), and decreased testosterone levels in men.

Hypothalamic-pituitary-adrenal axis. Dysregulation of the hypothalamic-pituitary-adrenal (HPA) axis in major depressive disorder remains one of the most consistent psychobiological findings. Since the association between HPA axis dysfunction and major depression was made, neuroendocrine function tests have elucidated mechanisms that underlie the pathophysiology of depression. Individuals with major depressive disorder often present with hypercortisolemia, resistance of cortisol to suppression by dexamethasone, blunted ACTH responses to corticotropin-releasing factor (CRF) challenge as compared with controls, and elevated CRF concentrations in the CSF.

The pathophysiological mechanisms underlying HPA axis dysregulation in depression and other mood disorders remain to be seen. Two hypotheses have been advanced to account for the observed blunting of ACTH secretion in response to CRF challenge associated with major depressive disorder: (1) down-regulation of adenohypophyseal CRF receptors as a result of hypothalamic CRF hypersecretion, and (2) increased glucocorticoid-mediated negative feedback tone at the pituitary or central nervous system (CNS). In a series of studies, Nemeroff et al[16] demonstrated significant CRF elevation in the CSF of drug-free suicide victims who had major depression. Collection of postmortem cisternal CSF-CRF concentrations from postmortem depressed suicide victims and sudden death controls also revealed elevated CRF concentrations in the depressed groups. Such elevations of CRF concentrations have also been reported in patients with anorexia nervosa (see Chapter 8); these concentrations revert to the normal range as these patients approach normal body weight.[11] Interestingly, patients with depression and elevated CRF concentrations in the CSF show normalization of CRF concentrations 24 hours after a final electroconvulsive treatment, which indicates that CSF-CRF concentration defects, like cortisolemia, are a *state* rather than a trait marker. The treatment of depression with fluoxetine (and presumably other SSRIs) also reduces CRF concentrations in the CSF.[6]

Somatostatin Alterations

Clinical studies of somatostatin levels and depression have focused on neurological cases. Consistent decreases of somatostatin in tissues and CSF have been observed with Alzheimer's disease, Parkinson's disease, and multiple sclerosis during relapse. Patients with depression (and anorexia nervosa) have also shown decreased somatostatin concentrations. Rubinow, Gold, and Post[22] have shown that CSF somatostatin is significantly decreased in patients with depression, whether unipolar or bipolar. Although CSF somatostatin levels do not correlate with the severity of depression, somatostatin values in clinically improved patients rise toward the concentrations found in normal subjects. In patients with bipolar disorder, concentrations are significantly lower during the depressed state than during the improved or manic states. Although data are relatively limited, an overview of the literature suggests that decreases in CSF somatostatin are a consistent, state-dependent finding of depression. Along with hypercortisolemia, these somatostatin decreases may be one of the more consistent findings in mood disorder cases.

Thyroid Alterations

The use of thyrotropin-releasing hormone (TRH) as a provocative agent for the assessment of thyroid axis function evolved rapidly after its isolation and synthesis. Clinical use of the TRH stimulation test to assess HPA axis function reveals blunting of the response of thyroid-stimulating hormone (TSH) to TRH in approximately 25% of euthyroid patients with major depression.[15] Subpopulations of more severely depressed patients may be more likely to exhibit TSH blunting and elevations of thyroxine (T_4) before therapy. The relevance of TRH to depression and other mental disorders is reviewed thoroughly by Nemeroff et al.[16]

Sleep Alterations

Problems with sleeping, such as initial and terminal insomnia, fragmented sleep, and hypersomnia are classic symptoms of depression; a perceived decreased need for sleep is a classic symptom of mania. Researchers have long recognized abnormalities in the sleep electroencephalograms (EEGs) of many patients with depression. Common abnormalities are delayed sleep onset, shortened rapid eye movement (REM) latency (i.e., the time before falling asleep and the first REM period), increased length of the first REM period, and abnormal delta sleep.

Some investigators have attempted to use sleep EEG studies in the diagnostic assessment of patients with mood disorders. The abnormalities of sleep architecture in depression and the transient clinical improvement in depression associated with sleep deprivation have led to theories that depression reflects an abnormal regulation of circadian rhythms. Some animal studies indicate that many of the standard antidepressant treatments are effective in changing the "setting" of the internal biological clock.

Kindling

Another pathophysiological disturbance of mood disorders involves the concept of *kindling*. Kindling is an electrophysiological process in which the repeated subthreshold stimulation of a neuron eventually generates an action potential. At the organ level, repeated subthreshold stimulation of an area of the brain results in a seizure. The clinical observation that antiepileptic drugs (e.g., carbamazepine and valproic acid) are useful in the treatment of mood disorders, particularly bipolar I disorder, has given rise to the theory that the pathophysiology of mood disorders may involve kindling in the temporal lobes.

Other Alterations

Other findings that occur with reasonable consistency in mood disorders may be summarized as follows:

1. Patients with bipolar I (but not bipolar II) disorder can be separated from patients with unipolar depression on the basis of urinary 3-methoxy-4-hydroxyphenylglycol (MHPG) levels and other catecholamine and metabolite measures.
2. At least some patients with unipolar depression are characterized by elevated catecholamine and metabolite measures.
3. With depression, increased levels of catecholamine metabolites and elevated platelet monoamine oxidase activity are associated with increased levels of cortisol or dexamethasone suppression test nonsuppression.
4. Patients with low urinary MHPG levels respond more robustly to imipramine (and perhaps fluoxetine) than do patients with high MHPG levels.
5. Patients with depression demonstrate blunted growth hormone responses to clonidine during periods of depression and remission.

6. Patients with depression demonstrate decreased responsiveness of β-receptors to challenges by specific β-agonists.
7. Patients with mania demonstrate elevated catecholamine and metabolite levels.
8. The treatment of depressed and manic patients with antidepressants and lithium carbonate results in a decrease in norepinephrine turnover.[18] The significance of and explanation for these findings remain to be determined.

Although they point to alterations in catecholamine activity in patients with mood disorder, the exact roles of receptor activity and catecholamine synthesis, as well as the specific biological dysfunctions that may account for these findings, remain to be investigated. Imaging studies may define the key loci of catecholamine activity, underlying pathophysiology, and biological characteristics of mood disturbance.

Brain Imaging Techniques, Findings, and Research

A growing literature suggests that patients with mood disorders have structural brain abnormalities. The findings are neither as commonly reported nor as consistently replicated as with schizophrenia (see Chapter 5). Early studies using computerized tomography (CT) demonstrated that patients with mood disorders have both ventricular enlargement and prominent sulci. These findings appear to be somewhat more consistent in patients with bipolar disorder than with unipolar disorder. However, not all studies have characterized samples by polarity. Within the depressive groups, structural abnormalities are more likely to be associated with endogenous features, recurrence, or the presence of psychotic symptoms. As with schizophrenia, structural abnormalities in mood disorder are not diagnostic. The presence of similar abnormalities in both mood disorders and schizophrenia suggests a nonspecificity of structural abnormalities and possibly nonspecificity of the mechanisms that produce these changes. Unfortunately, techniques designed to illuminate pathophysiological mechanisms, such as the study of first-episode patients or twin studies, have not been systemically applied to mood disorders.

Brain imaging studies in patients with mood disorders have provided a number of clues regarding abnormal brain function. Although the findings are inconclusive, data indicate the following: (1) significant samples of patients with bipolar I disorder, predominantly male patients, have enlarged cerebral ventricles, and (2) ventricular enlargement is much less common in patients with major depressive disorder than in patients with bipolar I disorder. However, patients with major depressive disorder with psychotic features *do* tend to have enlarged cerebral ventricles.

Magnetic resonance imaging (MRI) studies have indicated that patients with major depressive disorder have smaller caudate nuclei and smaller frontal lobes than do control subjects; the patients with major depressive disorder show abnormal hippocampal T1 relaxation times as compared with control subjects. Temporal lobe volume reductions in the right hippocampus are seen in the MRI scans of patients with bipolar I disorder.[1,26] At least one MRI study reported that patients with bipolar I disorder have a significantly increased number of deep white matter lesions as compared with control subjects.[26]

Several functional brain abnormalities have been hypothesized to occur in patients with mood disorder. One view suggests that diffuse cerebral blood flow and hypometabolism occurs with depression, whereas increased cerebral metabolic activity occurs with mania. Another hypothesis stresses the possibility of cerebral asymmetries, which suggests that depression could be accounted for by hypometabolism in the left hemisphere, especially in the frontal regions. The primary support for this hypothesis is provided by lesion studies. Additional support is provided by the general catecholamine hypothesis and by related theories concerning serotonergic dysregulation in mood disturbance consistent with diffuse dysregulation of neurotransmitter systems.

Single photon emission computed tomography (SPECT) or positron emission tomography (PET)

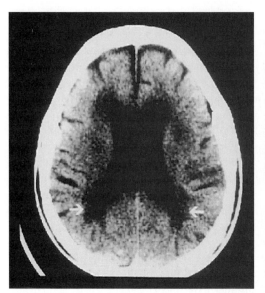

figure 6.2   CT of head. Substantial white matter loss from the periventricular zone, sometimes called leukoaraiosis, is common in the elderly and may be associated with vascular disease. This severe thinning of white matter suggests a significant pathological condition *(arrows)*. The density of affected white matter approaches that of CSF in the lateral ventricles and suggests substantial loss of neuropil. *(Courtesy Dr. Richard E. Powers, Director, University of Alabama at Birmingham Brain Resource Program.)*

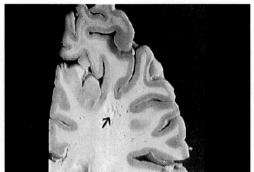

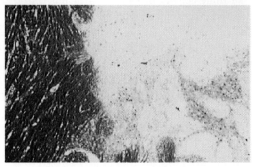

figure 6.3   Gross and microscopic appearance of Binswanger's disease. **A,** The appearance of punched-out white matter lesions *(arrow)*. **B,** Luxol fast blue stain of the same lesion. Densely stained blue tissue represents normal white matter. The pale area in the right half of the panel demonstrates the marked loss of myelin secondary to ischemia caused by small vessel occlusion. Fibers passing through this ischemic area are damaged. *(Courtesy Dr. Richard E. Powers, Director, University of Alabama at Birmingham Brain Resource Program.)*

studies (see Chapter 4) have reported decreased blood flow that generally affects the cerebral cortex, especially frontal areas. Magnetic resonance spectroscopy (MRS) studies of patients with bipolar I disorder have produced consistent data to support the hypothesis that the pathophysiology of this disorder may involve an abnormal regulation of membrane phospholipid metabolism. Animal studies using lithium treatment have shown the effects of lithium on phospholipids. Another application of MRS to bipolar I disorder is the use of radioactive-labeled lithium to study brain versus plasma concentrations of lithium. These studies have found that the brain concentrations of lithium are approximately 40% of plasma lithium concentrations after 1 week of treatment, which correlates with the onset of the therapeutic effect of lithium.

Some brain imaging studies have focused on comparing geriatric populations with late-onset depression to age-matched patients with early-onset depression. An association of greater sulcal widening and greater severity of subcortical white matter changes has been reported in geriatric patients with late-onset depression (Figures 6.2 and 6.3).[20] An MRI study in 29 normal volunteers and 20 patients with major depression also revealed particularly prominent shortened T1 relaxation times in the hippocampus of geriatric patients with depression, which suggests that major depression in the elderly may be associated with tissue changes in the aging hippocampus.[14]

Considerably more data on secondary mood disorders following CNS lesions have been obtained as compared with primary mood disorders. Reviews of new affective symptoms following stroke have shown that depression is much more common than mania, but manic symptoms are often observed in patients with a previous personal or familial history of mood disorder.[24] Several studies have attempted to establish a connection between the site of a lesion and depressive symptomatology. A CT study of patients with head injury has demonstrated that major depression develops more often in patients with left basal ganglia and left dorsolateral frontal lesions. Stroke patients with right temporal, right superior frontal, left inferior frontal, and left parieto-occipital lesions were found to have more sleep disturbances and greater dysphoria than patients with lesions in other areas of the brain.[25] Lesions associated with depression and mania often occur in the temporal and frontal lobes; right-sided lesions tend to be associated with mania, and left-sided lesions are associated with depression.

Mood disorders associated with Huntington's disease are well documented, and there are neuropathological correlations between clinical findings and the extent of the structural alterations. Approximately 40% of patients suffering from Huntington's disease develop symptoms of mood disorder; 10% have manic episodes.[7] Interestingly, affective symptoms associated with Huntington's disease sometimes precede the motor and cognitive symptoms by many years. Marked reductions in the volume of the putamen and caudate nucleus are noted in mild cases of Huntington's disease. Changes in the size of the putamen are correlated with neurological impairment, whereas changes in the size of the caudate nucleus are not.

Clinical Applications
Clinical Findings and Course

Depression is a part of the human condition and is characterized by an array of conditions such as demoralization, disappointment, or transient emotional responses to injury or loss. The complaint of depression may be seen in several major psychiatric syndromes. However, the diagnosis of depression as a mood disorder requires more than just the presence of depressive symptoms. A mood disorder must be accompanied by a variety of cognitive, psychological, somatic, and vegetative disturbances that cause significant disability in psychosocial functions and interpersonal relationships. Although numerous symptoms are associated with the syndrome of major depression, none are essential for the diagnosis.

Mania is the opposite of depression. Although a heightened sense of euphoria is typical, in many cases anger or irritability may be the predominant feature. The patient with mania may be hyperverbal, hyperactive, overconfident, adventuresome, and irrational. As with severely depressed individuals, patients experiencing mania may be delusional or psychotic.

Major Depressive Disorder and Subtypes

The hallmarks of major depressive disorder are depressed mood or a sense of dysphoria and/or a loss of interest or pleasure in all previously enjoyed activities and pastimes (anhedonia). The syndrome of major depressive disorder includes not only disturbance of mood but also associated symptoms such as appetite, sleep, or psychomotor disturbances; decreased energy; decreased libido; feelings of worthlessness or guilt; difficulty with concentration, memory, or thinking; and thoughts of death or suicide. Individuals with this disorder think of themselves in negative terms and often display self-reproach or believe that they or their families would be better off if they were dead. The thought processes of severely depressed individuals may become quite distorted and result in delusional and/or psychotic thinking. Physical activity may be significantly decreased (i.e., psychomotor retardation) or purposely increased (i.e., psychomotor agitation). Individuals with severe depression may find it difficult to motivate themselves to carry out even the most common activities of daily living.

Depressed mood is a common complaint in patients with depression. However, a subjective sense of depression may be absent, especially in geriatric patients who masquerade their depression with

box 6.1
Key Features of Major Depressive Episodes

At least a 2-week period of maladaptive functioning that is a clear change from previous levels of functioning. At least five of the following symptoms must be present during that 2-week period, one of which must be (1) or (2):
1. Depressed mood
2. Inability to experience pleasure or markedly diminished interest in pleasurable activities
3. Appetite disturbance with weight change (change >5% of body weight within 1 month)
4. Sleep disturbance
5. Psychomotor disturbance
6. Fatigue or loss of energy
7. Feelings of worthlessness or excessive or inappropriate guilt
8. Diminished ability to concentrate or indecisiveness
9. Recurrent thoughts of death or suicidal ideations
   The mood disturbance causes marked distress and/or significant impairment in social or occupational functioning.
   There is no evidence of a physical or substance-induced etiology for the patient's symptoms or of the presence of another major mental disorder that accounts for the patient's depressive symptoms.

Modified from American Psychiatric Association: *Diagnostic and statistical manual of mental disorders,* ed 4, Washington, DC, 1994, The Association.

complaints of weakness, somatization, or irritability. Somatic symptoms of depression may include a specific organ system, prominent pain symptoms (e.g., headache, backache), gastrointestinal complaints, neuromuscular complaints such as dizziness and numbness, or generalized fatigue and lethargy. The diagnostic criteria for a major depressive episode are listed in Box 6.1.

The course or natural history of major depressive disorder is variable. Although it may begin at any age, the average age at onset is the mid-20s.[2] Although some individuals have a single episode of major depression with full recovery to premorbid levels of functioning, most patients with depression (approximately 80%) eventually have recurrent episodes. Some individuals have episodes separated by many years of normal functioning, whereas others experience clusters of episodes followed by periods of remission. For other individuals, the episodes become increasingly frequent as they grow older.[21]

Patients who recover from major depressive episodes have a high probability of recurrence, and each new episode carries renewed risks of chronicity, psychosocial impairment, and suicide.

The clinical studies of the collaborative program on the psychobiology of depression for the National Institute of Mental Health—known as the Collaborative Depression Study (CDS)—found that one quarter of the patients who recovered during the first year of depression relapsed within 12 weeks of recovery. The most common predictor of relapse was a history of three or more previous episodes of major depression.[12] Psychosocial stressors are often but not always identifiable before the first affective episode and become increasingly less apparent with future episodes. Therefore relapses appear to occur independently of life events as the depressive illness evolves. In addition, major depressive disorder, which was once thought to consist of discrete episodes followed by full recovery, may become chronic in some individuals. Higher rates of persistent depression have been found in women, in individuals at least 30 years of age, in individuals with 10 or more prior episodes, and in individuals with a high comorbidity index.[10]

If possible, the diagnosis of depression should characterize the specific subtype, such as unipolar or bipolar, melancholic or nonmelancholic, psychotic or nonpsychotic, or a predominance of "atypical" features. Some depression subtypes tend to respond to different forms of treatment. Thus identifying the subtype may be useful in determining the most appropriate treatment plan. The presence of mania or hypomania defines bipolar disorder. Melancholia (40% to 60% of all hospitalized patients) is characterized by vegetative symptoms. Psychotic depressions are characterized by the presence of delusions and/or hallucinations and may be seen in patients with unipolar or bipolar disorder. Studies suggest that approximately 10% to 25% of hospitalized patients, especially geriatric patients, have psychotic symptoms.[26] Atypical depression is depicted by neurovegetative symptoms that are generally the opposite of those seen in melancholia, such as hypersomnia rather than insomnia; hyperphagia, including carbohydrate craving, rather than anorexia; and mood reactivity with environmental circumstances and a long-standing pattern of interpersonal rejection sensitivity. Many patients with atypical depression also report significant lethargy or "leadened paralysis" or commonly report anxious or irritable mood rather than dysphoria.[19]

Dysthymic disorder. Dysthymic disorder represents a distinct depressive entity in which depressed mood (or possibly an irritable mood in children or adolescents) is chronic, present for most of the day, and occurs on more days than not for at least 2 years (or 1 year for children or adolescents). The severity of the mood disturbance does not meet the criteria for major depressive disorder. Major depressive disorder may be superimposed on dysthymic disorder, but a diagnosis of dysthymic disorder is not made if there is clear evidence of major depressive episodes during the first 2 years of the disturbance. Although patients with dysthymic disorder may be socially or occupationally impaired, they are often able to function, and the severity of their symptoms rarely warrants hospitalization.

Adjustment disorder. Adjustment disorder with depressed mood usually occurs during an identifiable psychosocial stressor such as divorce, job loss, physical illness, or some significant disaster or event. The individual's response to the stressor is considered to be extreme or in excess of what would normally be expected or results in significant impairments in social, occupational, or interpersonal functioning. The symptoms remit in time, either when the stressor resolves or when a new level of coping is reached.

Other depressive disorders. Depressive symptoms may occur in medical or surgical patients. Patients with both a medical illness and depression usually have core issues that include loss of health, helplessness, chronic disability, pain, injuries to self-esteem, and financial and interpersonal strain secondary to the illness. Depressive illness may be a consequence of an underlying illness or may be induced by the medications used to treat the illness. Many depressive symptoms in medically or surgically ill patients do not meet the diagnostic criteria for a mood disorder. However, if the depressive symptoms do not resolve with an improvement in the medical condition, a diagnosis of major depressive episode is considered, with symptoms treated according to this diagnosis.

Women are at higher risk than men to develop depressive episodes during the reproductive years. Furthermore, women are vulnerable to depression associated with oral contraceptives, abortion, the premenstrual period, puerperium, and menopause. The phenomenological and biological mechanisms involved with these phenomena establish a link between depression and female reproductive functions.[17] Women are especially vulnerable to rapid-cycling bipolar disorder and hyperthyroidism, a factor associated with bipolar mood disorder. The postpartum period is also associated with impaired thyroid function and is linked to mood swings. Therefore alterations in thyroid hormones may be a prominent feature of both the postpartum and rapid-cycling forms of mood disturbance in women. A previous history of postpartum depression places women at a higher risk for the development of subsequent episodes. Difficulties during pregnancy may also predispose a woman to the development of other reproduction-related depressions. Understanding the role of reproductive hormones and the sensitization phenomenon will likely improve the understanding of the relationship between depression and the female reproductive cycle. Appropriately timed clinical psychopharmacological interventions may inhibit this sensitization phenomenon and benefit the long-term prognosis.[17]

Rates of suicide with major depressive disorder are between 15% and 30%. In general, women attempt suicide more often than men, but men more often complete the act. A number of factors that identify patients at high risk for suicide include increasing age, living alone, a recent major loss, chronic illness, substance abuse, a previous history of depression or suicide attempts, or symptoms of psychosis or mood cycling. Patients with low self-esteem, excessive guilt, or feelings of helplessness and hopelessness may be severely suicidal. Patients with schizophrenia, alcoholism, drug addictions, or cognitive impairment syndromes are much more likely to commit suicide because of impaired judgment and impulsivity.

Patients with significant suicidal risk may require involuntary hospitalization. The broad grounds of psychiatric "commitment" usually require that the patients have a severe mental illness and be immediately dangerous to themselves or others or so gravely incapacitated that they are unable to care for themselves. These commitment criteria and procedures vary from state to state, and psychiatric consultation is advised before pursuing this avenue.

Bipolar Disorder

The mean age at onset for a manic episode is the early 20s, but in some cases bipolar disorder begins in adolescence or after 50 years of age. Manic episodes occur with sudden onset and a rapid escalation of symptoms over a few days. Manic episodes often follow significant psychosocial stressors. Episodes usually last from a few weeks to several months and end more abruptly than major depressive episodes. In approximately half of the cases, a major depressive episode immediately precedes or follows a manic episode with no intervening period of euthymia. If the mania occurs during the postpartum period, there is an increased risk for recurrence in subsequent postpartum periods. Mixed episodes can evolve from a manic or depressive episode, or they may arise de novo. It is far less common for a mixed episode to evolve *into* a manic episode. Hypomania typically begins with a rapid escalation of symptoms within 1 or 2 days; 5% to 15% of individuals with hypomania ultimately develop a manic episode.

The presence of mania or hypomania generally defines bipolar disorder. Mania is a distinct period during which the predominant mood is either elevated, expansive, or irritable, with associated symptoms such as hyperactivity, pressured speech, racing thoughts, inflated self-esteem, decreased need for sleep, distractibility, and excessive involvement in potentially dangerous activity. Psychotic symptoms such as delusions or perceptual disturbances (i.e., hallucinations) may be seen in the patient with acute mania. With mania, the mood disturbance is severe and causes marked impairment in social or occupational functioning (Box 6.2). With hypomania many of the features of mania may be present, but the mood disturbance is less severe. At times it may be difficult to differentiate severe hypomania from mania.

Two major subtypes of bipolar disorder are bipolar I and bipolar II. Bipolar I disorder identifies a patient who has had at least one true manic episode. A history of depression or hypomania may also be present. Bipolar II disorder involves a history of hypomania and major depressive episodes but no history of mania. Many patients with bipolar disorder present acutely with both manic and depressive symptoms (mixed type). This dysphoric mania generally requires that mania and depression occur every day for at least a 1-week period. Dysphoria and mixed manic states tend to be more difficult to diagnose and treat than classic mania. Patients with dysphoric mania tend to be female or older and are generally nonresponsive to lithium.[13]

Cyclothymic disorder is conceptualized as a relatively less severe form of bipolar illness. It generally has an insidious onset, beginning in the late teens or early 20s. By definition, cyclothymic disorder is a chronic mood disturbance of at least 2 years' duration and involves numerous hypomanic

box 6.2
Key Features of Bipolar Disorder: Manic Episode

A distinct period of abnormally and persistently elevated, expansive, or irritable mood, lasting at least 1 week and of sufficient severity to cause marked impairment in social or occupational functioning. During the period of the mood disturbance, at least three of the following symptoms are also present:
1. Grandiosity
2. Decreased need for sleep
3. Hyperverbal or pressured speech
4. Flight of ideas or racing thoughts
5. Distractibility
6. Increase in goal-directed activity or psychomotor agitation
7. Excessive involvement in pleasurable activities that have a high potential for painful consequences
   There is no evidence of a physical or substance-induced etiology or the presence of another major mental disorder to account for the patient's symptoms.

Modified from American Psychiatric Association: *Diagnostic and statistical manual of mental disorders,* ed 4, Washington, DC, 1994, The Association.

or mild depressive episodes that do not meet the criteria for mania or major depression. No periods of euthymia greater than 2 months occur in the context of cyclothymic disorder. The mood disturbance is not severe enough to markedly impair the individual's social or occupational functioning.[2]

Clinical Consequences

Individuals with depressive disorders may present with tearfulness, irritability, brooding, obsessive rumination, anxiety, phobias, excessive worry over physical health, and complaints of pain. Approximately 30% of individuals with depressive disorders have panic attacks that occur in a pattern that meets the DSM-IV criteria for panic (see Chapter 7). Some individuals note difficulty in intimate relationships, less satisfying social interactions, or difficulties in sexual functioning. Marital, academic, or occupational problems commonly occur. Alcohol or other substance abuse or an increased use of medical services may result from depression. The most serious consequence of major depressive disorder is attempted or completed suicide. The risk for suicide is especially high for individuals with psychotic features, a history of previous suicide attempts, a family history of com-

pleted suicides, or concurrent substance abuse. Increased rates of premature death from general medical conditions have also been reported to be associated with major depressive episodes.

Clinical Management Implications

The clinical management of mood disorders is generally based on pharmacotherapy and/or psychotherapy that is designed to improve symptoms and general functioning. Disruptive behaviors, psychosocial problems, and core psychological issues may become a focus of treatment. Depending on the presentation and circumstances, psychotherapeutic approaches may involve the individual or the entire family constellation. Mood disturbances are etiologically heterogenous with overlapping symptoms; therefore no single treatment of choice exists. Formulating a treatment plan must first involve assessing whether the patient meets the diagnostic criteria as discussed; an effort is made to rule out the presence of a coexisting psychiatric disorder, substance abuse disorder, or general medical condition. Assessment of the psychosocial circumstances, degree of impairment, chronicity of disturbance, and presence of suicidal and homicidal ideations is essential. Patients with a mild mood disturbance or stress associated with interpersonal conflicts are best treated with psychotherapy. Moderate-to-severe depression and mania or hypomania often benefit from pharmacotherapy.

Psychosocial/Behavioral Implications

Regardless of the diagnosis, all psychiatric patients benefit from a positive therapeutic relationship. A wide range of psychotherapeutic interventions are useful in the treatment of mood disorders, particularly depressive mood disturbances. The establishment of a supportive therapeutic relationship is often crucial when treating patients with depression. Supportive therapy generally consists of providing an explanation for the patient's symptoms, as well as ongoing education, knowledge, and feedback in regard to the patient's illness, prognosis, and treatment. Supportive therapy may also include guiding the patient in reference to interpersonal relationships, work, and major life adjustments, as well as helping to bolster the patient's morale, setting realistic goals, and being available in times of crisis.

Psychodynamic psychotherapy may embrace issues in which the relationship to a highly ambivalent lost person is of central importance. Formulated psychodynamic themes are often declarations of love, affection, or guilt secondary to a harsh conscience and repressed fantasies, or frustration related to excessively high personal ideals. Psychodynamic therapy suggests that individuals improve as they become more aware of these issues; future difficulties can be anticipated and mastered, and future conflicts can be neutralized through the process of insight.

Interpersonal therapy seeks to recognize and explore depressive precipitants, role disputes, social isolation, or deficits in social skills. Cognitive therapy views a patient's symptoms as secondary to irrational beliefs and distorted attitudes about the self, environment, and future.

In general, research is sparse or inconclusive regarding the efficacy of various psychotherapies (either alone or in conjunction with pharmacotherapy) and the acute and maintenance phase of depression. However, it is generally agreed that patients with mild depressions or dysthymic disorders benefit from purely psychotherapeutic approaches. Psychotherapy can assist the patient in reversing the negative self-images, negative feelings about the future, and poor self-esteem that are ubiquitous features of depression.

Psychopharmacology

The pharmacological approach to depression generally uses antidepressants such as SSRIs; heterocyclic or newer agents such as nefazodone, bupropion, or mirtazapine; or older agents such as the monoamine oxidase inhibitors (MAOIs). Lithium, thyroid hormone, and many other agents are used as adjuncts in the treatment of depressive illness.[13]

Mirtazapine (Remeron) is a noradrenergic and specific serotonin agent that recently has been approved by the Food and Drug Administration. This tetracyclic compound enhances noradrenergic and serotonergic neurotransmission, but it does *not* accomplish this task through reuptake inhibition. Mirtazapine antagonizes α_2-adrenergic receptors and binding at $5HT_2$ and $5HT_3$ receptors, which accounts for its antidepressant mechanisms and is consistent with the previous discussion of neurotransmitter physiology. The adverse effects of mirtazapine include drowsiness, increased appetite, weight gain, and dizziness. Bone marrow suppression, including agranulocytosis and neutropenia, are possible in a small percentage of cases.

Because of the substantial differences among individuals and among the various antidepressants, no single medication can be recommended as optimal for all patients. In general, patients who are nonpsychotic respond well to most antidepressants, and atypical depressions seem to respond preferentially to MAOIs. Patients with bipolar disorder are treated with an antidepressant plus a mood stabilizer, and patients with psychotic depression require a combination of antidepressant and antipsychotic or electroconvulsive therapy.[23]

The choice of antidepressant is often predicated on such factors as the patient's age, general health status, and past history of antidepressant use; the side effect profile; and cost. A history of prior response to an antidepressant or a favorable response by a family member is generally a good predictor of a favorable response.

Symptoms such as sleep, appetite, or psychomotor disturbances are relatively clear target symptoms for antidepressant medications and are usually the first symptoms to improve. Cognitive symptoms of depression, such as low self-esteem, guilt, uncertainty, pessimism, and suicidal thoughts tend to improve more slowly. In general, a lag time of 3 to 4 weeks occurs before a mood-elevating effect is seen; patients are warned not to expect overnight results. In older patients, significant antidepressant responses occur later than in younger patients and generally require 6 to 12 weeks of therapy. Sleep disturbance, agitation, and anxiety may improve early in the treatment and precede the onset of true antidepressant efficacy. Tricyclic antidepressants have been replaced as first-line drugs in the treatment of depression by SSRIs and newer heterocyclic agents such as nefazodone. Newer generation antidepressants such as bupropion, venlafaxine, and mirtazapine are often used as second-line agents for patients who do not respond to the first trial of antidepressant medication.

A large armamentarium of clinically effective antidepressants is available to the clinician; patients with psychosis and melancholia tend to respond most predictably to electroconvulsive therapy (ECT). ECT remains the most effective treatment for all major depressive disorders and should be considered in patients who cannot tolerate the side effects of antidepressant medications. Other indications for ECT include refractory depression; depressions in frail, geriatric patients; and some cases of acute mania, schizoaffective disorder, or acute onset psychotic episodes presenting with a predominance of affective or catatonic symptoms. The only contraindications to ECT are the presence of CNS mass lesions, recent myocardial infarction, or a history of malignant ventricular arrhythmia.[21]

The treatment of bipolar disorder usually requires a combined pharmacological approach that involves an antidepressant medication and a mood stabilizer. Differentiating unipolar from bipolar depression is critical because most if not all antidepressants may precipitate a manic episode or increase the mood cycling in bipolar disorders. Thus a personal and family history of bipolar disorder should prompt a cautious approach in prescribing antidepressants alone. Ideally, the antidepressant therapy of a patient with bipolar disorder should occur in combination with a mood stabilizer such as lithium or sodium valproate. Lithium itself has some antidepressant properties that may be useful in some patients with bipolar depression and may allow some cases to be maintained by this one agent. Sodium valproate and carbamazepine may have similar antidepressant properties, but this effect has not yet been demonstrated.

The efficacy of lithium in preventing or attenuating the occurrence of depression and mania in patients with bipolar disorder is well established. Patients with mixed mania, rapid cycling, or mania induced by a general medical condition (secondary mania) are usually more responsive to alternative agents such as sodium valproate. Sodium valproate and carbamazepine have emerged significantly as agents in the treatment of bipolar disorder. Sodium valproate has demonstrated efficacy in the treatment of acute mania, mixed manic states, and rapid cycling. The mechanism by which antiepileptic drugs and lithium work in the treatment of mood disturbance is unclear. These drugs somehow stabilize dysregulated brain functioning and allow mood to progress toward normal ranges. The use of psychopharmacological agents in the treatment of bipolar mood disorders is more fully discussed in the companion text, *Psychotropic Drugs,* second edition.[13]

REFERENCES

1. Altshuler LL et al: Reduction of temporal lobe volume in bipolar disorder: a preliminary report of magnetic resonance imaging (letter), *Arch Gen Psychiatry* 48:482, 1991.

2. American Psychiatric Association: *Diagnostic and statistical manual of mental disorders,* ed 4, Washington, DC, 1994.

3. Beckmann H, Jakob H: Prenatal disturbances of nerve cell migration in the entorhinal region: a common vulnerability factor in functional psychoses? *J Neural Transm Gen Sect (Wien)* 84:155, 1991.

4. Bogerts B, Lieberman J: Neuropathology in the study of psychiatric disease. In Costa E, Silva J, Nadelson C, editors: *International review of psychiatry,* vol 1, Washington, DC, 1993, American Psychiatric Press.

5. Casanova M, Atkinson, Goldberg et al: A quantitative morphometric study of the corpus callosum and cingulate cortex in schizophrenia. In Racagni G et al, editors: *Biological psychiatry,* Amsterdam, 1991, Elsevier.

6. DeBellis MD, Gold PW, Geracioti TD et al: Fluoxetine significantly reduces CSF, CRH and AVP concentrations in patients with major depression, *Am J Psychiatry* 150:656, 1993.

7. Folstein SE, Chase GA, Wahl WE et al: Huntington disease in Maryland: clinical aspects of racial variation, *Am J Hum Genet* 41:168, 1987.

8. Goodwin FK, Jamison KR: *Manic depressive illness,* New York, 1990, Oxford University Press.

9. Jeste D, Lohr JB, Goodwin FK: Neuroanatomical studies of major affective disorders, *Br J Psychiatry* 153:444, 1988.

10. Katon W, Schulberg H: Epidemiology of depression in primary care, *Gen Hosp Psychiatry* 14(4):237, 1992.

11. Kaye WH, Gwirtsman HE, George DT et al: Elevated cerebrospinal fluid levels of immunoreactive corticotropin-releasing hormone in anorexia nervosa: relation to state of nutrition, adrenal function, and intensity of depression, *J Clin Endocrinol Metab* 64:203, 1987.

12. Keller MB, Baker LA: The clinical course of panic disorder and depression, *J Clin Psychiatry* 53(suppl 3):5, 1992.

13. Keltner N, Folks DG: *Psychotropic drugs,* St Louis, ed 2, 1997, Mosby.

14. Krishnan K et al: Hippocampal abnormalities in depression, *J Neuropsychiatry Clin Neurosci* 3:387, 1991.

15. Nemeroff CB: The relevance of thyrotropin-releasing hormone to psychiatric disorders. In Nemeroff CB, editor: *Progress in psychiatry, neuropeptides, and psychiatric disease,* Washington, DC, 1990, American Psychatric Press.

16. Nemeroff CB, Widerlov E, Bissette G et al: Elevated concentrations of CSF corticotropin-releasing factor–like immunoreactivity in depressed patients, *Science* 226:1342, 1984.

17. Parry BL: Mood disorders linked to the reproductive cycle in women. In Bloom FE, Kupfer DJ, editors: *Psychopharmacology: the fourth generation of progress,* New York, 1995, Raven Press.

18. Plotsky PM, Owens MJ, Nemeroff CB: Neuropeptide alterations in mood disorders. In Bloom F, Kupfer DJ, editors: *Psychopharmacology: the fourth generation of progress,* New York, 1995, Raven Press.

19. Preskorn SH, Burke M: Somatic therapy for major depressive disorder: selection of an antidepressant, *J Clin Psychiatry* 53(suppl 9):5, 1992.

20. Rabins P, Pearlson G, Aylward E et al: Cortical magnetic resonance imaging changes in elderly inpatients with major depression, *Am J Psychiatry* 148:617, 1991.

21. Risby ED, Risch C, Stoudemire A: Mood disorders. In Stoudemire A, editor: *Clinical psychiatry for medical students,* ed 2, Philadelphia, 1994, JB Lippincott.

22. Rubinow DR, Gold PW, Post RM: CSF somatostatin in affective illness, *Arch Gen Psychiatry* 40:409, 1983.

23. Schatzberg AF: Recent developments in the acute somatic treatment of major depression, *J Clin Psychiatry* 53(suppl 3):20, 1992.

24. Starkstein SE, Robinson RG: Affective disorders and cerebral vascular disease, *Br J Psychiatry* 154:170, 1989.

25. Stern RA, Bachmann DL: Depressive symptoms following stroke, *Am J Psychiatry* 148:351, 1991.

26. Swayze VW, Andreasen NC, Alliger RJ et al: Subcortical and temporal structures in affective disorder and schizophrenia: a magnetic resonance imaging study, *Biol Psychiatry* 31:221, 1992.

chapter seven
Anxiety Disorders

The anxiety disorders constitute a spectrum of clinical syndromes characterized by nervousness, apprehension, worry, tension, sleep difficulties, irritability, and somatic complaints that are significantly disabling with respect to psychosocial functioning or interpersonal relationships. Specific syndromes discussed in the *Diagnostic and Statistical Manual of Mental Disorders,* fourth edition (DSM-IV) include panic disorder with or without agoraphobia, specific phobia, social phobia, obsessive-compulsive disorder, posttraumatic stress disorder, acute stress disorder, and generalized anxiety disorder.[1] Other syndromes may include anxiety disorder due to a general medical condition, substance-induced anxiety disorder, or mixed anxiety-depressive disorder, all of which may constitute a focus of treatment. Because panic attacks and agoraphobia occur in the context of several of these disorders, their criteria are treated as separate entities in DSM-IV.

Epidemiology and Demographics

Anxiety is the most common mental disorder, with approximately 25% of the adult population suffering from a clinically diagnosable level of anxiety in their lifetime.

Panic Disorder With or Without Agoraphobia

The lifetime prevalence of panic disorder with or without agoraphobia is consistently found to be between 1.5% and 3.5%. Lifetime rates for agoraphobia are 2.5 to 4 times greater for women than for men. For panic disorder, lifetime rates are 1 to 3.5 times greater for women; however, 6-month prevalence rates for panic disorder are either similar between genders or increased in men.[13,17] The 1-year prevalence rate for panic disorder is between 1% and 2%. Approximately one third to one half of persons diagnosed with panic disorder in the community have agoraphobia, but some studies find a much higher rate. The age at onset for panic disorder varies but usually occurs between late adolescence and the mid-30s. A bimodal distribution may occur, with peak occurrence in late adolescence and a second smaller peak by the mid-30s.[1] A small number of cases begin during childhood or after 45 years of age.

Approximately 78% of patients with panic disorder describe their initial panic attacks as spontaneous and as occurring without an environmental trigger; the remainder of the attacks are precipitated by confrontation with a phobic stimulus or the use of a psychoactive drug.[9] Onset of the disorder may follow within 6 months of a major stressful life event such as marital separation, occupational change, or pregnancy. Panic disorder appears to be less prevalent among the elderly, but in this population possible underreporting, decreased survival with the disorder, or a cohort effect may occur. Prevalence rates are similar for blacks and whites, higher for noncollege graduates and unmarried individuals, and higher among family members of individuals with the disorder. Individuals with a family history of panic disorder are 4 to 7 times more likely to develop panic disorder; twin studies indicate a genetic factor.[1] A history of childhood separation disorder is reported in 20% to 50% of patients; therefore the disorder may have developmental antecedents.[13]

Specific Phobias

Phobias are generally common but rarely result in levels of impairment or distress that warrant the diagnosis of a specific phobia. The reported prevalence may vary depending on the phobias surveyed and on the thresholds of impairment or distress. Agoraphobia may be confused with specific phobia and may account for some of the errors in previous epidemiological studies. In epidemiological studies the presence of agoraphobia without history of panic disorder has been reported to be higher than that for panic disorder with agoraphobia. However, at least 95% of individuals who present with agoraphobia have a concurrent diagnosis of panic.[9]

Community samples have shown a 1-year prevalence rate of approximately 9% for specific phobias; lifetime rates range between 10% and 11.3%.[1] As reported in the Epidemiology Catchment Area studies, 6-month prevalence rates of specific phobias are between 4.5% and 11.8%; rates are higher for females than for males.[12,16] Age at onset for specific situational phobias tends to peak in early childhood, with a second peak in the mid-20s. Specific natural environment phobias tend to begin primarily in childhood, but many new cases of phobia develop in early adulthood (e.g., height phobia). Animal-type and blood-injection-injury–type phobias commonly have their onset in childhood. Age at onset may be more variable for other types.[1]

Traumatic events, unexpected panic attacks, and observing others undergoing trauma or demonstrating fearfulness may predispose an individual to the development of a specific phobia. A phobia may also develop from such events as media coverage of airplane crashes. The content and prevalence of phobias varies with culture and ethnic group. In some cultures the fear of magic or spirits is prominent in the etiology and development of specific phobias. The gender ratio varies across different types of specific phobias; 75% to 90% of individuals with animal-, natural environment–, or situational-type phobias are female. Approximately 55% to 70% of those with blood-injection-injury–type or a fear of heights are fe-

male. There may be an aggregate of families with blood-injection-injury–type phobia.[1] Many childhood-onset specific phobias may remit spontaneously. Specific phobias may coexist with social phobia or panic disorder but are believed to be unrelated.

Social Phobia

Social phobia has a lifetime prevalence of 3% to 13%. The prevalence may vary depending on the criteria used to determine stress or the number of times a situation precipitates distress. Estimates of 6-month prevalence rates of social phobia from the Epidemiological Catchment Areas (ECAs) are 1.2% to 2.2%.[12,16] Distribution is fairly even across the age span and slightly more common in women than in men. Onset is usually between 15 and 20 years of age, and the course tends to be chronic and unremitting.

Obsessive-Compulsive Disorder

Obsessive-compulsive disorder (OCD) occurs at a point prevalence rate of 0.05% of the population. The ECA studies found lifetime population prevalence rates to be 2% to 3% and 6-month prevalence rates to be 1.3% to 2.0%.[12,16] Rates of OCD and its traits are increased in family members of patients with OCD. Age at onset is usually in adolescence or early adulthood; most patients are unable to identify any environmental trigger or precipitant to the onset of this disorder. Once OCD is established, many individuals experience an increase in symptoms with stressful life events; the majority of patients with OCD report depressive symptoms. OCD may also coexist with panic disorder, eating disorders, Tourette's syndrome, or schizophrenia.

Posttraumatic Stress Disorder

Posttraumatic stress disorder (PTSD) has been recognized as an independent diagnosis since 1980, but descriptions of the syndrome date back to the U.S. Civil War. The lifetime rate of PTSD in male veterans is 31%; 15% of veterans currently have the disorder. A direct relationship exists between the level of combat and the risk of PTSD, even when premilitary factors are considered. Lifetime and current rates in females are 26.9% and 8.5%, respectively. Surveys of women with PTSD have revealed alarmingly high rates of traumatic events, particularly as crime victims, with lifetime and current prevalence rates at 13% and 3%, respectively.[10] Victims of sexual assault are at high risk for subsequent psychiatric disturbances and suicide.

Risk factors for exposure to traumatic events include a family history of psychiatric disorder, a history of conduct disorder, male gender, extroversion, and eroticism. Risk factors for PTSD following exposure to traumatic events include separation from parents during childhood, family history of anxiety, preexisting anxiety or depression, family history of antisocial behavior, female gender, and eroticism. Hispanic race has been associated with increased risk. Rates of comorbid psychiatric disorders are elevated with PTSD.

Generalized Anxiety Disorder

Generalized anxiety disorder (GAD) has a lifetime prevalence rate of approximately 5%.[1] Over the course of a lifetime, women (6.6%) are almost twice as likely as men (3.6%) to develop GAD. This disorder is manifested by unrealistic or excessive anxiety and worry about two or more life circumstances (e.g., children, financial situation). The state of excessive anxiety and worry persists for at least 6 months.

Psychobiological Considerations

Biological theories regarding anxiety have developed from animal models of anxiety, patients in whom biological factors have been ascertained, basic neuroscience, and the actions of psychotropic drugs. One school of thought suggests that biological changes with anxiety reflect the results of psychological conflicts, whereas another suggests that biological events *precede* the psychological conflicts. Both types of changes likely exist in specific individuals because a range of biological

sensitivities may exist with associated symptoms of anxiety disorders.

Microscopic Brain Alterations

The locus ceruleus and raphe nuclei project primarily to the limbic system and the cerebral cortex. These areas have become the focus of many hypotheses regarding the neuroanatomic substrates of anxiety disorders. In addition to receiving noradrenergic and serotonergic innervation, the limbic system contains a high concentration of γ-aminobutyric acid–A (GABA$_A$) receptors. Studies in primates have implicated the limbic system in the generation of anxiety and fear response. Two areas of the limbic system have received special attention as a result of increased activity: the septohippocampal pathway and the cingulate gyrus. A defect in the cingulate gyrus has been particularly important in the pathophysiology of OCD.

The frontal cerebral cortex is connected with the parahippocampal region, the cingulate gyrus, and the hypothalamus; therefore it may be involved in the production of anxiety disorders. The temporal cortex has also been implicated as a pathophysiological site in anxiety disorders. That association is based in part on the similarity in clinical presentation and electrophysiology between temporal lobe epilepsy (complex partial seizures) and OCD.

Neurophysiological Brain Alterations

Stimulation of the autonomic nervous system results in cardiovascular, neuromuscular, gastrointestinal, and respiratory responses. Clinical manifestations may include tachycardia, headache, diarrhea, and tachypnea; peripheral manifestations of anxiety are neither peculiar to anxiety disorders nor necessarily correlated with an individual's subjective experience of anxiety.

The Lange Theory suggests that subjective anxiety is a response to a peripheral phenomenon. It is generally thought that central nervous system anxiety precedes the peripheral manifestations of anxiety except when the specific peripheral cause is present, such as with pheochromocytoma (a hormonally active tumor). Some anxiety disorders (especially panic disorder) are associated with autonomic nervous system function that exhibits increased sympathetic tone, adapts slowly to repeated stimuli, and responds excessively to moderate stimuli.

The three major neurotransmitters associated with anxiety are norepinephrine (NE), serotonin (5HT), and GABA. Much basic neuroscience information about anxiety comes from animal studies involving behavioral paradigms and psychoactive agents. One such animal model is the *conflict test*, in which an animal is simultaneously presented with several negative stimuli. Anxiolytic drugs tend to facilitate adaption to that situation, whereas other drugs may disrupt the behavioral responses of the animals.[9]

The general theory regarding the role of NE in anxiety disorders presumes a poorly regulated noradrenergic system that results in occasional bursts of activity. The cell bodies of the noradrenergic systems are primarily located in the locus ceruleus in the rostral pons and project their axons to the cerebral cortex, limbic system, brainstem, and spinal cord.

Human studies have found that patients with panic disorder experience frequent and severe panic attacks when exposed to β-adrenergic agonists such as isoproterenol or to α-adrenergic antagonists such as yohimbine. Conversely, clonidine and α_2-adrenergic agonists reduce anxiety symptoms in some therapeutic situations. Glutamate and cholecystokinin systems, as well as norepinephrine, have been implicated. Subsensitivity of the α_2-adrenergic receptors has been noted in patients with GAD and is indicated by a blunted release of growth hormone after clonidine infusion. A less consistent finding is that patients with anxiety disorders, particularly panic disorder, have elevated cerebrospinal fluid (CSF) or urinary levels of 3-methoxy-4-hydroxyphenylglycol (MHPG), a noradrenergic metabolite.

The therapeutic efficacies of the benzodiazepines in GAD have led biological research to focus on the GABA neurotransmitter systems. Abnormalities in patients with GAD have been found in the occipital lobe, which has the highest concentration of benzodiazepine receptors. Other brain areas hypothesized to be involved include the basal ganglia, limbic system, and frontal cortex.

The role of GABA in anxiety disorders is most strongly supported by the undisputed efficacy of the benzodiazepines, which enhance the activity of GABA at the $GABA_A$ receptor. Low-potency benzodiazepines are most effective with symptoms of generalized anxiety, but benzodiazepines of the highest potency, such as alprazolam, are more effective in the treatment of panic disorder. Studies of alprazolam resulted in the discovery of the benzodiazepine-GABA receptor complex.

Studies in primates have found that the autonomic nervous system symptoms of anxiety disorders are induced when ethyl β-carboline-3-carboxylate (β-CCE), a benzodiazepine agonist, is administered; β-CCE also causes anxiety in normal controls. Flumazenil, a benzodiazepine antagonist, causes frequent and severe panic attacks in patients with panic disorder. These data have led researchers to hypothesize that some patients with anxiety disorders have abnormally functioning $GABA_A$ receptors, but this connection remains to be shown directly.

The identification of many 5HT receptor types has stimulated a search for the role of serotonin in the pathogenesis of anxiety disorders. The interest in 5HT was initially motivated by the observation that serotonergic antidepressants have therapeutic effects in some anxiety disorders (e.g., clomipramine in OCD). The agonist effect of buspirone in the treatment of anxiety disorders is also presumably a result of its receptor-specific action at the $5HT_{1A}$ receptor and suggests the possibility of an association between serotonin and anxiety.

Most cell bodies of the serotonergic neurons are located in the raphe nuclei in the rostral brainstem and project to the cerebral cortex, limbic system (especially the amygdala and hippocampus), and hypothalamus. Although the administration of serotonergic agents to animals results in behaviors suggestive of anxiety, data for similar effects in humans are less robust. Several reports indicate that anxiety in patients with anxiety disorders is increased by *M*-chlorphenylpiperazine (MCPP), a drug with multiple serotonergic and nonserotonergic effects, and fenfluramine, which causes the release of serotonin. Many "serotonergic" hallucinogens (e.g., LSD) are associated with the development of both acute and chronic anxiety.

Many clinical trials have supported the hypothesis that serotonin dysregulation is involved in the formation of OCD symptoms. Clinical studies have assayed CSF concentrations of serotonin metabolites, as well as the affinities and numbers of platelet binding sites to tritiated imipramine, which binds to serotonin reuptake sites. These studies have reported variable findings in OCD. Some researchers have also suggested that cholinergic and dopaminergic neurotransmitter systems are directly involved in OCD, which is an area for future research.

Biological theories regarding PTSD have developed from preclinical studies and measures of biological variables in clinical populations. Many neurotransmitter systems have been implicated. Models of learned helplessness, kindling, and sensitization in animals have led to theories involving NE, dopamine, endogenous opiate, and benzodiazepine receptors in the hypothalamic-pituitary-adrenal (HPA) axis. In clinical populations, data have supported hypotheses that the HPA axis and noradrenergic and endogenous opiate systems (see Chapter 8) are hyperactive in at least some patients with PTSD. Other major findings include abnormal sleep architecture (e.g., sleep fragmentation and increased sleep latency) and increased activity and responsiveness of the autonomic nervous system, which is evidenced by elevated heart rates and blood pressure. These findings have led many researchers to suggest psychobiological similarities between PTSD, major depression, and panic disorder.

The adenosine receptor may eventually prove to be a target for anxiolytic drugs. Adenosine is a purine neurotransmitter that decreases the release of many other neurotransmitters, such as NE, glutamate, dopamine, 5HT, and GABA. Caffeine, which affects this receptor, is an anxiogenic in many people but can induce frank panic attacks in individuals with panic disorder. Although it is generally accepted that all benzodiazepine actions are mediated through their binding sites on $GABA_A$ receptors, the interaction of the benzodiazepines and adenosine are a matter of interest. Adenosine and diazepam have synergistic actions, and caffeine may antagonize many of the behavioral effects of the benzodiazepines. The role of adenosine in human anxiety is unclear, but adenosine receptor agonists may prove to be useful in the treatment of various types of anxiety disorders.[8]

Brain Imaging Techniques, Findings, and Research

A range of brain imaging studies generally conducted with specific anxiety disorders has suggested several possibilities with respect to understanding anxiety. Some increase in the size of cerebral ventricles has occasionally been found. In one study the increase was correlated with the length of time that patients had been taking benzodiazepines.[3] Another MRI study showed a specific defect in the right temporal lobe of patients with panic disorders.[2] Other brain imaging studies of GAD have reported abnormal findings in the right but not the left hemisphere, which suggests that some type of cerebral asymmetry may be important in the development of anxiety symptoms in some patients.

Together with electroencephalograms (EEGs), functional brain imaging studies such as positron emission tomography (PET) and single photon emission computed tomography (SPECT) have variously reported abnormalities in the frontal cortex, occipital and temporal lobes and, in one study of panic, the parahippocampal gyrus.[14] One PET study reported a lower metabolic rate in the basal ganglia and white matter of individuals with GAD as compared with normal controls.[19] In panic disorder, several brain imaging studies have suggested abnormalities in brain regions around the hippocampus. Reiman et al[15] noted that, when compared with controls, lactate-induced panic attacks in 16 patients with panic disorder resulted in asymmetry of blood flow, blood volume, and metabolic rates for oxygen in the parahippocampal gyrus, with the left side being less than the right. In a follow-up study of these subjects and other patients who panicked with lactate infusion, physiological challenges showed increased cerebral blood flow near the left inferior cerebellar vermis and bilaterallly in the temporal poles, insular cortex, claustrum, lateral putamen, and superior colliculus.[15] In addition, studies using different functional imaging methods support the general finding of parahippocampal abnormalities in panic disorder.[18]

In OCD, many brain imaging studies have provided evidence for symptom-related functional activity in the orbital prefrontal cortex and caudate nucleus. The pattern of orbitostriatal dysfunction is different from that reported for panic, depression, or schizophrenia.[2] A variety of functional brain imaging studies have found increased activity in the frontal lobes, basal ganglia, and cingulate area of patients with OCD. Pharmacological and behavioral treatments have reportedly reversed such abnormalities.

Functional and structural brain imaging studies are consistent with the observation that neurosurgical procedures involving the cingulum are sometimes effective in the treatment of OCD. MRI studies have shown increased T1 relaxation times in the frontal cortex, a finding that is consistent with the location of the neurophysiological abnormalities found in PET studies. Together with animal studies, the results of neurosurgeries for OCD that interrupt tracts in the cingulum allow proposal of a model for the mediation of symptoms in treatment-responsive OCD. This model essentially suggests a dysfunctional cortical-limbic-basal ganglia-thalamic circuit in OCD.[3] This theory suggests inadequate sensory information, gating, sieving or, to use Freud's term, repressive functions in the basal ganglia, which allow cortical inputs to capture and drive a self-sustaining loop. This loop drives behavioral routines or rituals that are difficult to interrupt even when maladaptive. However, it is believed successful OCD treatment adequately restores the gating functions of the caudate and breaks up the driving circuitry. The involved neurotransmitter systems have not been es-

tablished, but further clarification may facilitate treatment response.

Clinical Applications

Anxiety disorders are among the most common problems in the general population and lead to high use of health care services, significant distress, and disability. Fortunately, anxiety disorders are among the psychiatric syndromes that are potentially the most amenable to treatment with respect to outcome and a return to a premorbid level of functioning.

Panic Disorder With or Without Agoraphobia
Clinical Findings and Course

Panic disorder is characterized by recurrent, discrete attacks of anxiety accompanied by several somatic symptoms such as palpitations, paresthesias, hyperventilation, diaphoresis, chest pain, dizziness, trembling, and dyspnea. This condition is usually accompanied by agoraphobia, which consists of an excessive fear of situations in which escape or obtaining help would be difficult, such as driving, crowded places, stores, or being alone. DSM-IV establishes diagnoses for panic disorder with or without agoraphobia, as well as agoraphobia without history of panic disorder.

Panic disorder usually begins with a spontaneous panic attack that often leads the individual to seek medical treatment, such as going to the emergency room believing that he or she is having a heart attack, stroke, losing his or her mind, or experiencing some serious medical event (Box 7.1). Subsequent attacks occur over time with varying degrees of regularity. A patient may feel constantly fearful or anxious anticipating additional attacks. Some individuals experience nocturnal attacks that awaken them from sleep. Patients usually become more fearful of situations as they associate situations with the attack, find that they are unable to flee if the attack occurs, or find themselves in situations in which help is not readily available or in which embarrassment occurs if others notice the attack. Clinical features of ago-

box 7.1
Symptoms of a Panic Attack

A discrete period of intense fear or discomfort in which at least four of the following symptoms develop abruptly and reach a peak within 10 minutes:
1. Palpitations, pounding heart, or accelerated heart rate
2. Sweating
3. Trembling or shaking
4. Sensations of shortness of breath or smothering
5. Feeling of choking
6. Chest pain or discomfort
7. Nausea or abdominal distress
8. Feeling dizzy, unsteady, lightheaded, or faint
9. Derealization (feelings of unreality) or depersonalization (being detached from oneself)
10. Fear of losing control or going crazy
11. Fear of dying
12. Paresthesias (numbness or tingling sensations)
13. Chills or hot flashes

Modified from American Psychiatric Association: *Diagnostic and statistical manual of mental disorders,* ed 4, Washington, DC, 1994, The Association.

raphobia may then develop (Box 7.2). Less commonly, a history of phobia may precede a panic attack. Individuals are often embarrassed about their symptoms and try to hide them from others, often making excuses not to attend functions or enter phobic situations.

The differential diagnosis of panic disorder and agoraphobia includes anxiety disorder due to a general medical condition, substance-induced anxiety disorder, withdrawal from substances, GAD, and psychosis. Medical disorders that may produce symptoms similar to panic attacks include endocrinopathy (e.g., pheochromocytoma, thyroid disease), hypoglycemia, gastrointestinal problems (e.g., colitis), and cardiorespiratory problems that are associated with tachycardia, palpitations, chest pain, or dyspnea. Some neurological conditions, such as complex partial seizure disorder, may also result in panic.

Clinical Consequences

Panic disorder is often associated with major depressive disorder, other anxiety disorders, or alcohol and substance dependence. Self-medication with alcohol occurs at a very high rate, but the onset of alcoholism precedes the first attack in almost all patients.[4] Panic disorder follows a chronic course but waxes and wanes. In some individuals episodic outbreaks alternate with years of remission, whereas in others the symptomatology is continuous and severe. The development of agoraphobia usually occurs within the first year of recurrent panic attacks; its relationship to panic attacks varies. Agoraphobia (see Box 7.2) may become chronic whether or not panic attacks are present.[1]

Clinical Management Implications

The pharmacological treatment of panic disorder is well established in the literature, with the selective serotonin reuptake inhibitors (SSRIs) being the drugs of choice. Paroxetine has recently received formal approval for the treatment of panic disorder; other reports suggest that other SSRIs, including fluvoxamine, fluoxetine, and sertraline may be quite effective. Despite their efficacy in depression, trazodone and bupropion appear to be ineffective in panic disorder. Studies of nefazodone and venlafaxine are in the preliminary stages and appear quite promising.

Among the older antidepressants, imipramine

box 7.2
Features of Agoraphobia

A. **Panic Disorder With Agoraphobia:** The patient experiences anxiety about being in places or situations in which escape might be difficult (or embarrassing) or in which help may not be available in the event of having an unexpected or situationally predisposed panic attack.
Agoraphobia Without History of Panic Disorder: The patient has never met criteria for panic disorder. The anxiety may occur in situations in which help may not be available in the event of suddenly developing panic-like symptoms that the individual fears could be incapacitating or extremely embarrassing (e.g., fear of going outside because of fear of having a sudden episode of dizziness or a sudden attack of diarrhea). If a general medical condition is present, this fear described in the latter diagnosis is clearly in excess of that usually associated with the condition.

B. Agoraphobic fears typically involve characteristic clusters of situations that include the following:

Travel	**Proximity of safety**
Airplane*	May have a safe perimeter†
Car	Far from medical help
Bus	Being home alone or outside the home
Subway	**Public places**
Train	Stores
Driving	Malls
Alone	Restaurants
Highways	Theaters
Bridges	Church/temple
Tunnels	Crowds
Heavy traffic	**Other**
Inner lane of highway	Sitting in a meeting
	Waiting in line
	Sitting far from an exit‡

C. Agoraphobic situations are avoided (e.g., restricts travel), endured with marked distress or anxiety about having a panic attack (or panic-like symptoms), or require the presence of a companion.

D. The anxiety or phobic avoidance is not better accounted for by another mental disorder, such as specific phobia (e.g., avoidance limited to a single situation such as elevators), separation anxiety (e.g., avoidance of school), obsessive-compulsive disorder (e.g., fear of contamination), posttraumatic stress disorder (e.g., avoidance of stimuli associated with a traumatic event), or social phobia (e.g., avoidance limited to social situations because of fear of embarrassment unrelated to panic attacks).

Modified from American Psychiatric Association: *Diagnostic and statistical manual of mental disorders,* ed 4, Washington, DC, 1994, The Association.
*Fear is of being trapped, not that the plane will crash.
†A specific distance from home; in severe form patient can become housebound.
‡Prefer last row, aisle seat in theater, auditorium, or classroom.

is the most well-established medication for the treatment of panic disorder. However, most tricyclic antidepressants, including clomipramine, probably have similar efficacy. Monoamine oxidase inhibitors (MAOIs) can be very effective for patients with anxiety but are not drugs of choice because of the dietary restrictions and safety issues relative to the risk of hypertensive crisis. With all SSRIs, tricyclic antidepressants, MAOIs, or other antidepressant agents, approximately 20% of patients with panic disorder experience a stimulant-like reaction during initial treatment. Therefore it is recommended that low dosing and slow titration occur with all antidepressant agents. Extra reassurance and encouragement are often needed when treating patients with panic disorder. Alprazolam is the best studied of the benzodiazepines in the treatment of panic disorder; other benzodiazepines, including lorazepam, clonazepam, and diazepam are also effective when adequate doses are used. The onset of therapeutic effect is fairly rapid; some individuals respond to low doses, but higher doses are often required. The use of benzodiazepines should be avoided in those with a history of alcohol or substance dependence or personality disorder.

Social Phobia

Clinical Findings and Course

The course of social phobia is often continuous. The condition commonly has a lifelong duration, but it may lessen in severity or remit during adulthood. The severity of this disorder may vary with life stressors.

Clinical Management Implications

Pharmacological treatments for social phobia have generally involved mixed phobic groups or have examined social anxiety in nonpatient populations. However, clinical studies of social phobia are beginning to be published. One study noted that 45 to 90 mg/day of phenelzine (an MAOI) was superior to both a 50- to 90-mg/day dosage of the β-blocker atenolol and a placebo. However, atenolol may have specific efficacy for discrete performance anxiety.[11] Another study suggests that phenelzine with exposure instructions may have a higher rate of full responders and greater maintenance of treatment 2 months after treatment discontinuation as compared with the use of benzodiazepines or cognitive behavioral therapy alone. However, all three treatment conditions demonstrate some level of improvement.[6]

Combining behavioral techniques and matching treatment to patient characteristics have been quite effective in treating social phobia. Exposure and cognitive restructuring techniques are superior to either treatment by itself, and patients are more likely to continue to improve after treatment. Anxiety management training with relaxation, distraction, and rational self-talk may also

augment exposure therapy. Other types of psychotherapeutic interventions, including psychodynamic treatment, have not been useful with social phobia, but systematic studies are lacking.

Obsessive-Compulsive Disorder

Clinical Findings and Course

OCD is defined as the presence of obsessions or compulsions that produce discomfort or impairment (Boxes 7.3 and 7.4). Obsessions are thoughts, impulses, or images that are recurrent, persistent, intrusive, and recognized as senseless (at least initially). Compulsions are behaviors or rituals that are repetitive, purposeful, and intentional; are in response to an obsession; are performed in a stereotypical fashion or according to certain rules to prevent discomfort or a dreaded event; and are initially recognized as excessive or unreasonable. Obsessions and compulsions are not in themselves pleasurable; patients usually attempt to ignore, suppress, or neutralize obsessions.

In general, OCD has a gradual onset, but there are some cases of acute onset. The course of OCD is usually chronic with waxing and waning, and there may be an exacerbation of stress-related

box 7.3

Common Obsessions and Compulsions

Obsessions
Contamination/illness
Violent images
Fear of harming others/self
Perverse/forbidden sexual thoughts, images, or impulses
Symmetry/exactness
Somatic
Religious

Compulsions
Checking
Cleaning/washing
Counting
Hoarding/collecting
Ordering/arranging
Repeating

box 7.4

Symptoms of Obsessive-Compulsive Disorder

A. Either obsessions or compulsions

Obsessions

1. Recurrent and persistent thoughts, impulses, or images that are experienced, at sometime during the disturbance, as intrusive and inappropriate and cause anxiety or distress (e.g., a parent's repeated impulses to kill a loved child, a religious person's recurrent blasphemous thoughts).
2. The thoughts, impulses, or images are not simply excessive worries about real-life problems.
3. The person attempts to ignore or suppress such thoughts or impulses or to neutralize them with some other thought or action.
4. The person recognizes that the obsessions are the product of his or her own mind (not imposed from without as in thought insertion).

Compulsions

1. Repetitive behaviors or mental acts that the person feels driven to perform in response to an obsession or according to rigid rules.
2. The behavior or mental act is aimed at preventing or reducing distress or preventing some dreaded event or situation; however, these behaviors or mental acts are either not connected in a realistic way with what they are designed to neutralize or prevent, or they are clearly excessive.
3. The person recognizes that his or her behavior is excessive or unreasonable (this may not be true for young children; it may no longer be true for people whose obsessions have evolved into overvalued ideas).

B. At some time during the course of the disorder, the person has recognized that the obsessions and compulsions are excessive and unreasonable (may not apply to children).

C. The obsessions or compulsions cause marked distress, are time consuming (take more than an hour a day), or significantly interfere with the person's normal routine, occupational functioning, or usual social activities or relationships with others.

D. If another Axis I disorder is present, the content of the obsessions or compulsions is not restricted to it (e.g., the ideas, thoughts, impulses, or images are not about food in the presence of an eating disorder, about drugs in the presence of a substance use disorder, or guilty thoughts in the presence of a major depressive disorder).

E. The disorder is not due to a substance-induced disorder or an anxiety disorder due to a general medical condition.

Modified from American Psychiatric Association: *Diagnostic and statistical manual of mental disorders,* ed 4, Washington, DC, 1994, The Association.

symptoms. There is progressive deterioration in occupational and social functioning in 15% of cases; in 5% of cases there are episodes with few or no symptoms in between.[1]

Because patients with OCD are often reluctant to spontaneously divulge their conditions, the clinical symptoms must be inquired about directly. Obsessions may include such themes as contamination, violent images, fear of harming others or self, perverse and forbidden sexual thoughts, symmetry or exactness, somatic obsessions, or religiosity. Compulsions may include checking, cleaning, washing, counting, hoarding, collecting, ordering, arranging, or repeating. Symptoms may result in lateness because of the time spent repeating rituals or in chapped and thickened skin from repeated washings.

Clinical Consequences

OCD may cause isolation from and dependence on others. Patients may make demands on families and clinicians to perform such tasks as decontaminating and checking for objects. Suicide risk must be considered, because death may be perceived as an escape from the chronic symptoms. Symptoms are generally present continuously from the time of onset until the patient seeks treatment. Occasionally there is chronic deterioration in which obsessions and compulsions become more pronounced and consume all of the individual's time. Other diagnostic considerations may include schizophrenia, depression, phobias, Tourette's syndrome, and substance abuse.

Although similar in nature to OCD, a compulsive personality involves ego-syntonic attitudes and behaviors that are not resistive or experienced as intrusive. Other repetitive behaviors such as gambling, addiction, sexual behavior, and eating are to some degree inherently pleasurable, are resisted only because of deleterious consequences, and lack the simplest, unrealistic nature of OCD symptoms.

Clinical Management Implications

A variety of behavioral techniques have been applied to OCD and are often beneficial. Specific elements for treatment are prolonged exposure to ritual-eliciting stimuli together with prevention of the compulsive response. Flooding is not as tolerated as gradual exposure and is no more effective. Home-based treatment administered by the patient or with the assistance of a partner may improve maintenance and therapeutic gains. Behavioral therapies are generally enhanced by pharmacological treatments and assertiveness training. Many treatment gains have been maintained for up to 6 years.

Clomipramine was the first medication to demonstrate a significant therapeutic effect on OCD symptoms. The serotonergic effects of clomipramine have a greater efficacy and more potent serotonergic activity than other tricyclic antidepressants.

SSRIs have become the treatment of choice for OCD and include drugs such as fluvoxamine, fluoxetine, paroxetine, and sertraline. Individuals who do not respond to a particular SSRI may be switched to another. Unlike for major depression, the onset of therapeutic effect with OCD usually takes longer than 3 to 4 weeks. A lower response rate of 40% to 60%, more gradual improvement,

and a significant reduction of symptoms and disability (usually without complete remission) are observed. Symptoms commonly return if the medication is decreased or discontinued. With OCD, dosage requirements of SSRIs are two to three times higher than those used to treat depression; lower maintenance doses are often adequate.

MAOIs may be helpful in treating individuals with OCD and a history of panic attacks. Lithium augmentation has also been used with varying results. Reports indicate that lithium added to clomipramine, trazodone, or fluvoxamine may further reduce obsessions and compulsions. In general, buspirone has not been useful when prescribed alone to treat OCD symptoms, but it has been used successfully to augment SSRIs in treating refractory patients. Although benzodiazepines may reduce the anxiety associated with OCD symptoms, they do not appear to alleviate the central symptoms of the disorder. In individuals with schizotypal symptoms or tics, the neuroleptic drug pimozide may be useful in combination with an antidepressant drug to treat OCD. Current evidence does not support the use of neuroleptics alone in the treatment of OCD.

For severe debilitating cases in which all conservative treatments have failed, psychosurgical techniques such as cingulotomy, subcaudate tractotomy, stereotactic leucotomy, or anterior capsulotomy can be beneficial. The effect of these procedures is believed to be the disruption of efferent pathways from the frontal cortex to the basal ganglia. In general, electroconvulsive therapy has not been effective in OCD, but symptom response has been reported in individual cases with associated symptoms of depression. Depression may be responsive generally.[7]

Posttraumatic Stress Disorder and Acute Stress Disorder
Clinical Findings and Course

The diagnosis of PTSD requires exposure to significant trauma or abuse. Traumatic events may include combat, serious accidents, natural disasters, physical assault, serious danger of death or severe injury to oneself, or witnessing the mutila-

box 7.5

Criteria for Posttraumatic Stress Disorder

A. The person has experienced or witnessed an event that involves death, threat to life, or serious injury to self or others and that was experienced with intense fear, helplessness, or horror.

B. The traumatic event is persistently reexperienced in at least one of the following ways:
   1. Recurrent and intrusive distressing recollections of the event (in young children, repetitive play in which themes or aspects of the trauma are expressed)
   2. Recurrent distressing dreams of the event
   3. Sudden acting or feeling as if the traumatic event were recurring (includes a sense of reliving the experience, illusions, hallucinations, or dissociative [flashback] episodes, even those that occur on awakening or when intoxicated)
   4. Intense psychological distress at exposure to events that symbolize or resemble an aspect of the traumatic event, including anniversaries of the trauma
   5. Physiological reactivity on exposure to internal or external cues that symbolize or resemble an aspect of the traumatic event (e.g., a woman who was raped in an elevator breaks out in a sweat when entering any elevator)

C. Persistent avoidance of stimuli associated with the trauma or numbing of general responsiveness (not present before the trauma), as indicated by at least three of the following:
   1. Efforts to avoid thoughts or feelings associated with the trauma
   2. Efforts to avoid activities, situations, or people that arouse recollections of the trauma
   3. Inability to recall an important aspect of the trauma (psychogenic amnesia)
   4. Markedly diminished interest in significant activities (in young children, loss of recently acquired development skills such as toilet training or language skills)
   5. Feeling of detachment or estrangement from others
   6. Restricted range of affect (e.g., unable to have loving feelings)
   7. Sense of a foreshortened future (e.g., does not expect to have a career, marriage, children, or a long life)

D. Persistent symptoms of increased arousal (not present before the trauma), as indicated by at least two of the following:
   1. Difficulty falling or staying asleep
   2. Irritability or outbursts of anger
   3. Difficulty concentrating
   4. Hypervigilance
   5. Exaggerated startle response

E. Duration of the disturbance (symptoms in B, C, and D) of at least 1 month.

F. The disturbance causes marked distress or significant impairment in social or occupational functioning.
   Specify delayed onset if the onset of symptoms was at least 6 months after the trauma.

Modified from American Psychiatric Association: *Diagnostic and statistical manual of mental disorders,* ed 4, Washington, DC, 1994, The Association.

tion, serious injury, or violent death of another person. Symptoms are clustered into three categories: (1) reexperiencing the trauma, (2) psychic numbing or avoidance of stimuli associated with the trauma, and (3) increased arousal (Box 7.5). The reexperiencing phenomenon includes intru-sive memories, flashbacks, nightmares, and psychological and physiological distress in response to trauma reminders. Intrusive memories are spontaneous, unwanted, and distressing recollections of the traumatic event. Repeated nightmares contain themes of the trauma or a highly accurate and detailed recreation of the actual event. Flashbacks are dissociative states in which components of the events are relived; for a few seconds—or as long as several days—the person feels as if he or she is reexperiencing the event. Reactivity to trauma-related stimuli can involve intense emotional distress or physical symptoms similar to those of a panic attack and can occur when the individual is exposed to the sights, sounds, smells, or events that were present during the traumatic event. Numbing may include amnesia, emotional detachment, restricted affect, or loss of interest in activities. Avoidance may include thoughts, feelings, situations, or activities that are reminders of the trauma. Increased arousal may include insomnia, irritability, hypervigilance, increased startle response, or impaired concentration. PTSD may have pervasive effects on the individual's interpersonal behavior and all aspects of his or her psychosocial life. The duration of the symptoms and the level of distress and impairment are critical to the diagnosis.

Acute stress disorder is a new addition to DSM-IV and adds to the diagnostic nomenclature.[1] This disorder includes symptoms that occur in the immediate aftermath of a trauma and are predictive of subsequent problems with PTSD symptoms.[5] As with PTSD, this syndrome is characterized by numbing or dissociative symptoms, one or more reexperiencing symptoms, and other symptoms of hyperarousal. The diagnosis is made when the level of distress is clinically significant, when impairment occurs with functioning, or when the individual fails to pursue a necessary task such as obtaining medical, legal, or social assistance. A diagnosis of PTSD must be considered if the symptoms persist beyond 4 weeks.

Symptoms of PTSD usually begin within the first 3 months of the trauma but may be delayed for months or years. Immediately after the trauma, PTSD meets the criteria for acute stress disorder. The symptoms and the predominance of reexperiencing, avoidance, and hyperarousal symptoms may vary over time. The symptoms vary in duration. Approximately half of the cases completely recover within 3 months, whereas other cases have symptoms that persist for longer than 12 months. Predisposing conditions for PTSD include social supports, family history, childhood experiences, personality variables, and preexisting mental disorders. However, individuals without any predisposing conditions may develop PTSD, especially if the stressor is extreme.[1]

Clinical Management Implications

Assessing and treating an individual immediately after a trauma is the best way to potentially prevent many of the complications and associated disabilities. As with other anxiety disorders, treatment is often best accomplished with a combination of pharmacological and nonpharmacological therapies. Pharmacological treatment may be required to control the physiological symptoms and enable the patient to work through the highly emotional material in psychotherapy.

Comorbid conditions, especially depression or alcohol and substance abuse, must often be addressed and may be a focus of treatment in PTSD. Even if coexisting depression is present, treatment should focus on PTSD because the course, biology, and treatment response are unlike those of major depression. Few controlled medication trials have been reported with PTSD. Trials of phenelzine and imipramine have proven effective, but there is some suggestion that greater efficacy is shown by the MAOIs. Alprazolam and the other benzodiazepines have not been found to be any more effective than placebos. This lack of efficacy, together with the high rate of alcohol and substance abuse problems in patients with PTSD, make benzodiazepines a poor choice for treatment.

Open trials and case reports continue to support that SSRIs, venlafaxine, and nefazodone are useful in treating PTSD; controlled trials are under way. Clonidine 0.2 to 0.4 mg/day and propranolol 120 to 180 mg/day relieve startle responses, explosiveness, nightmares, and intrusive reexperiencing in some patients.[17] In one study, lithium decreased autonomic arousal, reexperiencing of symptoms, and ethanol use in 64% of patients; carbamazepine had similar effects.[17]

Controlled studies of behavioral therapies, including systematic desensitization and flooding, produce a decrease in reexperiencing and hyperarousal but not avoidant numbing. A controlled trial of cognitive therapy found that stress inoculation training reduced PTSD symptoms early in treatment; long-term results were best when this therapy was combined with prolonged exposure.[17]

After successful cognitive behavioral treatment, subsequent relapse resulting from a new trigger of traumatic memories can respond to another course of therapy. A controlled study of the use of psychodynamic therapy, hypnotherapy, and systematic desensitization in individuals with PTSD compared with waiting list controls showed that hypnotherapy was similar to desensitization, with more improvement in reexperiencing symptoms and less improvement in avoidance; psychodynamic therapy had a greater effect on avoidance than on reexperiencing.[17]

Generalized Anxiety Disorder
Clinical Findings and Course

GAD is commonly overdiagnosed because many of the symptoms of anxiety are prominent in underlying conditions, including depression, psychosis, substance abuse, somatoform disorder, and many general medical conditions. GAD is characterized by chronic excessive worry about life circumstances and is accompanied by symptoms of apprehension, motor tension, autonomic hyperactivity, vigilance, and scanning (Box 7.6). The individual may awaken with apprehension and unrealistic concern about future misfortune. To differentiate the disorder from more transient forms of anxiety, symptoms must occur for 6

---

box 7.6
Major Features of Generalized Anxiety Disorder

A. Excessive anxiety or worry (apprehension expectation) about several life events or activities, such as worrying about possible misfortune to one's child (who is in no danger) or about finances (for no good reason) for a period of 6 months or longer, during which the person has been bothered more days than not by these concerns. In children and adolescents, this disorder may take the form of anxiety and worry about academic, athletic, and social performance.

B. The person finds it difficult to control the worry.

C. At least three of the following six symptoms are often present when anxious:
   1. Muscle tension
   2. Restlessness or feeling keyed up or on edge
   3. Easy fatigability
   4. Difficulty concentrating or "mind going blank" because of anxiety
   5. Trouble falling or staying asleep
   6. Irritability

D. If another Axis I disorder is present, the focus of the anxiety and worry is unrelated to it (e.g., the anxiety or worry is not about having a panic attack in the presence of panic disorder, being embarrassed in public in the presence of social phobia, being contaminated in the presence of OCD, gaining weight in the presence of anorexia nervosa, having an illness as in hypochondriasis or somatization disorder, and is not part of PTSD).

E. The anxiety, worry, or physical symptoms significantly interfere with the person's normal routine or usual activities or cause marked distress.

F. The disorder is not due to a substance-induced or anxiety disorder due to a general medical condition and does not occur only during a mood disorder, psychotic disorder, or pervasive developmental disorder.

Modified from American Psychiatric Association: *Diagnostic and statistical manual of mental disorders,* ed 4, Washington, DC, 1994, The Association.

months. The diagnostic criteria noted in Box 7.6 emphasize that worry is out of proportion to the likelihood of the impact of the feared events; the anxiety is pervasive, difficult to control, and unrelated to hypochondriacal concerns, PTSD, or another anxiety or a substance-related disorder. Tension and nervousness may be manifested as restlessness, fatigability, edginess, difficulty concentrating, or irritability. Significant functional impairment may result in marked distress and is required for diagnosis.

GAD may be associated with muscle tension, trembling, twitching, shakiness, and muscle aches/soreness. Many individuals have prominent somatic complaints such as cold, clammy hands, dry mouth, sweating, nausea, diarrhea, urinary frequency, trouble swallowing, or an exaggerated startle response; dysphoria is quite common.[1] GAD often occurs with a mood disorder or other anxiety disorders. Other conditions commonly associated with GAD include irritable bowel syndrome, headache, and substance-related disorders. The course is often chronic but fluctuates, and it often worsens with stress.

Clinical Management Implications

Psychotherapy may be indicated for cases of GAD in which the clinician feels that core psychological conflicts cause or perpetuate the patient's anxiety. Preliminary studies of behavioral treatments suggest positive results with progressive muscle relaxation and anxiety management techniques. Biofeedback does *not* appear to have specific value, and cognitive therapy alone is not effective unless combined with systematic desensitization or relaxation.

The most commonly used pharmacological agents for acute GAD are the benzodiazepines. Advantages include the rapid onset of efficacy and long-term safety. Disadvantages include memory impairment, sedation, difficulty with discontinuation because of dependence, and abuse potential. Antidepressant therapies appear to be ineffective in GAD.

Buspirone, the nonbenzodiazepine anxiolytic, represents the treatment of choice for persistent GAD. Buspirone has a serotonergic mechanism of action and affects the $5HT_{1A}$ system. In contrast to the benzodiazepines, the therapeutic effects are delayed from 1 to 4 weeks. Side effects include dizziness, nausea, diarrhea, headache, or nervousness. Buspirone does not cause pronounced drowsiness or impair driving skills, and appears to lack abuse potential or withdrawal symptoms with abrupt discontinuation. Buspirone is nonsedating and does not significantly interact with alcohol or other drugs.

As with other anxiety disorders, optimal treatment may involve a combination of psychotherapy, behavioral therapy, and/or pharmacotherapy. Trials comparing integrative treatments are needed to establish the relative efficacies of these treatment modalities alone or in combination.

REFERENCES

1. American Psychiatric Association: *Diagnostic and statistical manual of mental disorders,* ed 4, Washington, DC, 1994, The Association.
2. Baxter LR: Neuroimaging studies of human anxiety disorders. In Bloom FE, Kupfer DJ, editors: *Psychopharmacology: the fourth generation of progress,* New York, 1995, Raven Press.
3. Baxter LR, Schwartz JM, Bergman KS et al: Caudate glucose metabolic rate changes with both drug and behavior therapy for obsessive-compulsive disorder, *Arch Gen Psychiatry* 49:681, 1992.
4. Breier A, Charney DS, Heninger GR: Agoraphobia with panic attacks: development, diagnostic stability, and course of illness, *Arch Gen Psychiatry* 43:1029, 1986.
5. Cardena E, Spiegel D: Dissociative reactions to the San Francisco Bay area earthquake of 1989, *Am J Psychiatry* 150:474, 1993.
6. Gelernter CS, Uhde TW, Cimbolic P et al: Cognitive-behavioral and pharmacological treatments of social phobia: a controlled study, *Arch Gen Psychiatry* 48:938, 1991.
7. Goodman WK, McDougle J, Price LH: Pharmacotherapy of obsessive-compulsive disorder, *J Clin Psychiatry* 54(suppl 4):29, 1992.
8. Hyman SE, Nestler EJ: *The molecular foundations of psychiatry,* Washington, DC, 1993, American Psychiatric Press.

9. Kaplan HI, Sadock BJ, Grebb JA, editors: *Kaplan and Sadock's synopsis of psychiatry,* ed 7, Baltimore, 1994, Williams & Wilkins.

10. Kilpatrick DG, Best CL, Veronen LJ et al: Mental health correlates of criminal victimization: a random community survey, *J Consult Clin Psychol* 53:866, 1985.

11. Liebowitz MR, Schneider F, Campeas R et al: Phenelzine vs atenolol in social phobia: review of a neglected anxiety disorder, *Arch Gen Psychiatry* 49:290, 1992.

12. Myers JK, Weissman MM, Tischler GL et al: Six-month prevalence of psychiatric disorders in three communities: 1980 to 1982, *Arch Gen Psychiatry* 41:959, 1984.

13. Nagy LM, Krystal JH, Charney DS: Anxiety disorders. In Stoudemire A, editor: *Clinical psychiatry for medical students*, ed 2, Philadelphia, 1994, JB Lippincott.

14. Reiman EM, Raichle ME, Butler FK et al: A focal brain abnormality in panic disorder, a severe form of anxiety, *Nature* 310:683, 1984.

15. Reiman EM, Raichle ME, Robins E et al: Neuroanatomical correlates of a lactate-induced anxiety attack, *Arch Gen Psychiatry* 46:493, 1989.

16. Robins LN, Helzer JE, Weissman MM et al: Lifetime prevalence of specific psychiatric disorders in three sites, *Arch Gen Psychiatry* 41:949, 1984.

17. Solomon SD, Gerrity DT, Muff AM: Efficacy treatments for posttraumatic stress disorder: an empirical review, *JAMA* 268:633, 1992.

18. Teresa M, De Cristofaro DER, Sessarego A et al: Brain perfusion abnormalities in drug-naive, lactate-sensitive panic patients: a SPECT study, *Biol Psychiatry* 33:505, 1993.

19. Wu JC, Buchsbaum MS, Hershey TG et al: PET in generalized anxiety disorder, *Biol Psychiatry* 29:1181-1199, 1991.

c h a p t e r e i g h t

Consummatory Problems: Eating and Substance-Related Disorders

 ## Eating Disorders

Cases of anorexia have been reported for centuries and were first described in the late 1870s. Eating disorders are characterized by severe disturbances in eating behavior. Symptoms include body image distortion, an extreme fear of being fat that is out of proportion with health concerns, a desire to reduce body fat to levels below that ordinarily considered healthy, restrictive and fad dieting, amphetamine and cocaine use for anorectic effects, purging by means of vomiting or laxative or diuretic abuse, and obsessive or compulsive exercise among normal weight or underweight individuals.

Two specific disorders are addressed in this chapter: anorexia nervosa (AN) and bulimia nervosa (BN). AN is characterized by a refusal to maintain a minimally normal body weight. BN is characterized by repeated episodes of binge eating followed by inappropriate compensatory behaviors such as self-induced vomiting; misuse of laxatives, diuretics, or other medications; fasting; or excessive exercise. A disturbance in perception of body shape and weight is an essential feature of both disorders. Obesity is not included in the fourth edition of the *Diagnostic and Statistical Manual of Mental Disorders* (DSM-IV) because it is not consistently associated with psychological

or behavioral syndromes.[3] Other disorders of feeding and eating that are usually first diagnosed in infancy or early childhood are not addressed in this chapter.

Epidemiology and Demographics

The onset of AN is associated with a stressful life event. The mean age at onset for AN is 17 years; it rarely begins in women more than 40 years of age. Some data suggest that peaks in incidence occur at 14 and 18 years of age.[3] The prevalence of clinically significant eating disorders among adolescent and young adult women in high school and college settings is approximately 4%; for more broadly defined eating problems the prevalence may be as high as 8%.[17] Men with AN are in the minority; 90% to 95% of the cases are women. Contrary to popular belief, this disorder is well represented among all social classes and ethnic groups.

For presentations that meet the criteria for AN, studies have found prevalence rates in young women to be between 0.5% and 1%. It is more common for individuals to meet some but not all criteria for the disorder. Limited data are available for men.[3] First-degree relatives of individuals with AN are at an increased risk for developing AN or mood disorders. The risk for mood disorders is especially increased among those whose relatives have the binge-eating/purging type of AN. Concordance rates for monozygotic twins are significantly higher than for dizygotic twins.[3]

AN appears to have become more prevalent in recent years and is occurring at an alarming frequency among young women and men. Despite extensive research the mortality rate is unchanged at 6%, and patients often experience repeated cycles of recovery and relapse. The causes of AN are related to a complex interaction of social, psychological, and biological factors. Some of the characteristic features of AN (e.g., dieting, weight reduction, and hyperactivity) have been argued to be primary features; therefore subpopulations in whom weight loss and exercise are encouraged are at particular risk for developing AN.[28]

The prevalence of BN among young women is approximately 1% to 3%; men have a prevalence rate approximately one-tenth that of females. Studies suggest that first-degree biological relatives of those with BN are at an increased risk for BN, mood disorders, and substance abuse/dependence.[3]

Psychobiological Considerations
Neurophysiological Brain Alterations

Several biological theories have suggested that eating disorders result from hypothalamic or suprahypothalamic dysfunction with abnormal secretion of luteinizing hormone (LH), follicle-stimulating hormone (FSH), cortisol, arginine/vasopressin, and other hormone peptides. Abnormalities in opioid and catecholamine metabolisms are also involved.[6] Unfortunately, many neurophysiological studies of eating disorders are based exclusively on data from patients who are already nutritionally unbalanced. Other theories regarding the biological underpinnings of eating disorders point out that eating disorders, especially bulimic syndromes, are variants of mood disorders. This notion is supported by the frequent comorbidity of mood disturbance and by an increased prevalence of mood disturbance among first-

degree relatives of patients with bulimia.

The process of dieting and exercise produces an autointoxication with respect to endogenous opioids. This autointoxication is essentially an altered state of consciousness as a consequence of the starvation state; at a certain point, internally generated opioids result in autoaddiction. The subsequent starvation and exercise are maintained in an effort to continue generating these endogenous opioids and sustain the "aura of good feeling" initially produced.[21]

Diminished norepinephrine turnover and activity are suggested by low MHPG (3-methoxy-4-hydroxyphenylglycol) levels. The diminution of MHPG, a major metabolite of norepinephrine, in the urine and cerebrospinal fluid (CSF) of patients with AN supports the noradrenergic neurotransmitter origin of this disorder. An inverse relationship occurs between MHPG and depression (see Chapter 6) versus AN. In addition, measurements of urinary MHPG levels in individuals with BN also somewhat support the noradrenergic hypothesis.

A direct link between AN and serotonin is likely, especially in acute cases of AN. In the CSF of patients with AN, the serotonin metabolite 5-HIAA (5-hydroxyindoleacetic acid) is 20% lower than normal but increases above normal after weight restoration. Patients diagnosed with AN and BN often present with depressive and obsessive-compulsive symptoms that also result presumably from abnormalities in brain serotonin (see Chapters 6 and 7). Because obsessive-compulsive disorder is best treated with serotonin agonists, indirectly acting serotonin agonists could be used effectively in the treatment of AN. However, the potential benefit of serotonin agonists is paradoxical because of their well-documented anorectic effects. Further research will determine whether serotonin agonists retard or promote AN.

The role of serotonin in eating disorders has received much interest in recent years and is concurrent with the development of newer antidepressants such as clomipramine, fluoxetine, nefazodone, and mirtazapine. Many of the newer antidepressants are unique in their activities and are specifically targeted for certain brain neurotransmitter sites. Because serotonergic pathways are involved in sleep regulation, arousal, and sexual and aggressive activities, the significance of dysfunction in this system and the impact on subsequent eating disorder symptoms needs further study with respect to neuropharmacology.

Research on seasonal affective disorder syndrome has demonstrated a pattern of carbohydrate craving and bulimia. Thus this syndrome may have some biological relationship to BN. Seasonal depression and carbohydrate craving also display a therapeutic response to serotonergic antidepressants. Because carbohydrate consumption has been shown to increase brain serotonin, O'Rourke, Wurtman, and Wurtman[24] have suggested that the frequency of carbohydrate craving and bulimia may reflect an attempt by the body to modulate an unrecognized mood disorder. Other evidence of altered serotonin function has been reported by Jimerson, Brandt, and Brewerton.[13] Their review of related research supports the hypothesis that etiological factors associated with decreased serotonin activity serve as a common vulnerability in both AN and BN.

The role of the endocrine system in the development of eating disorders is illustrated by the essential role of neurohormones in stimulating the synthesis, release, reuptake, and/or metabolism of neurotransmitters. Interestingly, a number of neuroendocrine findings that are present in eating disorders have also been documented in bipolar and depressive mood disorders. Dysfunction in the hypothalamic-pituitary-adrenal (HPA) axis, which affects both cortisol pituitary rate and urinary free cortisol levels, is found in mood disorders and AN and, less conclusively, in BN.[10] In eating disorders the dysregulated state of circulating cortisol levels contributes to adrenergic arousal of the limbic system, thus producing symptoms associated with depression.[12]

Similar to research applied in depression, studies of individuals with eating disorders have shown blunted TSH (thyroid-stimulating hormone) responses to TRH (thyrotropin-releasing hormone). This blunted response of TSH is thought to adversely affect the modulation of adrenergic receptors. Metabolic abnormalities in BN have been studied through an investigation of resting metabolic rate and thyroid function, a major contributor to resting metabolism. Such studies show a disturbance in energy regulation, which may reflect the need of those with BN to restrict intake to avoid gaining weight, therein experiencing increased hunger, preoccupation with food, and vulnerability to binge eating.[12]

Another endocrinological disturbance that occurs in individuals with eating disorders, particularly those with AN, involves decreased secretion of LH and FSH in response to correspondingly low levels of gonadotropin-releasing hormone. These low levels resemble prepubertal levels and result in the menstrual irregularities or amenorrhea that often occurs before substantial weight loss has been achieved. Another neurohormone that has been under investigation is vasopressin. Significantly lower CSF levels of vasopressin have been found in the presence of depression; this lowering is believed to be a reaction to the alteration of biogenic amine levels. Vasopressin levels in patients with AN are abnormally low in both CSF and plasma, which complicates the reestablishment of optimum fluid electrolyte balance following the polyuria that occurs with AN. The most recent study of vasopressin levels in BN has shown lowered plasma levels. However, in contrast with cases of depression and AN, CSF levels of vasopressin are *elevated* in BN.

Brain Imaging Techniques, Findings, and Research

Several computed tomography (CT) studies have revealed enlarged CSF spaces with enlarged sulci and ventricles during starvation in patients with AN. Interestingly, this finding is reversed by weight gain. In one positron emission tomography (PET) scan study, caudate nucleus metabolism was higher in the anorectic state than after realimentation.[19]

box 8.1

Symptoms of Anorexia Nervosa and Bulimia Nervosa

Anorexia Nervosa
- The patient refuses to maintain body weight at a minimal normal weight for age and height, leading to maintenance of body weight 15% below expected, or fails to gain weight as expected during growth, leading to body weight 15% below expected.
- Even though underweight, the patient intensely fears gaining weight or becoming fat.
- The patient experiences body weight, size, or shape in a disturbed fashion (e.g., claiming to "feel fat" even when clearly underweight).
- In female patients, the lack or absence of at least three consecutive missed menstrual cycles that should otherwise be expected to occur (primary or secondary amenorrhea). (Women are considered to have amenorrhea if periods occur only following hormone administration.)
- Two subtypes are specified: restricting type and binge-eating/purging type.

Bulimia Nervosa
- Repeated episodes of rapidly binge eating much larger amounts of food than most people would eat under similar circumstances in brief periods of time (e.g., 2 hours). During these binges the patient believes that the eating is out of control.
- The patient regularly engages in severe compensatory behaviors to prevent weight gain (e.g., self-induced vomiting, misuse of large amounts of laxatives or diuretics, diet pills, fasts, very strict diets, and/or very vigorous exercise).
- At least two binge-eating and purging or severe compensatory behavior episodes per week for a minimum of 3 months.
- Unrelenting overconcern with weight and body shape.
- These episodes do not occur only during a course of anorexia nervosa.
- Two subtypes are specified: purging type and nonpurging type.

Modified from American Psychiatric Association: *Diagnostic and statistical manual of mental disorders,* ed 4, Washington, DC, 1994, The Association.

Clinical Applications

The clinical features of AN and BN are found in Box 8.1. The primary symptoms of both AN and BN are a preoccupation with weight and a desire to be thinner. The two disorders are not mutually exclusive. A continuum involving self-starvation and the binge/purge cycle exists among patients of the two symptom complexes; approximately 50% of outpatients with AN have BN, and many patients with BN may have had AN previously.

Eating disorders share similar addictive-like features. The focus on food takes on the quality of a fetish/addiction. The addictive use of food and the concurrent attachment of one's body works quite well, at least initially in the cycle and, albeit brief, results in control, predictability, self-soothing, and regulating.[19]

Although a diagnosis of AN requires a weight loss of at least 15% below normal, many patients have lost considerably more by the time they come to medical attention. Patients engage in a variety of behaviors designed to lose weight. Remarkable restrictions in caloric intake, usually in the range of 300 to 600 calories per day, and strange dietary rituals such as the refusal to eat in front of others, the avoidance of entire classes of foods, and unusual spice and flavoring practices have been observed. Some patients with AN exercise compulsively for hours or engage in non–eating-related compulsions such as cleaning and counting.

box 8.2

Medical Complications of Eating Disorders

Related to Weight Loss
- Cachexia: loss of fat, muscle mass, reduced thyroid metabolism (low T_3 syndrome), cold intolerance, and difficulty maintaining core body temperature
- Cardiac: loss of cardiac muscle, small heart, cardiac arrhythmias (including atrial and ventricular premature contractions), prolonged His bundle transmission (prolonged Q-T interval), bradycardia, ventricular tachycardia, sudden death
- Digestive/gastrointestinal: delayed gastric emptying, bloating, constipation, abdominal pain
- Reproductive: amenorrhea, infertility, low levels of luteinizing hormone (LH) and follicle-stimulating hormone (FSH)
- Dermatological: lanugo (fine, babylike hair over body), edema
- Hematological: leukopenia
- Neuropsychiatric: abnormal taste sensation (possibly zinc deficiency), apathetic depression, irritability, obsessional thinking, compulsive behaviors, mild organic mental symptoms
- Skeletal: osteoporosis

Related to Purging (vomiting and laxative abuse)
- Metabolic: electrolyte abnormalities, particularly hypokalemia, hypochloremic alkalosis, hypomagnesemia
- Digestive/gastrointestinal: salivary gland and pancreatic inflammation and enlargement with increase in serum amylase, esophageal and gastric erosion, bowel with haustral dilation
- Dental: erosion of dental enamel, particularly of front teeth, with corresponding decay
- Neuropsychiatric: seizures (related to large fluid shifts and electrolyte disturbances), mild neuropathies, fatigue and weakness, mild degrees of cognitive dysfunction

From Yager J: Eating disorders. In Stoudemire A, editor: *Clinical psychiatry for medical students,* ed 2, Philadelphia, 1994, JB Lippincott.

Many patients with AN initially seem cheerful and energetic, but approximately 50% develop an accompanying depressive disorder or become moody and irritable. Approximately 25% of individuals develop obsessive-compulsive disorder.[11] The medical complications of AN are summarized in Box 8.2.

Clinical Findings and Course

AN appears to have two subtypes: restricting and binge eating. Those with the restricting subtype exert maximal self-control regarding food intake and tend to be socially avoidant, withdrawn, and isolated, with an obsessional thinking style and ritualistic behavior in nonfood areas. By contrast, those with the binge-eating subtype are unable to restrain themselves from frequent food binges and purges. These patients are also commonly depressed, self-destructive, engage in alcohol or drug abuse, and may display emotional, dramatic, or erratic personality clusters.

The course and outcome of AN are highly variable. Full recovery from AN is seen within a few years in 30% to 50% of patients. Younger patients and those with the restricting subtype appear to have a better prognosis. Death from starvation, electrolyte imbalances, cardiac arrhythmias, and suicide occur in 5% to 10% of patients within 10 years and 20% of patients within 20 years.[34] Some recover fully after a single episode, some experience a pattern of weight gain and relapse. Others experience a chronically deteriorating course over many years. Hospitalization may be required for weight restoration and for correction of fluid and electrolyte imbalances.[3]

Two subtypes of individuals with BN are distinguished: (1) the purging type who uses self-induced vomiting or misuses laxatives or diuretics, and (2) the nonpurging type who engages in other inappropriate behaviors such as excessive exercise or fasting and does not ordinarily self-induce vomiting or misuse laxatives or diuretics.[3] A concurrent major depression or anxiety disorder is found in 75% of patients with BN.[14]

BN usually begins in late adolescence or early adult life, may be chronic or intermittent, and often persists for at least several years. Binge eating often begins during or after dieting. The long-term outcome is unknown.[3] The medical complications associated with BN are summarized in Box 8.2.

Clinical Management Implications

Regardless of orientation or theoretical framework, the clinical approach to AN and BN requires some appreciation of common themes.[33] First, AN and BN exist overwhelmingly in women. Second, social influences and role conflicts are quite relevant to the development of eating disorders, especially in cultures in which social influences early in life are different for women than for men.[25] Third, the link between eating disorders and mood disorders explains the varied presentations and the family and developmental psychopathology and psychodynamics.[29] Finally, eating disorders are addictions: AN is an addiction to food avoidance, to the pursuit of thinness, and to the feeling of a sense of control and mastery over the body; bulimia is an addiction to food binges and, perhaps, purging and laxative use.

The treatment of an eating disorder is generally based on a comprehensive assessment with attention to physical examination, psychological profile, and behavioral aspects of the eating disorder. Associated problems such as substance abuse, mood and personality disorder, and problems within the family constellation must be addressed simultaneously.

Each patient's problem list has unique aspects, and treatment components are targeted to each specific problem. Treatment usually includes attention to weight normalization, symptom reduction through cognitive and behavioral therapy programs, supportive nursing care, and dietary management and counseling. Individual and family issues are addressed through group, individual, or family therapy. Some mood disturbances and eating disorder symptoms are treated with pharmacological interventions. As with many types of disorders, self-help programs may be useful. Currently the best treatment approach integrates elements pragmatically.

Many controlled studies have dealt with short-term weight restoration rather than long-term treatment of AN. Weight restoration brings about psychological benefits, including a reduction in obsessional thinking and mood and personality disturbance. The large majority of severely emaciated patients require brief hospital treatment with a competent general hospital staff or specialized eating disorder unit. The solution is to "encourage, persuade, or benevolently coerce" the patient into gaining weight.[34] Carefully designed studies have demonstrated that behavioral programs can reliably encourage weight gain. Combining informational feedback regarding weight gain and caloric intake with large meals and a behavioral program that includes both positive and negative reinforcers has the best therapeutic effects on eating and weight gain. Some programs usually require a minimum of several weeks in the hospital or a suitable alternative such as intensive outpatient day hospital.

The role of individual and family psychotherapy in bringing about weight gain is difficult to evaluate. The patient's motivation may be increased by such therapies, and therefore they may be valuable. Families benefit from family therapy and counseling as soon as problems are identified. Patients appear to make the best of these therapies to deal with their own and their family's long-standing psychological problems after they have regained some weight and are better able to think clearly.

Medications are often avoided in the initial treatment of patients with AN. Cyproheptadine in doses of 32 mg/day have been used with modest benefit for lower-weight, nonbulimic patients. The mechanism of action of cyproheptadine is uncertain, but it does seem to increase hunger. Trials of fluoxetine have also been helpful in maintaining weight gain for 1 year following an initial weight gain.[15]

Controlled studies indicate that tricyclic antidepressants, fluoxetine (a selective serotonin reuptake inhibitor), and monoamine oxidase inhibitors are useful in reducing binge eating and purging.[34] Common problems include medication compliance and the maintainance of therapeutic levels in the face of persistent vomiting. Fluoxetine and the tricyclics have been best studied and used most often. The results of medication treatments are similar to those of cognitive behavioral psychotherapies. Many patients who do not respond to psychological approaches alone benefit from medication; symptoms are reduced in 70% to 90% of patients, and approximately one third become abstinent. Some evidence suggests that combining medication and cognitive behavioral psychotherapy is better than either treatment alone.

Hospitalization is rarely indicated for uncomplicated BN. Indications for hospitalization include a failure to respond to outpatient treatment, worrisome medical complications not managed in the outpatient setting, and a severe mood disorder with suicide ideation.

Nonpsychiatric clinicians play a major role in the prevention, detection, and management of patients with eating disorders. Primary care practitioners are alert to the excessive concerns about dieting and appearance in preteens and their families and educate them about healthy nutrition and the danger of unrealistic dieting and eating disorders. Primary care practitioners should routinely question young female patients about what they desire to weigh, their dieting and exercise practices, and their use of laxatives. Clinicians working in gynecology clinics or gastroenterology settings, as well as dentists, are likely to encounter large numbers of patients with eating disorders. With motivated patients, a multidisciplinary approach can be highly successful. Every patient with a serious eating disorder warrants consultation with a psychiatric specialist who is knowledgeable about eating disorders.

 Substance-Related Disorders

Psychoactive substances, including alcohol, continue to be widely used for medicinal, social, recreational, and religious purposes. Surveys suggest that approximately 90% of the American population consumes at least some alcohol, 80% consume caffeine-containing beverages or medications (not addressed in this chapter), and 25% use tobacco products. The 1988 national household survey of drug abuse estimated that 72.4 million Americans age 12 or older (30% of the population) have used an illicit psychoactive drug at least once in their lifetime.[16] Although the use of illicit drugs appears to have declined over the previous decade, substance-related disorders continue to represent an enormous problem. One study estimated that 14.5 million Americans (7% of the population) used at least one illicit psychoactive substance in the month before the survey. The annual total cost to society in the mid-1990s was estimated to be almost 200 billion dollars.[16]

Epidemiology and Demographics

A discussion of the epidemiology and demographics of substance-related disorders must begin with some definition of terms. Whereas DSM-IIIR referred to "psychoactive substances," DSM-IV refers to "substances" and "substance-related disorders."[2,3] The word *psychoactive* was dropped in DSM-IV because limited attention would have been given to substances that have brain-altering activity as a primary effect (e.g., cocaine). The word *substance* is generally preferable to the word *drug* because *drug* implies that a manufactured chemical is involved, whereas many substances of abuse are naturally occurring (e.g., opium) or are not meant for human consumption (e.g., inhalants) (Box 8.3). Substance-related disorders are further complicated by the ambiguity of the language used to describe substance use and by basic questions regarding whether addictive disorders constitute a medical or moral condition. For the purposes of this chapter, substance use disorders or addictive disorders are defined as compulsions to use substances that cause harm to self or others.

In a strict pharmacological sense, *dependence* is often defined as a state in which the specific withdrawal signs and symptoms of a drug follow the reduction or cessation of drug use. *Tolerance* refers to the state in which the physiological or behavioral effects of a constant dose of a substance decrease over time; a greater dose is necessary to achieve the same effect. *Withdrawal* is a physiological state that follows the cessation of drug use

or the abrupt reduction in the amount of the drug used. In general, the behavioral effects of withdrawal are opposite those that the drug produces; therefore withdrawal from depressants produces psychomotor activation, and withdrawal from stimulants produces psychomotor slowing. In the DSM-IV, the acute and chronic effects of psychoactive substances are classified under five major categories:[3]

- ***Substance dependence.*** A maladaptive pattern of substance use with adverse clinical consequences (Box 8.4)
- ***Substance abuse.*** A residual category that describes patterns of drug use that do not meet the criteria of dependence; a maladaptive pattern of substance use that causes clinically significant impairment
- ***Substance intoxication.*** Reversible, substance-specific physiological and behavioral changes resulting from recent exposure to a substance
- ***Substance withdrawal.*** A syndrome that develops following the cessation of drug use or the abrupt reduction in dosage of a regularly used substance
- ***Substance-persisting disorder.*** A substance-specific syndrome that persists long after acute intoxication or withdrawal states (e.g., flashbacks, memory impairments, or dementia)

---

box 8.3
Classes of Substances of Abuse

Alcohol
Amphetamines and related substances
Caffeine
Cannabis
Cocaine
Hallucinogens
Inhalants
Nicotine
Opioids
Phencyclidine and related substances
Sedatives, hypnotics, and anxiolytics
Other (e.g., steroids, nitrates)

---

box 8.4
Diagnosing Substance Dependence

At least three of the following occur over a 12-month period of time:
- Tolerance: the need for increased amounts of the substance to achieve intoxication or other desired effect, or markedly diminished effect with use of the same amount of substance
- Characteristic withdrawal symptoms (may not apply to cannabis, hallucinogens, or PCP) or the use of the substance (or a closely related substitute) to relieve or avoid withdrawal
- Substance often taken in larger amounts or over a longer period than the person intended
- Persistent desire or one or more unsuccessful attempts to cut down or control substance use
- A great deal of time spent in activities necessary to get the substance (e.g., theft), taking the substance (e.g., chain smoking), or recovering from its effects
- Important social, occupational, or recreational activities given up or reduced because of substance use
- Continued substance use despite knowledge of having a persistent or recurrent social, psychological, or physical problem that is caused or exacerbated by use of the substance

Modified from American Psychiatric Association: *Diagnostic and statistical manual of mental disorders,* ed 4, Washington, DC, 1994, The Association.

Disorders of mood, thought, cognition, sleep, and sexual functioning may be associated with substance use (e.g., drug-induced anxiety, depression, or psychosis).

A large recent survey found the lifetime prevalence of substance abuse or dependence among the U.S. population over 18 years of age to be 16.7%.[16] The lifetime prevalence for alcohol abuse or dependence is 13.8%, and for nonalcohol substances it is 6.2%.[16] The lifetime prevalence and use of substances in 1991 is presented in Table 8.1. Alcohol and nicotine are the most commonly used substances, but marijuana, hashish, and cocaine are also commonly used. In general, the use of all of these substances has gradually and consistently decreased from 1980 to the early 1990s. However, some evidence indicates that substance abuse is again increasing among children and adolescents under the age of 18.[16]

Substance abuse and dependence are more common in men than in women, with a more marked difference for nonalcohol substances. Substance abuse is higher among the unemployed and among some minority groups. Substance use is more common among medical professionals than nonmedical professionals of an equal level of training. The possible explanation for this difference is simply the relative ease of access to some classes of substances (e.g., sedatives, stimulants, and narcotics).

The prevalence of the use of illicit substances is highest among individuals between 18 and 25 years of age. Men are significantly more likely than women to use illicit substances, and blacks are more likely than whites and Hispanics to do so. Residents of large metropolitan areas are more likely than their nonmetropolitan counterparts to use illicit substances. In the past, illicit substance use has been significantly higher in the West than in the Northeast, South, and North Central regions. No differences in other regions have been statistically significant.

The factors that determine an individual's susceptibility to substance use disorders are not well understood. Studies of populations at risk have identified factors that foster the development and continuance of substance abuse, including ge-

netic, familial, environmental, occupational, socioeconomic, cultural, personality, life stress, psychiatric comorbidity, biological, social learning, and behavioral conditioning.[30] Substance abuse and dependence appear to cluster in families. The concurrent distribution of antisocial personality disorder in such families, which may predispose individuals to substance abuse, may provide a partial explanation for this clustering.[3]

Alcohol

Alcoholism is often a familial disorder. For children of alcoholics, an increased risk of alcoholism exists regardless of whether they are raised by their biological parents or by a nonalcoholic foster parent.[5,8] The concordance of alcoholism among identical twin pairs is twice that of fraternal twin pairs (70% versus 35%). Factors accounting for this genetic predisposition for alcoholism include genetic variations in the rate of metabolism of ethanol and acetaldehyde, differences in brain electrophysiology, differential subjective sensitivity to the intoxicating effects of alcohol, and altered brain cell membrane properties.[30] Environmental influences must also have some effect, because 30% of male identical twins of alcoholics do not themselves become alcoholic.

In the general population, alcohol dependence and abuse are among the most common mental disorders. From 1980 to 1985, approximately 8% of the U.S. adult population was alcohol dependent, and 5% abused alcohol at some point during their lives. During a 1-year period, approximately 7.5% had symptoms that met the criteria for alcohol-related disorders.[3]

The cultural tradition surrounding the use of alcohol in family, religious, and social settings, especially during childhood, affects both alcohol use patterns and the likelihood that alcohol problems will develop. Marked differences characterize the quantity, frequency, and pattern of alcohol consumption in various countries. For example, in Asian cultures the overall prevalence of alcohol-related disorders is relatively low, and the male-to-female ratio is high. These findings appear to relate to the absence—in perhaps 50% of Asian

table 8.1

Population Estimates of Lifetime and Current Substance Use, 1991

The following figures are estimates of the percentage of people, by age category, who reported that they have used substances nonmedically, Substances used under a physician's care are not included.

	12-17 YEARS (POP: 20,145,033)		18-25 YEARS (POP: 28,496,148)		26+ YEARS (POP: 154,217,972)		TOTAL (POP: 202,859,153)	
	% EVER USED	% CURRENT USERS	% EVER USED	% CURRENT USERS	% EVER USED	% CURRENT USERS	% EVER USED	% CURRENT USERS
Marijuana and hashish	13	4	51	13	33	3	33	5
Cocaine	2	*	18	2	12	1	12	1
Crack	1	*	4	*	2	*	2	*
Heroin	*	*	1	*	2	*	2	*
Hallucinogens	3	1	13	1	6	*	8	*
Inhalants*	7	2	11	2	4	*	6	1
Stimulants	3	1	9	1	7	*	7	*
Sedatives	2	1	4	1	5	*	4	*
Tranquilizers	2	*	8	1	6	*	6	*
Analgesics	4	1	10	2	6	1	6	1
Alcohol	46	20	90	64	89	53	85	51
Cigarettes	36	11	71	32	78	28	73	27
Smokeless tobacco	12	3	22	6	13	3	14	3

Developed by Jerome H. Haffe, M.D. Estimates were developed from the 1991 National Household Survey on Drug Abuse.

All figures are rounded to the nearest whole number.

Ever used: used at least once in a person's lifetime. Current users: used at least once in the 30 days before the survey.

*Low precision; no estimate shown.

individuals—of the form of aldehyde dehydrogenase that eliminates acetaldehyde, the first breakdown product of alcohol.

In the United States, blacks and whites have nearly identical rates of alcohol abuse and dependence. Latino men have somewhat higher rates, but the rates are lower among Latino women than among other women.[3] Alcohol abuse and dependence are more common in men than in women, with a ratio that varies with age but can be as high as 5 to 1. Low educational level, low socioeconomic status, and unemployment are also associated with alcohol-related disorders. Conduct disorder and repeated antisocial behavior often co-occur among adolescents.[3]

Cocaine

In the United States, cocaine use affects individuals without regard to race, age, gender, or socioeconomic level. Cocaine-related disorders are most common in individuals between 18 and 30 years of age. Recently, more rural areas have been affected. Unlike most other substance-related disorders, cocaine-related disorders occur at equal rates in men and women. According to a 1991 community survey in the United States, 12% of the population had used cocaine at least once; 3% had used it within the last year, and less than 1% within the last month.[3]

Amphetamines

Amphetamine dependence and abuse can be found at all levels of society. Individuals from lower socioeconomic groups are more likely to use amphetamines intravenously, with a male-to-female ratio of 4 to 1.

Opioids

Opioid dependence is disproportionately represented by minority groups who live in economically deprived areas. This dependence can begin at any age, but problems most commonly occur during the late teens or early twenties. The prevalence of opioid use appears to decrease with increasing age (usually after age 40) in a phenomenon called "maturing out." Nevertheless, a subset of individuals remain opioid dependent for at least 50 years. Men are affected three to four times more often than women. Opioid dependence usually continues for many years, but there may be frequent, brief periods of abstinence.[3]

Cannabis

Probably the most commonly used illicit substance, cannabis has been used since ancient times and is used to treat certain medical conditions. For all cultural groups in the United States, it is one of the first drugs of experimentation. Cannabis use is more common in men and between 18 and 30 years of age. The dependence on and abuse of this substance typically develops over an extended period. With chronic heavy use, the pleasurable effects are diminished or lost.[3]

Phencyclidine

The prevalence of phencyclidine (PCP)-related problems appears to occur twice as often in men and ethnic minorities and is more common in those between 20 and 40 years of age. PCP accounts for 3% of substance-related deaths and for 3% of substance-related visits to emergency departments.[3]

Hallucinogens

There are regional differences in the use of hallucinogens in the United States; some established religious practices involve the use of hallucinogens. Typically, hallucinogen intoxication is initially experienced during adolescence; younger users may experience more disruptive emotions. Hallucinogen use and intoxication occur three times more often among men. According to community surveys conducted in 1991 in the United States, 8% of the population has used hallucinogens at least once. Hallucinogen use was found to

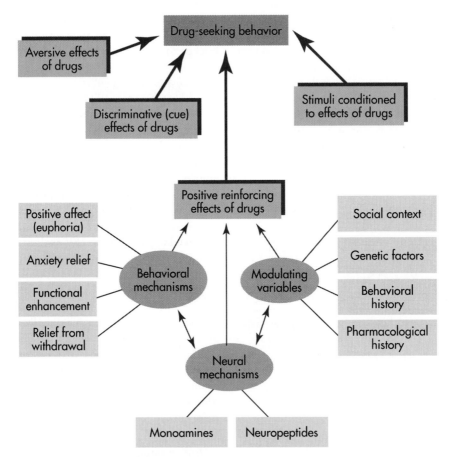

figure 8.1   A psychopharmacological model of substance-seeking behavior controlled by four main variables. The **positive reinforcing effects** of the substance begin with its initial use. **Reinforcing behavioral, neural,** and **modulating mechanisms** contribute to its continued use, whereas **aversive effects** contribute to a reduction in substance abuse. The **discriminative effects** of a drug allow for differentiation by the abuser. Other **reinforcing stimuli** (e.g., enjoying the effects of drinking in a lounge) also strengthen substance-seeking behavior. *(From Stolerman I: Drugs of abuse: behavioural principles, methods, and terms,* Trends Pharmacol Sci *13:171, 1992.)*

be most common in individuals between 18 and 25 years of age. [3]

Comorbidity

The comorbidity of substance use in a psychiatric illness is called "dual diagnosis." The National Institute of Mental Health Epidemiologic Catchment Area (ECA) studies have identified associations between alcohol use and anxiety disorders, depression, and schizophrenia.[26] Other studies of alcohol comorbidity have found associations between depressive disorders and cocaine and opioid use, as well as associations between depression and nicotine use. As discussed previously, there also appears to be a relationship between substance use and eating disorders.

A recent community survey found that 76% of men and 65% of women with a diagnosis of substance abuse or dependence had an additional psychiatric diagnosis. The most common comorbidity involves two substances of abuse—usually alcohol and some other substance. Other diagnoses commonly associated with substance-related disorders include antisocial personality, phobias, major depressive disorder, and dysthymic disorder. Various studies have found that between 35% and 60% of patients with substance abuse or dependence also meet the diagnostic criteria for antisocial personality disorder.[16] Patients with antisocial personality disorder are more likely to use more illegal substances, to have more psychopathology, and to be less satisfied with their lives, more impulsive, more isolated, and more depressed than patients with antisocial personality disorders alone.

Substance use is also a major precipitating factor for suicide. Compared with their counterparts in the general population, individuals who abuse substances are approximately 20 times more likely to die by suicide. Approximately 15% of individuals with alcohol abuse or dependence are reported to commit suicide. The frequency of suicide among substance abusers is second only to the frequency in patients with major depressive disorder.[26]

Psychobiological Considerations

The causes of substance abuse are complex and involve social, psychological, genetic, pharmacological, and other factors (Figure 8.1). The phenomenon of substance abuse has many implications for brain research, clinical medicine, and society in general (Table 8.2). Substances affect both internal perceived mental states and external observable behavior and activities. As with all mental disorders, the initial causative theories have grown from psychodynamic models; subsequent models have invoked behavioral, genetic, and neurobiological explanations, and recent studies include neuropathological and neuroimaging studies of selected conditions of substance abuse.

With the exception of alcohol and inhalants, researchers have identified particular neurotransmitter receptors at which the substances of abuse have specific effects. Even with normal endogenous receptor function and neurotransmitter concentrations, the long-term use of a particular substance may eventually modulate the brain receptor systems so that the brain requires the presence of the exogenous substance to maintain homeostasis. Such a process at the receptor level may be the mechanism for the development of tolerance within the central nervous system (CNS).

Major neurotransmitters involved in substance abuse and dependence are the opiate, dopamine (DA), and γ-aminobutyric acid (GABA) systems (Figure 8.2). The dopaminergic neurons are of particular importance in the ventral tegmental area (VTA), which projects to the cortical and limbic regions, especially the nucleus accumbens. This particular pathway is thought to be involved in the sensation of reward and to be the major mediator of the effects of most substances. The locus ceruleus, the largest group of adrenergic neurons, is also thought to be involved in mediating the effects of the opioids.

Activation of a single DA-modulated circuit is implicated regardless of the substance used. Repeatedly dosing the brain with addictive drugs alters the circuitry for pleasure. These changes

table 8.2   Substances Associated with Substance-Related Disorders

SUBSTANCE	BEHAVIORAL EFFECTS	PHYSICAL EFFECTS	LABORATORY FINDINGS	TREATMENT
Opioids	Euphoria, drowsiness, anorexia, decreased sex drive, hypoactivity, change in personality	Miosis; pruritus; nausea; bradycardia; constipation; needle tracks on arms, legs, groin	Detected in blood up to 24 hours after last dose	For gradual withdrawal: methadone 5-10 mg q6h for 24 hours, then decrease for 10 days For overdose: naloxone (Narcan) 0.4 mg IM q20 min for 3 doses, keep airway open, give O$_2$
Amphetamine and other sympathomimetics, including cocaine	Alertness, loquaciousness, euphoria, hyperactivity, irritability, aggressiveness, agitation, paranoid trends, impotence, visual and tactile hallucinations	Mydriasis, tremor, halitosis, dry mouth, tachycardia, hypertension, weight loss, arrhythmias, fever, convulsions, perforated nasal septum (with cocaine)	Detected in blood and urine	For agitation: diazepam (Valium) IM or by mouth 5-10 mg q3h For tachyarrhythmias: propranolol (Inderal) 10-20 mg by mouth q4h Vitamin C 0.5 g qid by mouth may increase urinary excretion by acidifying urine
CNS depressants, barbiturates, methaqualone, meprobamate, benzodiazepines, glutethimide (Doriden)	Drowsiness, confusion, inattentiveness	Diaphoresis, ataxia, hypotension, seizures, delirium, miosis	Detected in blood	For barbiturates: substitute 30 mg liquid phenobarbital for every 100 mg barbiturates abused and give in divided doses q6h; then decrease by 20% every other day May also substitute diazepam (Valium) for barbiturate abused; give 10 mg q2-4h for 24 hours and then reduce dose For benzodiazepines: gradual reduction of diazepam every other day over 10-day period

Alcohol	Poor judgment, loquaciousness, mood change, aggression, impaired attention, amnesia	Nystagmus, flushed face, ataxia, slurred speech	Blood level between 100 and 200 mg/dL	For delirium, diazepam (Valium) 5-10 mg IM or by mouth q3h, IM vitamin B complex, hydration. For hallucinosis: haloperidol (Haldol) 1-4 mg q6h IM or by mouth
Hallucinogens: LSD, psilocybin (mushrooms), mescaline (peyote), DET (diethyltryptamine), DOM or STP (2,5-dimethoxy-4-methylamphetamine), MDA (methylenedioxyamphetamine)	8- to 12-hour duration with flashbacks after abstinence, visual hallucinations, paranoid ideation, false sense of achievement and strength, suicidal or homicidal tendencies, depersonalization, derealization	Mydriasis, ataxia, hyperemic conjunctivae, tachycardia, hypertension	None	Emotional support (talking down); for mild agitation: diazepam (Valium) 10 mg IM or by mouth q2h for 4 doses; for severe agitation: haloperidol (Haldol) 1-5 mg IM and repeat q6h as needed; may have to continue haloperidol 1-2 mg a day by mouth for weeks to prevent flashback syndrome; *phenothiazines may be used only with LSD* **Caution:** phenothiazines can produce fatal results if used with other hallucinogens (e.g., DET, DMT), especially if they are adulterated with strychnine or belladonna alkaloids
Phencyclidine (PCP)	8- to 12-hour duration, hallucinations, paranoid ideation, labile mood, loose associations (may mimic schizophrenia), catatonia, violent behavior, convulsions	Nystagmus, mydriasis, ataxia, tachycardia, hypertension	Detected in urine up to 5 days after ingestion	Phenothiazines contraindicated for first week after ingestion; for violent delusions: haloperidol (Haldol) 1-4 mg IM or by mouth q2-4h until patient is calm

Modified from *Desk reference on drug misuse and abuse*, New York, 1984, New York State Medical Society.

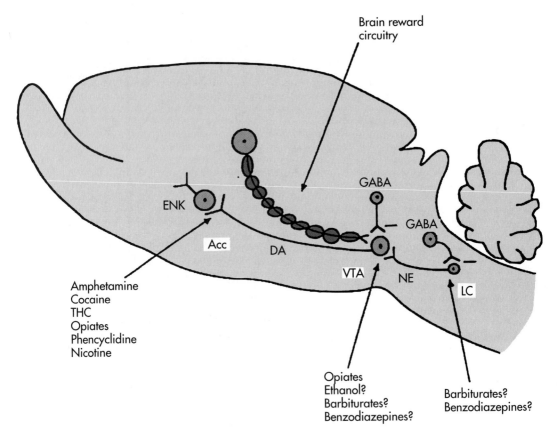

figure 8.2   Schematic diagram of the brain-reward circuitry of the rat brain, with sites at which various abusable substances appear to act. Neurotransmitters that may be involved in the development of substance abuse include the opioid, catecholamine (particularly dopamine), and GABA systems. Dopaminergic *(DA)* neurons that project from the ventral tegmental area *(VTA)* to the cortical and limbic areas (particularly to the nucleus accumbens *[Acc]*) are thought to be involved in reward mechanisms and seem to have a major role in stimulant abuse. CNS depressant abuse appears to be mediated by areas at which GABA inhibitory fibers synapse with locus ceruleus *(LC)* noradrenergic *(NE)* fibers. *ENK,* Enkephalin. *(From Gardner E: Brain reward mechanism. In JH Lowinson, P Ruiz, RB Millman, editors: Substance abuse: a comprehensive textbook, ed 2, Baltimore, 1992, Williams & Wilkins.)*

"starve" the brain cells of DA and trigger the craving for addictive drugs that will once again replenish the brain's supply. PET scans have shown that when an individual who is addicted to a substance has a craving for that substance, a high level of activation occurs in the limbic region and involves the amygdala to the anterior cingulate gyrus to the tip of both temporal lobes. This system seems to ordinarily play a part in the sense of pleasure, regardless of the reward: sex, chocolate, or a job well done. The mesolimbic DA system connects with other structures in the brain, especially the orbito-frontal cortex and the nucleus accumbens, and it appears to be active with the use of heroin, morphine, cocaine, amphetamines, marijuana, and alcohol.

Clinical Applications

The proper treatment and clinical management of substance-related disorders can be implemented only after an accurate diagnosis has been assigned. Box 8.4 lists the criteria for the diagnosis of substance dependence; Table 8.3 depicts diagnoses associated with various classes of substances. The recognition and diagnosis of a substance-related disorder, including alcoholism, is often complicated by a denial of the problem by both the patient and family or by efforts to conceal use because of fear of legal or other societal consequences. To recognize and treat substance-related disorders, the clinician must do the following: [30]

1. Know the pharmacokinetics and pharmacodynamics of the substance
2. Be able to identify the presence of substance abuse or dependence despite efforts by the patient to deny or conceal its use
3. Know the therapies for acute management of intoxication and withdrawal
4. Know the options for short-term treatment and long-term rehabilitation
5. Be aware of attitudes and possible negative biases toward such patients

To have psychoactive effects, a drug must be present as a free drug in a high enough concentration at its active site in the brain. A small amount of total administered drug is delivered to the site of action, whereas the rest is bound to serum or tissue proteins, is metabolized or excreted, or is otherwise unavailable. Although brain capillaries prevent the passage of many molecules into the brain via the blood-brain barrier, most psychoactive substances are lipid soluble.

Pharmacokinetic processes determine the availability of the active drug. The potency, duration, and mode of administration can be predicted by understanding these pharmacokinetic properties. The way the drug acts at the active site is known as a pharmacodynamic action. Many substances such as stimulants, sedatives, and hallucinogens bind to specific receptors. Cocaine and other stimulants appear to bind to specific neurotransmitter transporters, whereas other substances such as alcohol or inhalant solvents may nonspecifically dissolve in cell membranes and disrupt cellular functions and neurotransmitters.

Clinical Findings and Course

The assessment of individuals with dual diagnoses is particularly complex. The effects of substances may be similar to symptoms of psychiatric disorders or, alternatively, may mask the symptoms of an underlying psychiatric disorder. The physical, psychological, and social consequences of substance use may impair treatment of the other disorder. Most experts would agree that substance-related disorders must receive top priority in the treatment process if more than one psychiatric diagnosis is present.

Clinical Management Implications

Patients presenting for treatment of alcoholism and substance abuse do so in the context of a family structure that is often dysfunctional. Although family influences may motivate an individual to seek treatment, family members more often enable or facilitate the substance abuse and may or may not be aware of their contribution to the perpetuation of the problem. The clinician should try

table 8.3
Diagnoses Associated with Classes of Substances

	DEPEN-DENCE	ABUSE	INTOXI-CATION	WITH-DRAWAL	INTOXI-CATION DELIRIUM	WITH-DRAWAL DELIRIUM	DEMENTIA
Alcohol	X	X	X	X	I	W	P
Amphetamine	X	X	X	X	I		
Caffeine			X				
Cannabis	X	X	X		I		
Cocaine	X	X	X	X	I		
Hallucinogens	X	X	X		I		
Inhalants	X	X	X		I		
Nicotine	X			X			
Opioids	X	X	X	X	I		
Phencyclidine	X	X	X		I		
Sedatives, hypnotics or anxiolytics	X	X	X	X	I	W	
Polysubstance	X						
Other	X	X	X	X	I	W	

Note: X, I, W, I/W, and P indicate that the category is recognized in DSM-IV.
I, The specifier With Onset During Intoxication may be noted for the category (except for Intoxication Delirium); *W*, the specifier With Onset During Withdrawal may be noted for the category (except for Withdrawal Delirium); *I/W*, either With Onset During Intoxication or With Onset During Withdrawal may be noted for the category; *P*, the disorder is Persisting.
*Also Hallucinogen persisting perception disorder (flashbacks).

to involve the family members in the patient's treatment, using self-help organizations such as AlAnon, NarcAnon, AlaTeen, and Adult Children of Alcoholics. These groups provide valuable emotional support and education for family members. Family therapy is as essential as individual treatment for the patient.

Effectively confronting patients with their alcohol or drug problem before entry into treatment requires special skills and techniques. Presenting the problem as a disease is often the most effective approach. The individual is told that the alcohol or drug represents a serious threat to his or her health and well-being; the evidence by history or medical examination is pointed out in an objective and nonjudgmental manner. The clinician emphasizes the effects that the alcohol or substance has had on the health, behavior, and family. The clinician should not focus on the amount consumed because denial, excuses, rationalizations, and promises to stop are often obtained in response.

The clinician may further explain that the alcohol or drug has affected the brain and CNS, that the individual can no longer control his or her intake, and that he or she has lost sight of the negative effects that are occurring. Blaming, lecturing, cajoling, and threatening rarely work and may only heighten a patient's defensiveness, denial, and evasiveness. Frightening patients into treatment is not usually successful in the long run. Careful follow-up is generally required, and a referral to self-help groups is a valuable resource for consultations.

AMNESTIC DISORDERS	PSYCHOTIC DISORDERS	MOOD DISORDERS	ANXIETY DISORDERS	SEXUAL DYSFUNC- TIONS	SLEEP DISORDERS
P	I/W	I/W	I/W	I	I/W
	I	I/W	I	I	I/W
			I		I
	I		I		
	I	I/W	I/W	I	I/W
	I*	I	I		
	I	I	I		
	I	I		I	I/W
	I	I	I		
P	I/W	I/W	W	I	I/W
P	I/W	I/W	I/W	I	I/W

Members of Alcoholics Anonymous (AA) and similar groups will usually visit a prospective patient if the patient initiates a call. To maintain the family equilibrium, families develop rigid systems of denial to cope with drinking and substance abuse. The spouse may play a co-dependent role by enabling the drinking and by collaborating in a system of denial and rescue. Alcoholism may be the family secret that the family believes would be socially humiliating and embarrassing to acknowledge. Therefore effective intervention means working with the entire family, not just confronting the alcoholic. The best strategy often involves conferring with an addiction nurse specialist, psychiatrist, or other mental health professional with special expertise in alcoholism or addiction before direct confrontation occurs. The practitioner and specialist can then plan a coordinated intervention that includes follow-up.

 Specific Abused Substances

Alcohol
Macroscopic and Microscopic Brain Alterations

Alcohol consumption is toxic to the brain. Structural (and neurochemical) findings of alcohol disorders are characterized by the Wernicke-Korsakoff syndrome. In the small percentage of patients with Wernicke's encephalopathy, punctate hemorrhagic lesions have been found on brain autopsy in the hypothalamus, mamillary bodies, reticular formation, periaqueductal areas of the midbrain, floor of the fourth ventricle, and periventricular areas of the thalamus (Figure 8.3).

Quantitative studies of the cerebellum in alcoholism reveal a significant loss of cerebellar Pur-

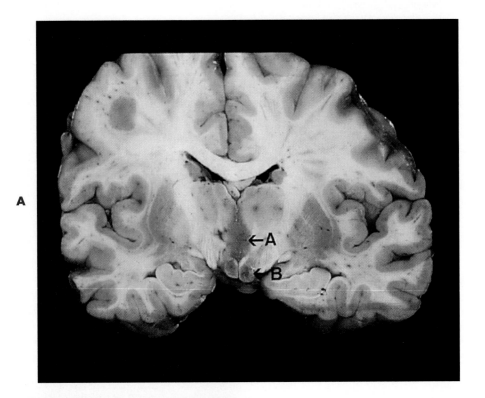

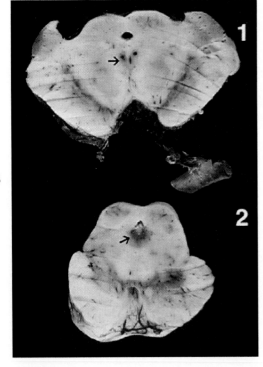

figure 8.3 **A,** Coronal section shows brain of a 65-year-old confused patient with alcoholism. Hemorrhagic necrosis is present in both the hypothalamus *(arrow A)* and the mamillary bodies *(arrow B)*. The normal light tan-brown appearance of brain tissue is replaced by the brownish-grey discoloration of punctate hemorrhages and parenchymal necrosis. **B,** Wernicke's encephalopathy also damages the brainstem. *1* and *2,* Sequential midbrain sections in which hemorrhagic necrosis *(arrow)* is present in the periaqueductal grey region. Damage to the oculomotor nucleus in this area causes ophthalmoplegia in Wernicke's encephalopathy. Patients with alcoholism who present with confusion and ophthalmoplegia need immediate thiamine replacement to prevent further complications. *(Courtesy Dr. Richard E. Powers, Director, University of Alabama at Birmingham Brain Resource Program.)*

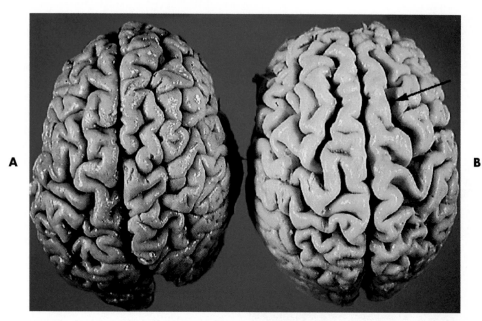

figure 8.4   The effects of long-term polysubstance abuse on the brain. **A,** Normal brain. **B,** Brain of a 40-year-old polysubstance abuser who used alcohol, cocaine, and intravenous heroin. This individual had multiple drug-related health problems, including cardiac, liver, and pancreatic disease. The conspicuous atrophy of the frontal lobes with widening of the superior frontal sulcus *(arrow)* results from toxic, anoxic, and metabolic damage to the brain. Microscopic examination of this brain shows nonspecific gliosis and neuronal loss. *(Courtesy Dr. Richard E. Powers, Director, University of Alabama at Birmingham Brain Resource Program.)*

kinje cells (approximately 10% to 30%) and shrinkage of the cerebellar molecular and granular cell layers. Alcohol alone may cause cerebellar atrophy, but with Wernicke's encephalopathy, thiamine deficiency may contribute. Abnormalities in thiamine metabolism have been postulated as a contributory factor in the development of severe thiamine deficiency with alcoholism.

Cerebellar atrophy has been reported to occur in approximately 40% of patients with chronic alcoholism (Figures 8.4 and 8.5). Brain shrinkage is somewhat reversible after prolonged periods of abstinence. This reversibility most commonly occurs in younger individuals and in those with the shortest drinking history. However, the loss of cerebellar and cortical neurons and the diencephalic and midbrain damage caused by Wernicke's encephalopathy is irreversible.

Neurophysiological Brain Alterations

The memory disruption of Korsakoff's psychosis may result from a breakdown of the functional anatomic linkages between the reward reinforcement and memory systems. Unlike patients with Alzheimer's disease, patients with Korsakoff's psychosis may have access to semantic memory. Decreases in CSF levels of norepinephrine, DA, and serotonin have been found, with the greatest decrements involving norepinephrine levels. One hypothesis suggests that norepinephrine systems are selectively damaged in Korsakoff's psychosis, which results in memory deficits but not global dementia.

Deficits in the acetylcholine system have also been suggested to cause a milder form of damage to the nucleus basalis of Meynert that is comparable to what is found in Alzheimer's disease. Direct

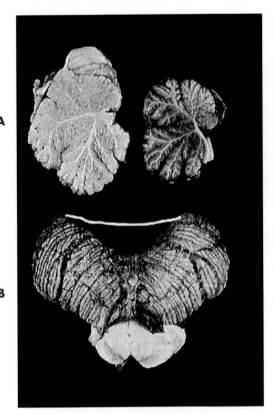

figure 8.5 The anterior cerebellar vermis in a patient with alcoholic cerebellar disease. **A,** Sagittal section of the anterior vermis of a normal individual *(left)* and a subject with alcoholic vermal atrophy *(right)*. **B,** Superior surface of the cerebellum with severe atrophy of the midline anterior vermis. The vermis coordinates truncal movement, and patients with alcoholism develop truncal ataxia, which predisposes them to falls. The white line emphasizes the degree of cerebellar atrophy. *(Courtesy Dr. Richard E. Powers, Director, University of Alabama at Birmingham Brain Resource Program.)*

alcohol neurotoxicity to this structure may also play a role in Korsakoff's psychosis. Cholinergic blockade produces anterograde amnesia similar to the pattern seen in patients with Alzheimer's disease. This amnesia has been characterized as a basal forebrain rather than a diencephalic amnesia. However, Korsakoff's psychosis cannot be attributed to damage of any one structure.[7]

In contrast to most other substances, no single receptor site or molecular target has been identified as the mediator of the effects of alcohol. The latest findings support the hypothesis that alcohol produces its effects by *intercollating* itself into membranes, resulting in increased fluidity of the membrane with short-term use. Long-term use results in membrane stiffness. Membrane fluidity is critical to the normal functioning of receptors, ion channels, and other membrane proteins. Alcohol ion channel activities are associated with nicotine, nicotinic acetylcholine, serotonin-3 ($5HT_3$), and $GABA_A$ receptors, all of which are enhanced by alcohol.

The net result of the molecular activities of alcohol is that of a depressant, much like the barbiturates and benzodiazepines that are cross-tolerant and cross-dependent. At blood levels of 0.05%, thought, judgment, and restraint are loosened and sometimes disrupted; motor disturbances are also seen. Legal intoxication ranges from 0.08% to 0.15% in most states. At 0.2% the function of the entire motor area of the brain is measurably depressed; at 0.3%, confusion or stupor are commonly present. At 0.4% to 0.5%, an individual generally becomes comatose, with abnormal breathing, abnormal heart rate, and the potential for death. Individuals with long-standing histories of alcohol abuse may falsely appear to be less intoxicated than they really are because of their ability to tolerate higher concentrations of alcohol. It is a myth that drinking alcohol aids sleep; alcohol is associated with decreased rapid eye movement sleep, decreased deep sleep, and increased sleep fragmentation, including more and longer episodes of awakening.

The diagnostic criteria for alcohol withdrawal are listed in Box 8.5. Several studies have tried to explain withdrawal from alcohol. Observed autonomic hyperactivity during withdrawal, which is mediated by the sympathetic nervous system, has resulted in a focus on the noradrenergic neurotransmitter system. Increased CSF norepinephrine has been associated with the intensity of withdrawal symptoms. Alcohol by-products include acetaldehyde, which may have an inhibitory effect on the adrenergic receptors. Increased cyclic adenosine monophosphate (cAMP) in neurons

box 8.5

Diagnostic Criteria for Alcohol Withdrawal

A. Cessation of (or reduction in) alcohol use that has been heavy and prolonged.
B. Two (or more) of the following, developing within several hours to a few days after criterion A:
    (1) Autonomic hyperactivity (e.g., sweating or pulse rate greater than 100)
    (2) Hand tremor
    (3) Insomnia
    (4) Nausea or vomiting
    (5) Transient visual, tactile, or auditory hallucinations or illusions
    (6) Psychomotor agitation
    (7) Anxiety
    (8) Grand mal seizures
C. The symptoms in criterion B cause clinically significant distress or impairment in social, occupational, or other important areas of functioning.
D. The symptoms are not due to a general medical condition and not better accounted for by another mental disorder.
    Specify if:
    With perceptual disturbances

From American Psychiatric Association: *Diagnostic and statistical manual of mental disorders,* ed 4, Washington, DC, 1994, The Association.

with long-term alcohol exposure may increase norepinephrine receptor sensitivity and norepinephrine turnover.

A kindling model developed in rats has shown that repeated mild withdrawal from alcohol increases subcortical neuronal spiking. This increased spiking may serve as a kindling focus for the limbic, hypothalamic, and thalamic areas, thereby increasing the severity of withdrawal and the potential for seizures.

Brain Imaging Techniques, Findings, and Research

Enlargement of cortical sulci, fissures, and ventricles is commonly observed in the CT scans of many patients with alcoholism. Reduction in the brain volumes of these patients results from the loss of white matter in the cerebral hemispheres rather than from volume changes in the cortex. Advances in the use of PET scans now provide potential for the further study of the functional metabolic effect of alcohol on the brain.

Clinical Findings and Course

Alcohol abuse and dependence are characterized by periods of remission and relapse. An individual may decide to stop drinking, often in response to a crisis. Weeks (or longer) of abstinence may follow this decision; this abstinence is often followed by periods of controlled drinking. However, once the individual begins to drink, consumption usually escalates rapidly, and severe problems recur. Fortunately, the typical alcoholic has a much better prognosis. More than 65% of the more highly functioning individuals demonstrate a 1-year abstinence rate following treatment, and perhaps at least 20% achieve long-term sobriety without treatment.[3]

Withdrawal syndrome is characterized by the symptoms found in Box 8.6. Withdrawal may include perceptual disturbances such as hallucinations with intact reality testing, in which the individual knows that the hallucinations are alcohol-induced, not real. Auditory, visual, or tactile illusions without delirium may also occur during withdrawal.[3] Other alcohol-induced disorders include intoxication delirium, withdrawal delirium,

box 8.6
Commonly Reported Signs and Symptoms of Withdrawal

Mood Changes
Depression
Hostility
Impatience

Physiological Symptoms
Drowsiness
Fatigue
Decreased alertness
Lightheadedness
Headaches
Tightness in chest
Body aches and pains
Tingling sensation in limbs
Stomach distress

Physiological Signs
Increase in peripheral circulation
Drop in urinary adrenalin, noradrenaline, cortisol
Changes in EEG
Changes in endocrine function
Neurotransmitter changes
Performance deficits
Sleep disturbance
Constipation
Sweating
Mouth ulcers
Increased coughing

persisting dementia, persisting amnestic disorder, psychotic disorder, mood disorder, anxiety disorder, sexual dysfunction, or sleep disorder. A diagnosis of these disorders is made when the symptoms exceed those usually associated with alcohol intoxication or withdrawal.[3] Because withdrawal can be unpleasant and intense, individuals may continue to consume alcohol, despite the adverse consequences, to avoid or relieve the symptoms.

Clinical Consequences

The clinical consequences of alcoholism are characterized by the neuropsychiatric findings found in Table 8.4.

table 8.4 **Neuropsychiatric Signs and Symptoms Induced by Alcohol**

SYNDROME	KEY SIGNS AND SYMPTOMS	KEY NEUROPSYCHIATRIC SIGNS AND SYMPTOMS	TIME OF ONSET	TREATMENT
Alcohol intoxication	Disinhibition, sedation at high doses	Acute organic brain syndrome	Rapid; depends on tolerance of individual	Time, protective environment
Alcohol idiosyncratic intoxication	Marked aggressive or assaultive behavior	Absence of focal neurological signs and symptoms	Erratic occurrence	None
Alcohol withdrawal	Tremulousness, irritability, nausea, vomiting, insomnia, malaise, autonomic hyperactivity	Transient sensory disturbances possible	Several hours; peak symptoms 24-48 hours after last drink or relative drop in level	

Disorder				Treatment
Alcohol seizures	Grand mal seizures, in bursts of 2-6 seizures; rarely status epilepticus	Loss of consciousness, tonic-clonic movements, urinary incontinence, post-ictal confusion; look for focal signs	7-38 hours after cessation of alcohol	Diazepam, phenytoin; maintenance phenytoin if underlying seizure disorder is present; prevent by Librium detoxification
Alcohol withdrawal delirium	Confusion, disorientation, fluctuating consciousness, perceptual disturbances, autonomic hyperactivity	Marked changes in levels of consciousness and disorientation; may be fatal	Gradual onset 2-3 days after alcohol cessation; peak intensity at 4-5 days	Librium detoxification; haloperidol 2-5 mg po bid
Alcohol hallucinosis	Vivid auditory hallucinations with affect appropriate to content (often threatening)	Clear sensorium	Usually within 48 hours or less of last drink; may last several weeks	Haloperidol 2-5 mg po bid for psychotic symptoms
Wernicke's encephalopathy	Oculomotor disturbances, cerebellar ataxia	Mental confusion	Abrupt onset; ataxia may precede mental confusion	Thiamine 100 mg IV; $MgSO_4$ 1-2 ml in 50% solution IV diluted before glucose loading
Korsakoff's psychosis	Alcohol stigmata possible	Retrograde and anterograde amnesia; confabulation early; intellectual function generally spared	Several days following occurrence of Wernicke's encephalopathy	No effective treatment; institutionalization often needed
Alcohol dementia	Absence of other causes for dementia	Nonprogressing dementia if alcohol free	Associated with greater than 10-year history of drinking	None

From Franklin JE, Francis RJ: Alcohol-induced organic mental disorders. In Yudofsky SC, Hales RE, editors: *The American Psychiatric Press textbook of neuropsychiatry,* ed 2, 1992, American Psychiatric Press.

Delirium Tremens

Alcohol withdrawal delirium, or delirium tremens (DTs), can range from quiet confusion, agitation, and peculiar behaviors that last several weeks to marked abnormal behavior, vivid terrifying delusions, and hallucinations. Hallucinations may be auditory and of a persecutory nature, or they may be kinesthetic with tactile sensations of crawling insects. The level of consciousness may fluctuate. Patients tend to show similar patterns of behavior each time they withdraw from alcohol.

DTs generally occur in alcoholics with a history of 5 to 15 years of heavy drinking and markedly decreased blood alcohol levels. A major physical illness such as infection, trauma, liver disease, or metabolic disorder predisposes an individual to DTs. Useful predictors include a past history of alcohol withdrawal delirium or seizures. Fortunately, most cases of DTs are benign and short-lived and subside after 3 days; however, DTs may last up to 5 weeks. The delirious state may be fatal and/or be characterized by several relapses separated by lucid intervals, but this occurrence is less common. The syndrome may be modified and masked by sedatives, analgesics, or trauma. Death may be related to infections, fat emboli, or cardiac arrhythmia associated with hyperkalemia, hyponatremia, hypophosphatemia, alcoholic ketoacidosis, hyperpyrexia, poor hydration, rhabdomyolysis, and hypertension.

Alcoholic Hallucinosis

Alcoholic hallucinosis is characterized by vivid auditory hallucinations that occur shortly after the cessation or reduction of heavy drinking. The onset classically occurs after the cessation of drinking but has been reported to occur during drinking bouts. The differential diagnosis includes DTs, paranoid psychosis, borderline transient psychotic episodes, or other substance-related disorders. Withdrawal-induced hallucinosis is not a predictor of DTs. In contrast to alcohol-induced delirium and DTs, the hallucinations associated with this syndrome occur in a clear sensorium with a paucity of autonomic symptoms. Hallucinations may range from sounds such as clicks, roaring, humming, or ringing bells to chanting or

threatening/maligning voices of friends or enemies.[20] Remission of symptoms is not expected after a period of 6 months.[7]

Wernicke-Korsakoff Syndrome

Wernicke-Korsakoff syndrome is a spectrum of neurological disorders associated with thiamine deficiency. It is most often associated with alcoholism but can occur in any condition that causes thiamine deficiency. Thiamine deficiency produces a diffuse decrease in the use of glucose and results in neurotoxicity, perhaps as a result of the release of excitatory neurotransmitters such as glutamic acid. Repeated bouts of marginal thiamine deficiency can lead to the same pathological changes induced by a single episode of severe thiamine deficiency. Wernicke-Korsakoff syndrome constitutes 3% of all alcohol-related disorders.[23]

Classically, Wernicke's encephalopathy has an abrupt onset, with oculomotor disturbances, cerebellar ataxia, and mental confusion. The oculomotor disturbances range from various types of nystagmus to complete gaze palsy and truncal ataxia. These symptoms and signs may precede the mental confusion by days. In 10% to 80% of cases, a general confusional state with disorientation and slowed mental response may proceed to frank stupor and coma.[23] Wernicke's encephalopathy is associated with a 17% mortality rate and should be considered a medical emergency. If a patient does not respond quickly to treatment, the development of Korsakoff's psychosis is likely. Approximately 80% of patients with Wernicke's encephalopathy who survive develop Korsakoff's psychosis.[27]

Acute treatment of Wernicke's encephalopathy consists of parenteral thiamine 100 mg, with titration of thiamine upward until ophthalmoplegia has resolved. Resistance to thiamine replacement may result from hypomagnesemia. Magnesium sulphate 1 to 2 mL IM or diluted IV in a 50% solution should be administered. Thiamine must be given before any glucose loading. Ophthalmoplegia usually responds quickly, but truncal ataxia may persist.

Alcohol-induced persisting amnestic disorder, or Korsakoff's psychosis, is classically a chronic condition with both retrograde and anterograde amnesia. The retrograde amnesia may evolve a few years before the onset of illness. Confabulation is quite typical in the early stages but may not be present. Korsakoff's psychosis may also involve behavior changes such as apathy, inertia, and loss of insight, all of which are indicative of frontal lobe damage.

Treatment of Korsakoff's psychosis is symptomatic. Clonidine 0.3 mg bid has been reported to improve recent memory and recall, perhaps as a result of hypothesized damage to the ascending, norepinephrine-containing neurons in the brainstem and diencephalon. Propranolol, up to 20 mg/kg/day, has been used for the rage attacks often associated with Korsakoff's psychosis, which are possibly a result of a chronic catecholamine supersensitivity. Fluvoxamine recently has been shown to reduce the long-term memory deficits; this action is hypothesized to occur through the serotonergic effects of fluvoxamine. Further trials of serotonergic agents are needed to confirm their treatment utility.[22]

Fetal Alcohol Syndrome

Fetal alcohol syndrome (FAS) is the leading cause of mental retardation in the United States and results from the exposure of embryos to alcohol in utero. The presence of alcohol inhibits intrauterine growth and postnatal development. Microencephaly, craniofacial malformations, and limb and heart defects are common in affected individuals. Short stature as adults and the development of a range of adult maladaptive behaviors are associated with FAS. The risk of an alcoholic woman having an affected child is as high as 35%. Fetal alcohol effects such as borderline mental retardation, attention deficit hyperactivity disorder, or other behavioral sequelae may be observed in children, adolescents, or adults.

Clinical Management Implications

Patients presenting for alcohol treatment show various types of impairment. Many have profound social and financial problems that the health care system is ill equipped to handle. Acute alcohol intoxication is essentially treated with supportive measures that consist of maintaining physiological homeostasis by supporting vital functions. Alcohol withdrawal syndrome requires evaluation of the severity of withdrawal and may require behavioral or pharmacological intervention. Many alcohol treatment facilities achieve excellent results with social-setting detoxification, a nondrug method that includes intensive peer and group support in a nonmedical environment. This method is amazingly effective in reducing withdrawal signs and symptoms, with no reported increased incidence of medical complications.

Associated mood disturbances may be directly related to alcohol and can resolve within 2 to 3 weeks after detoxification. Depressive symptoms that persist beyond this period should be treated with antidepressant therapy; benzodiazepines and other dependence-producing agents should not be used chronically in patients with alcoholism. Patients who have chronic anxiety may be treated with nonpharmacologic approaches or with buspirone. Buspirone, an anxiolytic agent, is not known to be habit forming and has no abuse potential.

Many patients with acute alcohol intoxication require medical detoxification and intervention. Interviewers should be tolerant and nonthreatening and accept the intoxicated patient's insults and rudeness as part of the illness. Food and support often calm the patient. Security personnel can deter the belligerent patient and prevent violent outbursts while also reassuring the interviewer. Most patients respond more calmly if placed in a quiet room with minimal stimulation. Physical restraints may be necessary to prevent the individual from harming himself or herself or others. A physical examination is mandatory to rule out other medical conditions.

Hospital management of alcohol dependence, withdrawal, and DTs may require the use of medication. Benzodiazepines are clearly the treatment of choice because of their high therapeutic safety index; the option of oral, intramuscular (IM), or intravenous (IV) administration; and their anticonvulsant properties. Barbiturates have fallen into disuse because of the high incidence of respiratory depression and the low therapeutic safety index. Because of their long half-lives, chlordiazepoxide and diazepam have the advantage of a smooth introduction and a gradual decline in blood levels; thus fewer symptoms occur with dosage alterations. Chlordiazepoxide provides greater sedation, whereas diazepam has greater anticonvulsant activity and may be preferable for patients with a history of seizures. Geriatric patients or those with liver disease are better off with agents with short half-lives, such as lorazepam or oxazepam. Lorazepam has the advantage of being rapidly and completely absorbed following IM administration. The standard regimen for alcohol withdrawal is described in detail in *Psychotropic Drugs,* second edition, a companion text.[16]

Drugs that reduce alcohol consumption or result in pharmacological prophylaxis include disulfiram and naltrexone. Antidepressants, lithium carbonate, and other serotonergic agents may also be useful in reducing alcohol consumption. A detailed discussion is found in *Psychotropic Drugs,* second edition.[16]

Cocaine
Neurophysiological Brain Alterations

The primary pharmacodynamic effect of cocaine is related to its behavioral effects. It competitively blocks DA reuptake through the DA transporter system and also blocks the reuptake of the other major monoamines, norepinephrine and serotonin. The behavioral effects of cocaine last for only 30 to 60 minutes, which necessitates repeated administration to maintain the effects of intoxication. Although the behavioral effects are short-lived, metabolites may be present in the blood and urine for as long as 10 to 21 days.

Cocaine is a potent stimulant of the CNS and results in sympathomimetic potentiation of sympathetically innervated organs, including the mesolimbic system, which is related to the expression of mood, and the reticular activating system, which is related to cerebral arousal. Psychological dependence may occur after a single use of cocaine; repeated administration results in tolerance and sensitivity to various effects. Psychological de-

pendence does develop, but cocaine withdrawal is mild compared with the effects of opiate withdrawal.

No single neurotransmitter is responsible for the clinical manifestations of cocaine because these neurotransmitters are similarly affected by pharmacological agents that do not have the prominent characteristics of cocaine. Central dopaminergic, α-adrenergic, and β-adrenergic receptor supersensitivity induced by chronic cocaine administration has been demonstrated in animals and inferred in humans.

As discussed, the DA-containing neurons have cell bodies that are part of the ventral tegmentum. The reinforcing effects of cocaine (and amphetamines) result from the ability of the substance to elevate the synaptic concentrations of DA that affect these systems. The raphe nuclei of the dorsal pons contain serotonin cell bodies that project fibers to various aspects of the forebrain that are responsible for mood and arousal. Serotonin input to the met-enkephalin system synapses on DA neurons in the ventral tegmentum, which modulates the "reward center" (see Figure 8.2). Noradrenergic cell bodies are located in the locus ceruleus and project to various aspects of the limbic system and cerebral cortex. Although these neurons have been implicated in withdrawal from opiates and alcohol and are stimulated during cocaine intoxication, they have been shown to play only a minor role in the addictive behaviors associated with cocaine.

Clinical Findings and Course

Cocaine is a naturally occurring substance that is produced by the coca plant. Several forms of cocaine exist, each of which differs in purity and speed of onset of action. Cocaine hydrochloride powder is usually snorted or dissolved in water and injected intravenously. When mixed with heroin, it forms a drug known as "speedball." Crack cocaine is common in the United States and has extremely rapid effects because it is easily vaporized and inhaled. Crack is formed by mixing cocaine with sodium bicarbonate and allowing it to dry into small rocks. The problems associated with crack are identical to those encountered with

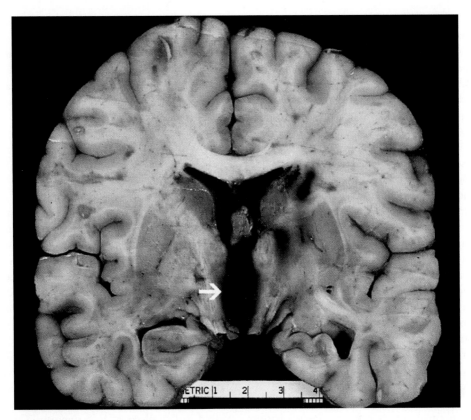

figure 8.6   Brain with a hemorrhage in the third ventricle and periventricular area *(arrow)* resulting from rupture of a small arteriovenous malformation. The patient was a chronic user of cocaine. *(Courtesy Dr. Richard E. Powers, Director, University of Alabama at Birmingham Brain Resource Program.)*

other cocaine preparations. Before crack was developed, "free base" cocaine was prepared by heating cocaine with ammonia or some other volatile solvent; this preparation was dangerous because the solvents could ignite and harm the user.[3]

A number of acute clinical effects occur with cocaine use. An immediate and intense euphoria analogous to a sexual orgasm occurs and may last seconds or minutes. Other alterations arise from mood elevation, including enhanced self-confidence and forceful boisterousness. Subsequently, the mood becomes mildly euphoric and mixed with anxiety for as long as 60 to 90 minutes. Thoughts typically race, and speech becomes pressured, with tangential and incoherent aspects. Appetite is suppressed, and arousal is elevated such that hypervigilance tends to persist as insomnia. Motor activity is commonly increased, with

agitated and fidgety behavior accompanying subjective sensations of restlessness and perpetual motion.

Activation of the cardiovascular system results in tachycardia, hypertension, and diaphoresis; CNS activation results in lowered seizure threshold, tremors, cerebral arousal, emesis, and hyperpyrexia. Peripheral nervous system stimulation results in bladder and bowel muscular contractions and cutaneous flushing.

Chronic cocaine intoxication may result in insomnia, anorexia, and increased motor activity and may produce ferocious hunger, fatigue, and eventual physical and mental exhaustion. Blood pressure may be elevated, sometimes to the point at which spontaneous hemorrhage, stroke, or myocardial infarction occur (Figure 8.6). Libido is depressed and sexual performance is impaired, with consequent impotency in men and anorgasmia in women.

As with amphetamines, cocaine dependence is associated with two patterns of self-administration: episodic or daily use. "Binges" are a form of episodic use. Dependence is commonly associated with progressive tolerance in which the desirable effects of cocaine require increasingly large doses. Tolerance resulting from continued use leads to a diminution of pleasurable effects and an increase in dysphoric effects.

Cocaine dependence can lead to financial disaster because thousands of dollars of expense can occur within a very short time. Individuals may turn to crime to obtain money for cocaine. Long-term dependence can lead to erratic behavior, social isolation, aggressiveness, violence, and sexual dysfunction. Promiscuous sexual behavior because of increased desire or for the purpose of obtaining cocaine has played a role in spreading sexually transmitted diseases such as human immunodeficiency virus (HIV).[3]

Clinical Management Implications

The optimal treatment for cocaine use has not been established. The cessation of cocaine use is not followed by physiological withdrawal syndromes as is seen with opioids or alcohol. However, dysphoria, depression, and drug craving are often intense and make abstinence difficult. Psychotherapy, group therapy, and behavior modification appear to be useful in maintaining abstinence.

Several pharmacological agents have been tried as adjunctive treatments for cocaine abuse, but the efficacy of pharmacotherapy remains an open question. Antidepressants, lithium, and dopamine agonists such as bromocriptine and amantadine have been used with varying degrees of success.

Many hospitals now offer short-term inpatient treatment for cocaine abusers. Long-term residential drug-free programs or therapeutic communities may also be available. Self-help groups such as Narcotics Anonymous may be useful as a primary treatment modality or as an adjunct to other treatments. The recognition and treatment of comorbid psychiatric disorders, most notably depression

and attention deficit disorder, may be necessary to stop the cocaine use. Many individuals who use cocaine also use alcohol or other drugs, particularly sedatives and heroin; the use of these substances also requires intervention. A more detailed discussion of treatment options is available in *Psychotropic Drugs,* second edition.[16]

Amphetamines
Neurophysiological Brain Alterations

Classic amphetamines such as dextroamphetamine or methamphetamine have their primary effects by causing the release of catecholamines, particularly DA, from presynaptic terminals. The effects are potent for the dopaminergic neurons that project from the VTA to the cerebral cortex and limbic areas. This reward pathway is probably the major addicting mechanism for the amphetamines.

"Designer" amphetamines such as MDMA, MDEA, MMDA, and DOM cause the release of catecholamines and serotonin. Serotonin is implicated as the major neurochemical pathway involved in the effects of hallucinogens. Therefore the clinical effects of the "designer" amphetamines are a cross between classic amphetamines and hallucinogens. The pharmacology of MDMA (3,4-methylenedioxymethamphetamine) is the best understood among the designer amphetamines. Once in the neuron, MDMA causes a rapid release of serotonin and inhibits the activity of serotonin-producing enzymes. As a result, individuals taking selective serotonin reuptake inhibitors (SSRIs) such as fluoxetine do not experience the effect of MDMA because the specific reuptake inhibitor properties of fluoxetine prevent MDMA from being taken up into the serotonergic neurons.

One of the primary effects of amphetamines and related compounds is CNS stimulation, which results in the characteristic activation of behavior. Amphetamines are potent anorectics and have been used extensively as appetite suppressants.

Table 8.5 illustrates the phases, symptoms, and behaviors of amphetamine abuse, as well as the

table 8.5

Phases of Development of Amphetamine Abuse: Factors Mediating Abuse Dependence, Proposed Mechanisms

PHASE	ABUSE DEPENDENCE	MECHANISM
Single dose	Conditioned cues High-dose rush	Mesolimbic dopamine release Classical conditioning Operant conditioning Enhancement of social/sexual activity Antifatigue properties
Dose escalation	Acute tolerance results in increasing dose and frequency of use	Rapid routes of administration, resulting in fast delivery to CNS with resulting dopamine release and euphoria Onset of neurotransmitter depletion
Binge	Compulsive frequent use that may be related to stereotypical patterns of use	Neurotransmitter depletion Neuronal destruction Impulsivity due to serotonin depletion Conditioned urges and memories of drug effects Drug acquisition behaviors become stereotyped
Crash		
Early	Depression Agitation Anxiety High drug craving	Neurotransmitter depletion Dopaminergic autoreceptor supersensitivity Memories of drug effects and conditioned urges
Middle	Fatigue No drug craving Insomnia with a high desire for sleep	
Late	Hyperphagia Hypersomnolence	
Withdrawal		
Intermediate	Reemergence of conditioned drug urges/cravings	Impulsivity due to serotonin depletion
Late	Gradual extinction of conditioned drug urges and cravings	Possible restoration of neurotransmitter functioning

Based on data from Gawin FH, Ellinwood EH: Cocaine and other stimulants, *N Engl J Med* 318:1173, 1988; and Ellinwood EH, Lee TH: Dose- and time-dependent effects of stimulants, in *NIDA monograph no. 94,* Pharmacology and toxicology of amphetamine and related designer drugs, pp 323-340, 1989.

toxic side effects and mechanisms associated with each phase. The chronic use of amphetamines results in permanent depletions of DA from a variety of brain regions. This depletion may mediate some of the tolerance and anhedonia experienced by individuals who use amphetamines.

Clinical Findings and Course

Amphetamines such as dextroamphetamine and methamphetamine have a substituted phenylethylamine structure. Other substances in this class (e.g., methylphenidate, appetite suppressants, diet pills) are structurally different but have amphetamine-like actions. "Ice," so named because of the appearance of its crystals when magnified, is a pure form of methamphetamine that can be smoked to produce an immediate and powerful effect such as occurs with crack cocaine. The substances in this class are usually taken by mouth or intravenously; methamphetamine is sometimes ingested nasally. The effects of these substances are usually similar to those of cocaine, but the effects last longer and may involve more intense peripheral sympathomimetic effects. Because these substances *do not* have local anesthetic effects, the risk for certain general medical conditions is significantly lower. Amphetamine-induced disorders may include psychosis, mood disturbance, anxiety, sexual dysfunction, sleep disorder, or intoxication withdrawal or delirium.[3]

Individuals who abuse or become dependent on amphetamines often begin using them in an attempt to control weight, whereas others are introduced to the drugs illegally. Dependence may occur rapidly, especially when used intravenously or smoked. Both episodic use and daily use may be observed. Periods of intensive, high-dose use are often called "speed runs" or "binges" and are associated with IV use. Runs tend to terminate only when drug supplies are depleted. Chronic users tend to escalate their dose over time, which often becomes unpleasant because of sensitization and the emergence of dysphoric and other negative effects. Adverse mental and physical effects emerge in association with long-term dependence. Individuals who have become dependent on amphetamines tend to decrease their use or stop using them after 8 to 10 years.[3]

Clinical Consequences

Amphetamine psychosis may occur with manifestations of agitation, paranoia, delusions, or hallucinosis. Paranoid states may persist even after detoxification; chronic amphetamine use may result in paranoid psychosis that is diagnostically similar to schizophrenia. Severe hypertension seen in overdose may be treated with α-adrenergic blockade. A withdrawal syndrome does not follow abstinence, but marked dysphoria, fatigue, and restlessness may occur. Amphetamine-like substances sold as appetite suppressants, decongestants, or bronchodilators may result in intoxication similar to the amphetamines, but there tends to be less CNS stimulation and greater autonomic effects.

Clinical Management Implications

The clinical management of amphetamine-related disorders includes physical examination, general support, identification and treatment of associated psychiatric disorders, and the use of many of the support mechanisms described generally with alcohol.

Opioids
Neurophysiological Brain Alterations

Heroin, the most commonly abused opioids, is more potent and lipid soluble than morphine and crosses the blood-brain barrier quite rapidly. It was first introduced as a treatment for morphine addiction but in fact is more dependence-producing than morphine. Codeine, which occurs naturally, is absorbed easily through the gastrointestinal tract and is subsequently transformed into morphine in the body.

The physiological effects of opioids result from the stimulation of receptors or endogenous hormones, enkephalins, endorphins, and dynorphins. Five distinct opioid receptors are designated by the Greek letters mu, kappa, sigma, delta, and epsilon. Morphine, heroin, and methadone act primarily through mu receptors and produce analgesia, euphoria, and respiratory depression. Drugs such as butorphanol and pentazocine are mediated through the kappa receptor and induce a so-called mixed agonist-antagonist effect. This effect produces analgesia but less respiratory depression. The sigma receptor appears similar to the receptor for PCP. The delta receptor binds endogenous opiate peptides. In high doses, the opioid drugs lose their receptor specificity and have agonist or antagonist properties at multiple receptor sites.

A large number of regions in the CNS are rich with opioid receptors. The dorsal root ganglion, dorsal horn of the spinal cord, periaqueductal grey matter, and thalamus have been implicated in the analgesic effect of opioids. These and other brain regions such as the locus ceruleus and amygdala have been implicated in the physical dependence on opioids and in the production of the physical symptoms of opioid withdrawal. Dopaminergic neurons in the VTA and their target neurons, most notably the nucleus accumbens, are also rich in opioid receptors and appear to play a critical role in an individual's physiological dependence on and craving for opioids. Various findings support the view advanced by Koob and Bloom[18] and Wise.[32] Along with other researchers, they believe that the VTA and nucleus accumbens, as well as certain inputs and outputs of these neurons, are critical "brain-reward regions" that mediate the positively reinforcing properties (see Figure 8.2). Other studies are being conducted to identify other, more specific mediators involved in opioid tolerance and dependence.

Clinical Findings and Course

The opioids consist of three classes: (1) natural opioids such as morphine, (2) semi-synthetics such as heroin, and (3) synthetics with morphine-like action such as codeine, methadone, oxycodone, meperidine, and fentanyl. Although they have both agonist and antagonist effects, medications such as pentazocine and buprenorphine are characterized as opioids because they produce similar physiological and behavioral effects.

Opioid-related disorders may include abuse, dependence, intoxication, or withdrawal. Opioid-induced disorders may include psychosis, mood disturbance, sexual dysfunction, sleep disorder, or opioid intoxication delirium. Routine urine toxicology tests are often positive for opioid drugs in individuals with opioid dependence.

Opioid overdose is a life-threatening emergency and should be suspected in patients who present with coma and respiratory suppression. Treatment includes emergency support of cardiorespiratory function. Administration of the antagonist nalox-

one, 0.4 to 0.8 mg IV, rapidly reverses coma and respiratory suppression; however, it does not affect depression caused by other sedatives such as alcohol or barbiturates. Naloxone can precipitate opioid withdrawal, causing the patient whose life has just been saved to be extremely ungrateful.

The opioid withdrawal syndrome is unpleasant but not life threatening. It is characterized by increased sympathetic nervous system activity coupled with nausea, vomiting, cramps, and diarrhea. Patients may report myalgias and arthralgias, restlessness, increased anxiety, insomnia, and a craving for opioids.

Clinical Consequences

At all socioeconomic levels, opioid dependence is often associated with drug-related crimes, divorce, unemployment, or irregular employment. Health care professionals and other addicted individuals with access to opioids often develop a pattern of illegal activities, which affects their relationship with professional boards and other administrative agencies.[3]

Individuals who are opioid dependent are at risk for brief, depressive symptoms or episodes of mild-to-moderate depression. Antisocial personality and posttraumatic stress disorder are more prevalent in individuals with opioid dependence.[3]

Many medical conditions result from acute and chronic opioid use. A dry mouth and nose, slowed gastrointestinal activity, and constipation result from a lack of secretions. Pupillary constriction may result in impaired vision. IV opioid use may lead to sclerosed veins or tracks and punctate marks on lower portions of the upper extremities. Difficulties in sexual functioning are common, with erectile dysfunction during intoxication or chronic use among men and erratic reproductive function and irregular menses among women. Although usually not severe or associated with serious adverse consequences, low–birth weight infants can be born to mothers with opioid dependence.[3]

Tuberculosis and HIV are particularly serious problems with opioid use and dependence. The incidence of HIV is high among individuals who use any type of IV drug—as high as 60% among those dependent on heroin in some areas of the United States.[3] Death, at an annual rate of approximately 10 out of every 1000 untreated individuals, often results from overdose, injuries, accidents, or other medical complications. Accidents and injuries often result from the violence associated with buying or selling drugs.[3]

Clinical Management Implications

Opioid detoxification is performed by readministering an opioid until withdrawal symptoms cease, then gradually decreasing the dosage of opioid over a period of 21 days as specified by federal law. Methadone is most often used for detoxification because of its long half-life and daily oral administration. Patients are given 10 to 20 mg every 2 to 4 hours until withdrawal symptoms are suppressed; the total initial dose is typically 20 to 40 mg. The dosage is tapered over time. Clonidine, an α_2-adrenergic agonist, may also be used to suppress many of the signs and symptoms of withdrawal.

Methadone maintenance is a major modality of the long-term treatment of opioid abuse and dependence. Approximately 100,000 patients are currently maintained on methadone.[21] The demand for treatment exceeds the availability; many programs have a waiting list as long as several months. A physician may apply to the Drug Enforcement Agency to maintain a patient on methadone outside of an established methadone program. Individuals who are dependent on opioids may also benefit from opioid antagonist therapy with naltrexone. Innovative treatments are described in *Psychotropic Drugs,* second edition.[16]

Drug-free treatment modalities are also useful in treating opioid addictions. Such programs emphasize total abstinence from opioids, alcohol, and other drugs, as well as social and psychological rehabilitation. Programs differ widely in intensity and theoretical orientation. Therapeutic community programs usually require a long-term commitment of at least several months, during which the addict is taken out of his or her usual environment and involved in intensive psycholog-

ical and behavioral individual and group therapy. Long-term residential treatment may be most useful for the chronic abuser who requires a lifestyle change. Self-help groups such as Narcotics Anonymous use the 12-Step philosophy and stress total abstinence; they may be useful as a primary treatment modality or as an adjunct to other treatments.

Cannabis

Neurophysiological Brain Alterations

Delta-9-tetrahydrocannabinol (THC) is the element responsible for the psychoactive effects of cannabis. A specific receptor for the cannabinoids has been identified, cloned, and characterized. This receptor is a member of the G protein–linked family of receptors. It is found in highest concentrations in the basal ganglia, hippocampus, and cerebellum, with lower concentrations in the cerebral cortex. It is not found in the brainstem, a fact that is consistent with the minimal effects that cannabis has on respiratory and cardiac functions.

Animal studies have shown that cannabinoids affect monoamine and GABA neurons. Unlike with other substances of abuse, most studies with cannabis do not suggest self-administration. Thus debates occur as to whether cannabinoids stimulate the so-called "reward centers" of the brain.

Clinical Findings and Course

The euphoric effects of cannabis appear within minutes, peak in 30 minutes, and last 2 to 4 hours; some motor and cognitive effects last for 5 to 12 hours. Cannabis can be taken orally when it is prepared in food such as brownies and cakes. Approximately three to four times as much cannabis must be taken orally to be as potent as that taken by smoke inhalation. Many variables affect the psychoactive properties of cannabis, including potency, route of administration, smoking technique, dose, setting, and past experience. Each user appears to display a unique biological vulnerability to the effects of cannabinoids. THC content, which is responsible for the psychoactive effects, has increased significantly since the late 1960s—from 1% to 5% to as much as 10% to 15%.

Cannabis-related disorders include dependence and abuse, as well as induced disorders such as intoxication, intoxication delirium, psychotic disorder with delusions or hallucinations, and cannabis-induced anxiety disorder. Cannabis is often used with nicotine, alcohol, cocaine, opioids, PCP, or other hallucinogens. Regular users of cannabis experience lethargy and mild forms of depression, anxiety, or irritability.[3]

High doses of cannabinoids can produce psychoactive effects similar to those produced by hallucinogens. Cannabis intoxication is characterized by tachycardia, muscle relaxation, euphoria, and a sense of well-being. Time sense is altered, and emotional lability, particularly inappropriate laughter, may be seen. Psychomotor tasks, including driving, are impaired. With high doses, depersonalization, paranoia, and anxiety reactions occasionally occur. Paranoid ideations ranging from suspiciousness to delusions and hallucinations may occur. Urine tests generally identify cannabinoid metabolites and can be positive for 7 to 10 days.

Cannabis has several medicinal uses and was used as medicine before the Marijuana Tax Act of 1937. Cannabis may be used to relieve asthma, to treat glaucoma, in the treatment of cancer as an appetite stimulant, and for the prevention of nausea and vomiting during chemotherapy. Although THC is a good antiemetic, many patients reject it because the psychoactive effects are unpleasant.[9] In addition, cannabis may not be legally prescribed—a topic of controversy in the United States.

Clinical Consequences

Chronic cough, as well as other nasopharyngeal pathological conditions, can occur in individuals who use cannabis because the smoke is highly irritating to the nasopharynx and bronchial lining. Weight gain resulting from overeating and reduced activity also occurs. Because the smoke from cannabis contains larger amounts of carcinogens than does tobacco, the risk for cancer may be

increased with heavy use.[3] Chronic cannabis use has been associated with an apathetic, amotivational state that improves when the drug is discontinued.

Tolerance to cannabis does develop, and psychological dependence has been found. However, there is no significant evidence of physiological dependence. Withdrawal symptoms are limited to irritability, restlessness, insomnia, anorexia, and mild nausea, all of which are seen only when a person abruptly stops taking high doses of cannabis.

Clinical Management Implications

Treatment of cannabis dependence is similar to the treatment of other drug dependencies. Initial assessment begins with complete psychiatric and medical examinations. Short-term goals focus on reducing or stopping the use and on interventions to ensure compliance. Inpatient treatment may be necessary to achieve abstinence. Because many patients are adolescents or young adults, it is important to involve the family in assessment and treatment. A change in social situation is often necessary to decrease drug availability and reduce peer pressure. Individual and group psychotherapy may be useful. Self-help groups such as Narcotics Anonymous can also provide group and individual support.

Phencyclidine

Neurophysiological Brain Alterations

PCP and its related compounds are variously sold as a crystalline powder, paste, liquid, or drug-soaked paper. The primary pharmacodynamic effect of PCP is antagonism of the N-methyl-D-aspartate (NMDA) subtype of glutamate receptors. PCP binds to a site within the NMDA-associated calcium channel and prevents the influx of calcium ions. Another effect of PCP is the activation of dopaminergic neurons of the VTA, which project to the limbic system. The activation of these neurons is usually involved in mediating the reinforcing qualities of PCP.

Clinical Findings and Course

The phencyclidines include PCP (the most commonly abused of this class) and similar compounds (e.g., ketamine, analogs of PCP). Initially developed to be dissociative anesthetics, these substances became street drugs by the 1960s. They can be smoked, taken orally, or injected.[3] Phencyclidine-related disorders include dependence and abuse. Induced disorders include intoxication, delirium, delusions, psychotic disorder, mood disorder, and anxiety disorder.

Tolerance to the phencyclidines does occur in humans, but physical dependency generally does not occur. Psychological dependence is more common. Physical withdrawal symptoms include lethargy, depression, and craving. However, withdrawal is rare in humans and is probably a function of dose and duration of use.

Individuals with PCP intoxication usually are alert and oriented but may be violent, agitated, or display bizarre behavior. Delirium, psychosis, or catatonic mutism with posturing may also be evident, and repeated intoxications may lead to personal and legal problems. Intoxication-induced hospitalizations, visits to the emergency department, and arrests for bizarre behavior may occur.[3]

PCP is found in the urine of acutely intoxicated individuals and may be detectable for several weeks. Rhabdomyolysis with renal impairment occurs in approximately 2% of individuals. PCP intoxication produces cardiovascular toxicity (cardiac arrest is rare), neurological toxicity (e.g., seizures, dystonias, dyskinesias, catalepsy, hypothermia, hyperthermia), and respiratory problems (e.g., apnea, bronchospasm, aspiration during coma, hypersalivation). Vertical and horizontal nystagmus, myoclonus, ataxia, and autonomic instability commonly occur. Individuals who take PCP intravenously are at risk for hepatitis, HIV infection, and bacterial endocarditis.[3]

Clinical Management Implications

Treatment of PCP intoxication generally involves supportive measures, efforts to maintain cardiovascular and respiratory functions, and efforts to ameliorate psychotic symptoms. Both haloperidol and the benzodiazepines have been useful for decreasing agitation and psychosis.[16] Psychiatric hospitalization may be necessary for patients with prolonged psychosis.

Hallucinogens

Neurophysiological Brain Alterations

Hallucinogenic substances vary in their pharmacological effects; D-lysergic acid diethylamide (LSD) is discussed as a general prototype. The fundamentals of LSD remain controversial, but it is well accepted that the principal effects involve the serotonergic system. It is unknown whether LSD acts as an antagonist or agonist, but most data suggest that it is a partial agonist at postsynaptic serotonin receptors.

The hallucinogenic effects are likely a result of LSD-induced decreases in serotonin turnover (synthesis and release) in the brain. In support of this hypothesis, Aghajanian, Foot, and Sheard[1] found that LSD inhibits the firing of serotonergic neurons in the dorsal raphe nucleus, most likely by interacting with presynaptic autoreceptors. Other indole-type hallucinogens such as psilocin and dimethyltryptamine (DMT) also show this effect. However, some studies refute the link between the presynaptic effects of LSD and its hallucinogenic activity. Certainly, both indole- and phenolethylamine-type hallucinogens have been found to bind to the serotonin-2 ($5HT_2$) receptor subtype,[31] and this agonist activity appears to underlie the mechanism of action for this drug class. The commonality of interactions with the $5HT_2$ receptor suggests that selective $5HT_2$ receptor antagonists could be useful in blocking the behavioral effects of the hallucinogens in humans.

The hallucinogens also promote significant autonomic activity. LSD causes marked pupillary dilation, blood pressure and body temperature increases, tremors, piloerection, and tachycardia. Some of these autonomic effects are variable and may partly result from the anxiety state of the user. LSD can also cause nausea; vomiting is especially noteworthy after the ingestion of mescaline. There is no generally accepted evidence of brain cell damage, chromosome abnormalities, or teratogenic effects following the use of indole-type hallucinogens or mescaline.

Clinical Findings and Course

The hallucinogens include ergot, LSD, morning glory seeds, mescaline, MDMA, psilocybin, and DMT. They are generally taken orally but can be injected; DMT is smoked. Hallucinogens may result in dependence or abuse; induced disorders include intoxication, flashbacks, intoxication delirium, psychotic disorder with delusions, psychotic disorder with hallucinations, mood disturbance disorder, and anxiety disorder.

Flashbacks are transient, recurrent perceptual disturbances that are reminiscent of those experienced during one or more earlier hallucinogen intoxications. For a diagnosis of flashbacks to be made, individuals must have had no recent hallucinogen intoxication and must show no current drug toxicity when reexperiencing the perceptual symptoms. Some individuals report no impairment or distress during flashbacks, but others experience significant impairment and distress.

Individuals with hallucinogen intoxication may demonstrate rapidly changing moods and may be volatile or discursive. They may be fearful, anxious, or dread insanity or death. Perceptual disturbances and impaired judgment may result in injuries or fatalities from accidents, fights, or attempts to "fly." The personality and expectations of each individual may define the type and severity of the intoxication.[3]

Hallucinogen intoxication may be brief and isolated or may occur repeatedly. Peak effects occur within minutes to hours and end within a few hours or a few days; the length of the effect varies with the drug used and the method of administration. Individuals tend to stop using hallucinogens as they get older.[3]

No physical dependence or withdrawal symptoms occur with the use of hallucinogens. Tolerance develops rapidly and is virtually complete within 3 to 4 days of continuous use. However, tolerance also reverses quickly (usually within 4 to 7 days).

Clinical Management Implications

Treatment of hallucinogen intoxication includes reducing agitation in psychosis, preventing patients from harming themselves or others, and maintaining vital functions. Agitation and psychosis usually respond to verbal reassurance and decreased sensory stimulation, but treatment with benzodiazepines or high-potency neuroleptics is sometimes required. Most hallucinogen intoxications are short-lived, but prolonged drug-induced psychoses may occur in patients who are predisposed to psychiatric illness.[4]

REFERENCES

1. Aghajanian GK, Foote WE, Sheard MH: Lysergic acid diethylamide: sensitive neuronal units in the midbrain raphe, *Science* 161:706-708, 1968.

2. American Psychiatric Association: *Diagnostic and statistical manual of mental disorders,* ed 3, Washington, DC, 1990.

3. American Psychiatric Association: *Diagnostic and statistical manual of mental disorders,* ed 4, Washington, DC, 1994.

4. Bowers MB, Swigar ME: Vulnerability to psychosis associated with hallucinogen use, *Psychiatry Res* 9:91, 1983.

5. Cloninger CR: Neurogenetic adaptive mechanisms in alcoholism, *Science* 236:410, 1987.

6. Fava M, Copeland P, Schweiger U et al: Neurochemical abnormalities of anorexia nervosa and bulimia nervosa, *Am J Psychiatry* 146:963, 1989.

7. Franklin JE, Frances RJ: Alcohol-induced organic mental disorders. In Yudofsky SC, Hales RE, editors: *The American Psychiatric Press textbook of neuropsychiatry,* ed 2, Washington, DC, 1992, American Psychiatric Press.

8. Goodwin DW: Alcoholics and genetics: the sins of the fathers, *Arch Gen Psychiatry* 42:171, 1985.

9. Grinspoon L, Bakalar J: Marijuana. In Lowinson JH, Ruiz P, Millman RB, editors: *Substance abuse: a comprehensive textbook,* ed 2, Baltimore, 1992, Williams & Wilkins.

10. Gwirtsman HE, Kaye WH, George DT et al: Central and peripheral ACTH and cortisol levels in anorexia nervosa and bulimia, *Arch Gen Psychiatry* 46:61, 1989.

11. Halmi KA, Eckert E, Marchi P et al: Comorbidity of psychiatric diagnosis in anorexia nervosa, *Arch Gen Psychiatry* 48:712, 1991.

12. Irwin EG: A focused overview of anorexia nervosa and bulimia. Part I. Etiological issues, *Arch Psychiatr Nurs* 7(6):342-346, 1993.

13. Jimerson DC, Brandt HA, Brewerton TD: Evidence for altered serotonin function in bulimia and anorexia nervosa: behavioral implications. In Pirke KM, Vandereycken W, Ploog D, editors: *The psychobiology of bulimia nervosa,* 1989, Berlin, Springer-Verlag.

14. Johnson C, Connors ME: *The etiology and treatment of bulimia nervosa,* New York, 1987, Basic Books.

15. Kaye WH, Weltzin TW, Hsu LKG et al: An open trial of fluoxetine in patients with anorexia nervosa, *J Clin Psychiatry* 52:464, 1991.

16. Keltner N, Folks DG: Alcohol and other substance abuse disorders. In *Psychotropic Drugs,* ed 2, St Louis, 1997, Mosby.

17. Kendler KS, Maclean C, Neale M et al: The genetic epidemiology of bulimia nervosa, *Am J Psychiatry* 148:1627, 1991.

18. Koob FF, Bloom FE: Cellular and molecular mechanisms of drug dependence, *Science* 242:715, 1988.

19. Krueger DW: Eating disorders. In Lowinson JH, Ruiz P, Millman RB, editors: *Substance abuse: a comprehensive textbook,* ed 2, Baltimore, 1992, Williams & Wilkins.

20. Lishman WA: Alcohol and the brain. *Br J Psychiatry* 156:635, 1990.

21. Marrazzi MA, Luby ED: An auto-addiction opioid model of chronic anorexia nervosa, *Int J Eating Disord* 5:191, 1986.

22. Martin PR, Adinoff B, Eckhardt MJ et al: Effective pharmacotherapy of alcoholic amnestic disorders with fluvoxamine, *Arch Gen Psychiatry* 46:617, 1989.

23. Nakada T, Knight RT: Alcohol and the central nervous system, *Med Clin North Am* 68:121, 1984.

24. O'Rourke D, Wurtman JJ, Wurtman RJ: Serotonin implicated in the etiology of seasonal affective disorder with carbohydrate craving. In Pirke KM, Vandereycken W, Ploog D, editors: *The psychobiology of bulimia nervosa,* Berlin, 1989, Springer-Verlag.

25. Pyle RL, Halvorson PA, Newman PA et al: The increasing prevalence of bulimia in freshman college students, *Int J Eating Disord* 4:631, 1986.

26. Regier DA, Farmer ME, Rae DS et al: Comorbidity of mental disorders with alcohol and other drug abuse, *Am J Med Assoc* 264:2511, 1990.

27. Reuler JB, Girard DE, Cooney TG: Wernicke's encephalopathy, *N Engl J Med* 312:1035, 1985.

28. Rieg TS, Maestrello AM, Aravich PF: Weight cycling alters the effects of D-fenfluramine on susceptibility to activity-based anorexia, *Am J Clin Nutr* 60:494-500, 1994.

29. Strober M, Katz JL: Depression in the eating disorders: a review and analysis of descriptive, family, and biological findings, *Diagn Issues* 34:107, 1990.

30. Swift RM: Alcoholism and substance abuse. In Stoudemire A, editor: *Clinical psychiatry for medical students,* ed 2, Philadelphia, 1994, JB Lippincott.

31. Titeler M, Lyon RA, Glennon RA: Radiologic and binding evidence implicates the brain 5-HT$_2$ receptor as a site of action for LSD and phenylisopropylamine hallucinogens, *Psychopharmacology* 94:213-216, 1988.

32. Wise RA: The role of reward pathways in the development of drug dependence, *Pharmacol Ther* 35:227, 1987.

33. Yager J: The treatment of eating disorders, *J Clin Psychiatry* 49(suppl): (9):18-25, 1988.

34. Yager J: Eating disorders. In Stoudemire A, editor: *Clinical psychiatry for medical students,* ed 2, Philadelphia, 1994, JB Lippincott.

Alzheimer's Dementia

Dementia comes from the Latin *de mens,* or "out of mind." Dementia is the loss of multiple intellectual functions as a result of the death or permanent dysfunction of neurons.[4,72,106] This definition distinguishes dementia from isolated cognitive losses, such as aphasia following a stroke. Patients with dementia experience two broad categories of symptoms: cognitive and psychiatric. Cognitive symptoms involve intellectual functions that are learned over time (e.g., language, complex motor skills, ability to abstract). Psychiatric manifestations include a range of psychotic and behavioral problems (e.g., hallucinations, delusions, assaultiveness). Dementia may be static (e.g., head trauma) or progressive (e.g., Alzheimer's disease).

Patients with dementia develop a myriad of cognitive symptoms that appear confusing to clinicians, health care professionals, and family caregivers.[52,109,110] The four most common and troublesome cognitive deficits manifested by patients with dementia are referred to as the four *A*s of Alzheimer's disease (AD): amnesia (memory problems), aphasia (communication problems), apraxia (inability to perform previously learned motor tasks), and agnosia (inability to recognize previously learned sensory input). Recognition of these symptoms prevents unnecessary behavioral problems in the patient with dementia and eases the burden of care for health professionals and family.[9] The basic principles of clinical management of AD described in this chapter also apply to most other types of dementia.[95] Other dementias and AIDS-related neuropsychiatric disorders are discussed in Chapters 10 and 11, respectively. Delirium associated with other dementias, as well as the general aspects of delirium, are addressed in Chapter 12.

Epidemiology and Demographics

Dementia is a common disorder that afflicts 10% of all individuals over age 65. All clinicians who care for elderly patients must understand dementia because the number of patients with dementia will increase dramatically as society's population ages. The basic assessment for dementia is a mental status examination, but primary care physicians perform this important clinical test on fewer than 1% of patients over age 60.[22,76] Primary care physicians describe patients with dementia as complex and difficult.[109,110] Clinicians who identify patients with dementia can reduce delirium, falls, patient injury, inaccurate reporting of clinical symptoms, and noncompliance with medications.[9] Forgetful, confused patients cannot accurately remember symptoms such as angina or comply with complicated medical regimens. Elderly patients with mild dementia may awaken from anesthesia with marked confusion that the family attributes to the surgery rather than to the unrecognized, preexisting AD.

Alois Alzheimer first described the condition that later assumed his name in 1907 when he reported a case involving a young woman in her 50s with a 4½-year course of progressive dementia.[4] Between 1907 and 1960 to 1970, most dementia was attributed to vascular disease, or "hardening of the arteries" (see Chapter 10; Figures 10.2 and 10.3).[12] It is now known that AD is a primary degenerative disorder of the brain and affects neurons.[12,13,98,102,103] AD is the single most common dementing illness among older adults and afflicts between 3 and 5 million individuals in the United States. The prevalence of AD increases with age, particularly after age 75. The incidence increases with age up until 90 years, after which it begins to decline.[75] A small but significant number of AD cases develop before 50 years of age. In addition to increasing age, risk factors for AD include Down's syndrome, a family history of the illness, head injury, and low educational levels. AD is slightly more common in women than in men. AD is subtyped as either early onset (i.e., before age 65) or late onset (i.e., after age 65), depending on the age at which the patient first manifests cognitive decline.

Compared with the general population, first-degree biological relatives of individuals with dementia of the Alzheimer's type, especially those with early onset, are more likely to develop the disorder.[75] Late-onset cases also have significant hereditary components. In some families AD is inherited as a dominant trait, with linkage to several chromosomes. However, the proportion of cases that are related to specific inherited abnormalities is unknown and remains a subject for further study. Current estimates suggest that the percentage of AD cases with direct genetic linkage defects is quite small and accounts for less than 1%.

Dementia is a major health problem; in 1991 the United States spent 67.3 billion dollars on patients with cognitive loss.[41,105] Most (60%) nursing home residents have some type of cognitive impairment. Clinicians may be less interested in dementia than are other health care professionals for several reasons, such as lack of diagnostic precision, lack of effective treatment, and many time-consuming complaints and problems.[6] Caregiver families are often unhappy with the quality of medical care provided by the health care system to patients with dementia.[4,9]

AD represents the fourth leading cause of death among older adults in the United States, with approximately 120,000 deaths per year. On the average, mortality occurs in approximately one third of all diagnosed individuals 5 years after diagnosis; most die from pneumonia or sepsis. The average life expectancy is 7 to 8 years, although prolonged

figure 9.1   Comparison of the superior aspects of a normal *(left)* versus an Alzheimer's *(right)* brain, including frontal and parietal cortices. The normal brain has full gyral volume with narrow sulci. The atrophic Alzheimer's brain exhibits diffuse cortical atrophy with shrinkage of the gyri and marked widening of the sulci. *(Courtesy Dr. Richard E. Powers, Director, University of Alabama at Birmingham Brain Resource Program.)*

survival—as much as 18 years—has been reported. With the rapid increase in the number of Americans over age 85, it is estimated that approximately 10 million individuals will have AD by the year 2050. Most patients are managed at home by family caregivers, who become physically, emotionally, and financially exhausted over the 5 to 7 years of patient care.

Psychobiological Considerations
Macroscopic Brain Alterations

The clinical symptoms of AD are best explained through the gross and microscopic alterations that occur as part of the brain pathology. The external examination of brains from patients with AD can be unremarkable or can demonstrate atrophy in the temporal, frontal, parietal, or occipital cortices.[1,47] Atrophy, a nonspecific brain change that indicates loss of cerebral brain tissue, is defined as a reduction in the volume of the gyri with widening of the sulci. Cerebral atrophy may result from loss of cortex, white matter, or both (Figure 9.1). The external surfaces of normal brains typically have a plump appearance, but brains with AD often resemble walnuts. Brain imaging such as computerized axial tomography (CT) scans or magnetic resonance imaging (MRI) (see Chapter 4) readily demonstrates the severity and distribution of cerebral atrophy.[3]

The uncinate and parahippocampal cortices of the mesial temporal cortex are usually atrophic in AD (Figures 9.2 and 9.3, *B*).[62,83] Frontal, parietal,

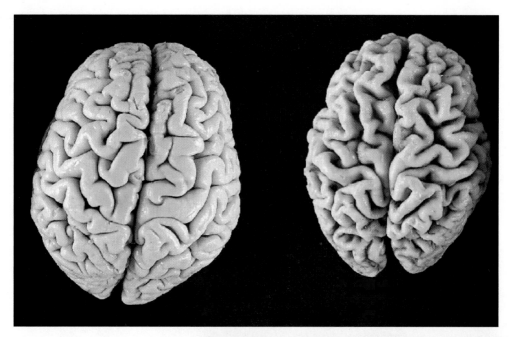

figure 9.1 For legend see opposite page.

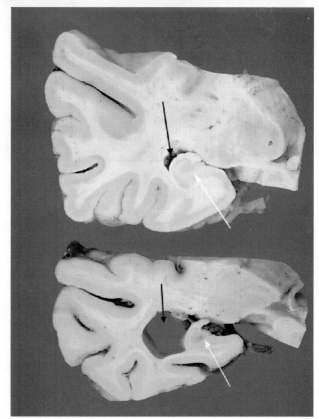

figure 9.2 Coronal sections of temporal lobes *(top normal, bottom AD)*, with a markedly atrophic hippocampus and parahippocampal cortex in the patient with AD *(white arrow)*, producing dilation of inferior horn of lateral ventricle *(black arrow)*. This atrophy explains short-term memory deficits (i.e., amnesia). *(Courtesy Dr. Richard E. Powers, Director, University of Alabama at Birmingham Brain Resource Program.)*

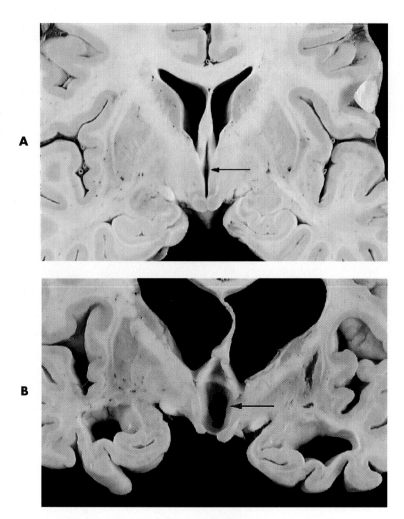

figure 9.3   Subcortical structures are also damaged in AD. In contrast to the normal brain (A), the Alzheimer's brain (B) has atrophy of hypothalamic structures and marked widening of the third ventricle *(arrow).* The amygdala, hippocampus, and entorhinal cortex are also atrophic, with marked dilation of the inferior horn of the lateral ventricle. *(Courtesy Dr. Richard E. Powers, Director, University of Alabama at Birmingham Brain Resource Program.)*

and occipital atrophy can vary. Mild cortical atrophy is present in many cognitively intact, aged individuals; severe atrophy is indicative of dementia.[12,98] The cranial nerves are not affected except for the olfactory nerves, which are often atrophic and demonstrate neurofibrillary tangles and dystrophic neurons on microscopic examinations.[37] The brains of patients with AD manifest selective atrophy of the association cortex, with relative sparing of both the primary motor and primary sensory cortices. Consequently, the motor strip is often spared, whereas adjacent frontal and parietal areas are atrophic. In the temporal lobe, the transverse temporal gyrus (the primary auditory cortex) is spared, and the association cortex (the superior temporal gyrus) is damaged (Figure 9.4).

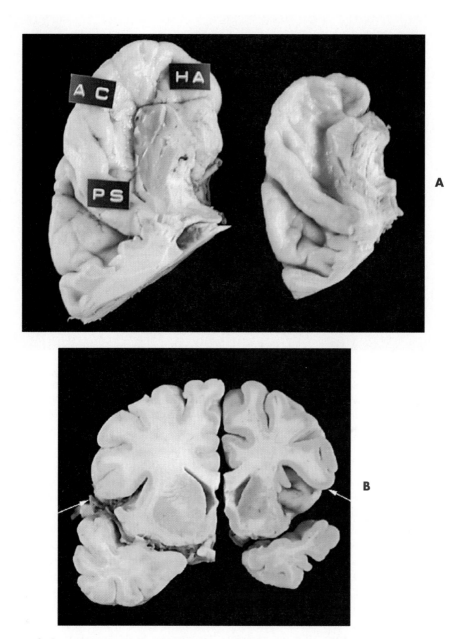

figure 9.4   The language areas are severely damaged in AD. **A,** A normal *(left)* versus Alzheimer's temporal lobe *(right)*. The transverse temporal gyrus (i.e., primary sensory cortex) *(PS)* is relatively spared, but the unimodal association cortex *(AC)* and heteromodal *(HA)* association cortex are severely atrophic in the Alzheimer's brain, which causes receptive aphasia. **B,** Coronal sections through normal *(left)* versus Alzheimer's *(right)* frontal lobes. Damage to the motor speech cortices (i.e., Broca's area) *(arrow)* produces expressive aphasia. *(Courtesy Dr. Richard E. Powers, Director, University of Alabama at Birmingham Brain Resource Program.)*

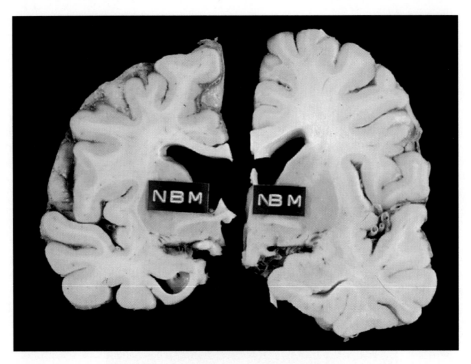

figure 9.5　The nucleus basalis of Meynert *(below NBM label)* beneath the curving anterior commissure. The NBM has sustained neuronal loss in the Alzheimer's brain hemisphere *(left)* as compared with a normal elderly brain *(right)*, which results in the cholinergic deficit. The amygdalae are also markedly atrophic, and the corpus callosum is thin. *(Courtesy Dr. Richard E. Powers, Director, University of Alabama at Birmingham Brain Resource Program.)*

The degree of cortical atrophy with dementia varies from individual to individual. Most patients with AD also have atherosclerosis of cerebral vessels that is similar to other patients in this age group.[12,98] The brainstem and cerebellum may appear normal or may be atrophic in severely damaged brains (see Figure 9.10, *B*).

When a brain with AD is sectioned in the coronal plane, the ventricular system (i.e., the lateral and third ventricles) is usually dilated. The inferior horns of the lateral ventricle are usually widened secondary to severe loss of volume in the hippocampus, amygdala, and temporal cortices (see Figure 9.3, *B*). The corpus callosum is often thinned, which reflects the loss of cortical neurons and fibers that traverse this white matter structure. The volume of the anterior commissure is often reduced, which reflects the atrophy of the amygdalae and hippocampi. The basal ganglia, including the caudate nucleus, putamen, and globus pallidus, are usually normal in size; however, the nucleus basalis of Meynert, which is located immediately beneath the anterior commissure, may be reduced in volume (Figure 9.5).[3,6,107] The thalami can be of normal volume or atrophic. In normal individuals, the third ventricle is usually slit-like but is bowed in cases of severe dementia from loss of tissue in the hypothalamic region and cortex (see Figure 9.3). Sections of brainstem often demonstrate some depigmentation of the substantia nigra and severe depigmentation in the locus ceruleus. The brainstem usually appears normal in size except in severely atrophic brains, in which the brainstem may be atrophic. The cerebellum and spinal cord usually appear normal. AD does not damage peripheral nerves or muscle.

Microscopic Brain Alterations

The microscopic features of AD are quite variable.[21,30,61,62] The human brain undergoes a variety of anatomical and neurochemical changes beginning at approximately age 40.[70] Beginning between 40 and 50 years of age in normal subjects, neurons are lost in selected subcortical nuclei such as the substantia nigra, locus ceruleus, and raphe.[60] Previous authors have suggested that cortical neurons are depleted with aging, but more recent studies indicate that the total number of neurons remains unchanged.[39,54-56] The overall cross-sectional diameter of neurons is reduced with aging, which causes large-diameter cortical neurons to be counted as small-diameter neurons and explains the decreased number of large-diameter neurons and the slightly increased number of small-caliber neurons.[55,56] Hippocampal pyramidal neurons are lost with aging, and cytoplasmic inclusions such as Hirano bodies or granulovacuolar degenerations (GVD) begin to appear in hippocampal pyramidal neurons.[34,82]

Neuronal plasticity is the ability of neurons to regenerate dendrites or synapses and reinnervate the neural network. Some plasticity, such as the ability to innervate regions with neuron loss, remains in aging human neurons.[24,43] For example, the dendritic arborization territory of some hippocampal neurons in the dentate gyrus becomes larger with aging because surviving neurons attempt to cover areas left vacant by granule cell neurons that begin to disappear between 50 and 60 years of age. Consequently, human brain aging includes a complex mixture of neuron atrophy, neuron loss, and attempts at reinnervation by surviving neurons.[24,43,53,82]

Senile Plaques

The senile plaque (Figure 9.6, *A* and *B*) is the pathological hallmark of AD.[88] A senile plaque is a spherical disruption of the normal woven fabric of the brain tissue; this disruption contains swollen, abnormal processes (dystrophic neurites), astrocytes, microglial cells, and amyloid deposits. The term *neurite* is used because scientists cannot determine whether these fibers are axons or dendrites. The dystrophic neurites in senile plaques contain a variety of chemical transmitters, including catecholamines, neuropeptides, trophic factors, and other substances.[97] The precise significance of senile plaques is unclear because scientists are unsure whether the plaque represents a degenerative or regenerative process. Senile plaques are not pathognomonic of AD because most individuals over age 65 (and some individuals under age 65) have small numbers of senile plaques and dystrophic neurites in the neocortex and hippocampus.[16,62,73,83,101] The pathological diagnosis of AD is confirmed by the number of senile plaques rather than by their mere presence.

Neurofibrillary Tangles

The neurofibrillary tangle (Figure 9.6, *D*) is the second type of pathological change in AD.[15,48] Neurofibrillary tangles are massive collections of abnormal straight and paired helical filaments that accumulate within the cytoplasm of neurons.[50,96] Most forms of neuronal disease contain cytoskeletal components (i.e., the delicate meshwork of tubules and filaments within a neuron that sustain neuronal structure and transport within the neuron).[50] The neuron constantly assembles and metabolizes filaments and tubules that are visible only with the electron microscope.[79] Neurofibrillary tangles, Hirano bodies, GVD, Pick's bodies, and Lewy bodies contain abnormal collections of cytoskeletal components.[98] Neurofibrillary tangles are less common in normal aging; high densities of tangles signify a neurodegenerative disease.[83] Neurofibrillary tangles are present in several neurodegenerative diseases, including AD, progressive supranuclear palsy,[2] and dementia pugilistica (punchdrunk syndrome).[28] The pathogenesis of neurofibrillary tangles is unclear, but the basic building block is the paired helical filament (PHF). Theories suggest that abnormal phosphorylation of tau, a microtubule-associated protein, may lead to inappropriate assembly of

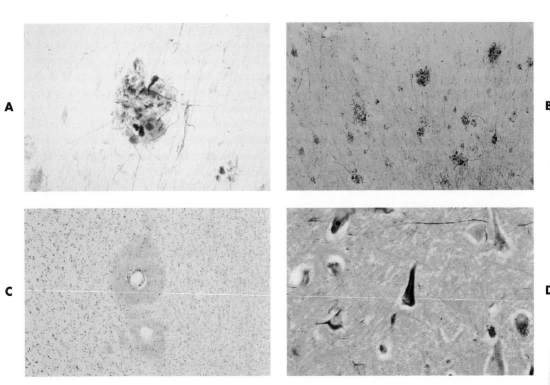

figure 9.6   The microscopic alterations of aging and AD, including senile plaques (**A** and **B**), amyloid (**C**), and neurofibrillary tangles (**D**). **A,** A single senile plaque (i.e., silver-stained collection of abnormal processes or glia that disrupt the neuropil). **B,** Demonstration of enough senile plaques to warrant a diagnosis of AD. **C,** Amyloid deposits (light-brown material) around blood vessels stained with antibody to the beta amyloid. **D,** Flame-shaped, silver-stained neurofibrillary tangle within a neuron *(center)*. Other neurons in the corners of the field lack tangles. *(Courtesy Dr. Richard E. Powers, Director, University of Alabama at Birmingham Brain Resource Program.)*

these molecules into PHFs and thus to the generation of neurofibrillary tangles. This molecular biological observation is of immense importance, and therapeutic interventions may inhibit the phosphorylation of tau and the assembly of tangles.[81] Although most research on AD focuses on neuronal abnormalities, white matter alterations are also reported.[21]

Neuritic Pathological Changes

Dystrophic neurites or neuropil threads are the third common type of pathological change in AD. These thickened, swollen, tortuous neuronal processes are readily seen with silver stains and contain abnormal cytoskeletal components.[15,16]

Dystrophic neurites are present in other diseases, including diffuse Lewy body disease[36] and Pick's disease.[114]

Amyloid

Amyloid is the fourth major pathological change in AD and consists of β-pleated sheets of abnormal fibrillary material that are deposited within senile plaques, around the blood vessels, and within the neuropil (Figure 9.6, *C*). Amyloid appears birefringent when Congo red stains are examined under polarizing light and fluorescent when thioflavin stains are illuminated with ultraviolet light.[49] Amyloid is minimally stained with silver preparations and is difficult to detect with standard histological preparations. Amyloid is easily detected using immunohistochemical techniques.[111] Amyloid deposits are common in the brains of elderly subjects, and quantity is more significant than the mere presence of occasional deposits.[35] Amyloid may be neurotoxic, and such deposits may precipitate neuronal damage.

Synaptic Loss

Synapses are the specialized contacts between axons and dendrites; information is transferred at the synapses via the delivery of packets of neurotransmitters. Synapses are too small to visualize with the microscope but are readily identified with the electron microscope and contain specialized proteins. Studies indicate substantial reduction in the number of synapses and alterations of basic synaptic proteins in AD.[69] The loss or incapacitation of synapses leads to neuronal dysfunction.

Neurophysiological Brain Alterations

Neurotransmitter alterations in AD include marked reductions of choline acetyltransferase (CHAT) and somatostatin, as well as more variable losses of serotonin (5HT), γ-aminobutyric acid (GABA), and norepinephrine (NE).[32,51,68,71] The neurochemical change most characteristic of AD is a severe deficiency of CHAT, the enzyme that catalyzes the synthesis of acetylcholine (ACh). This deficiency follows neuropathological degeneration in the nucleus basalis of Meynert (NBM), a basal forebrain nucleus containing neurons that manufacture CHAT (see Figure 9.5).[6,107] Norepinephrine, serotonin, GABA, substance P, corticotropin-releasing factor, somatostatin, and other transmitters are also significantly reduced in AD. Brainstem neurons in both the locus ceruleus (norepinephrine) and raphe (serotonin),[60,68,71] as well as dopamine-producing neurons in the ventral tegmental area[99] and substantia nigra,[100] are damaged by AD.

Neurochemical Alterations

The neurotransmitters most implicated in the pathogenesis of AD are ACh and norepinephrine,

both of which are hypothesized to be deficient in AD. Several studies suggest specific degeneration of cholinergic neurons in the NBM of patients with AD (see Figure 9.5).[6,107] Other data supporting a cholinergic deficit in AD include decreases in ACh and CHAT concentrations in the brain. CHAT is the key enzyme for the synthesis of ACh; a reduction in its concentration suggests a decrease in the number of cholinergic neurons. Additional support for this "cholinergic deficit hypothesis" comes from the observation that cholinergic antagonists such as scopolamine and atropine impair cognitive abilities, whereas cholinergic agonists such as physostigmine and arecoline enhance cognitive ability.

The cholinergic system has been implicated in a number of behaviors affected by AD, including motor function, sleep and arousal, mood and affect and, particularly, attention and memory. The importance of the cholinergic system for emotion and memory is consistent with higher concentrations of cholinergic innervation in limbic and paralimbic regions of the brain. The relationship of central cholinergic systems to learning and memory has been the subject of extensive research. Considerable interest has been generated by the possibility that cognitive deficits in AD are caused by cholinergic denervation of the cerebral cortex. A negative correlation exists between cortical CHAT activity and the degree of dementia as determined by neuropsychological tests, whereas cortical levels of other neurochemicals do not appear to show a relationship to the degree of dementia. The extent of cholinergic neuron loss has also been shown to be correlated with the degree of dementia. Despite this positive correlation, it is unlikely that cholinergic denervation constitutes the only or even the major determinant of the behavioral deficits in AD; virtually all sectors of limbic and association cortices also exhibit significant cell loss and contain a high density of plaques and tangles. Therefore cholinergic replacement therapy can be expected to have effects that are modest at best. In support, many trials of cholinesterase inhibitors, cholinergic precursor substances, and cholinergic receptor agonists have been undertaken, but only a few have produced modest—and mostly transient—improvements of patient function.

Molecular Genetics

Amyloid is a fibrillar material with extensive genetic linkage to AD. It is a major research focus because it is overabundant in AD, and some scientists believe that blocking its deposition may prevent damage (see Figure 9.6, C). The gene for the amyloid precursor protein is found on the long arm of chromosome 21, the causative chromosome in Down's syndrome. The process of differential splicing can result in one of four forms of the amyloid precursor protein. The beta amyloid type four (βA4) protein, a major constituent of senile plaques, is a 42–amino acid peptide that is a breakdown product of amyloid precursor protein. Many research groups are actively studying both the normal metabolic processing of amyloid precursor protein and the processing that occurs in patients with AD to determine whether abnormal amyloid precursor protein processing is of primary significance in AD.

Several family lines have been identified in which the early onset of AD appears to segregate in an autosomal dominant pattern. Mutations of the amyloid precursor protein gene appear to be responsible for the disease in a subset of early-onset familial AD kindreds.[90] Present data suggest that AD is a genetically heterogeneous disease caused by two or more genes located on two or more chromosomes; chromosomes 1, 14, 19, and 21 have been most consistently implicated to date.

It is possible to estimate the morbid risk among first-degree relatives of patients with AD in families with a genetic contributor to AD. One method involves the "life table method," which estimates the age-specific cumulative incidence of a disease in a manner that adjusts for the fact that individuals die of other causes before the onset of that disease.[17,75,114] Using this technique, the morbid risk among first-degree relatives of patients is as high as 50% by age 90.[75] These calculations have been used to suggest the dominant mode of inheritance for the AD gene, although it appears

that genetic predisposition to the illness shows variable penetrance. AD is probably not a single disease entity but rather a heterogeneous disorder with varying degrees of behavioral, neurochemical, and neuropathological differences.

Deposition of amyloid (see Figure 9.6, C) in the brain may be facilitated by apolipoprotein E4 (Apo-E4), a cholesterol-bearing protein.[93] There are at least three forms of Apo-E produced in humans. The presence of the Apo-E4 allele on chromosome 19 is a risk factor for late-onset familial and sporadic AD.[25] In the brain, Apo-E is synthesized by astrocytes and macrophages and upregulated in response to neuronal damage. This process allows the redistribution of cholesterol and lipid breakdown products in denervation and reinnervation.[85] The following three findings led to the scrutiny of this molecule as an important piece of the AD puzzle:

1. Apo-E is an amyloid-binding protein.
2. Apo-E is localized in senile plaques, neurofibrillary tangles, and within blood vessel walls that demonstrate congophilic angiopathy.
3. Apo-E has its genetic focus on chromosome 19, the chromosome linked to familial late-onset AD.

An allele is a segment of a gene that codes for a specific substance. The Apo-E genotype has three paired alleles: E2, E3, and E4. The Apo-E4 allele appears to be strongly associated with the development of AD. It is estimated that 80% of familial late-onset AD and 64% of sporadic late-onset AD cases have at least one E4 allele in contrast to 31% of controls. The E4 allele appears to have a gene-dosage effect on the expression of AD; 40% of the E2 or E3 subjects develop AD, whereas 91% of the E4 subjects develop the disease. The proposed mechanism whereby Apo-E4 leads to AD is indirect, with Apo-E2 and E3 offering protection against AD by binding amyloid protein. Apo-E2 and E3 enhance the stability of microtubules via a slowing of the abnormal deposition and self-assembly into the PHFs characteristic of AD. Individuals who inherit the Apo-E4 gene lose all or part of this protection.[94] This hypothesis has been criticized because it does not sufficiently allow for the proven role of amyloid in the development of AD. However, Apo-E4 does strongly enhance binding to the β-amyloid peptide fragment seen in AD.[93] The subsequent stable complexes form to promote amyloid aggregation, which compromises the lipid metabolism essential for neuronal survival. In contrast, Apo-E may act as an intracellular transporter for toxic β-amyloid fragments. These findings may prove useful for developing pharmacotherapy for AD to mimic or enhance the functions of Apo-E2 or E3. In addition, once therapy becomes available there is also the prospect of testing presymptomatic individuals at risk for AD. Apo-E genotype testing is currently available but is *not* recommended routinely.

The molecule βA4 is known to be neurotoxic, but the exact mechanism of toxicity remains obscure. It appears that βA4 is capable of assuming a molecular shape that can enter the lipid bilayer of neuronal membranes and form ion-selected channels. This channel-forming property of βA4 molecule has the potential to create membrane lesions, which results in the disruption of calcium homeostasis. These data now form the basis of the potassium ion channel hypothesis for βA4 neurotoxicity.[7]

During the course of a large statistical analysis of elderly twin pairs with AD, an inverse relationship was found between AD and reports of antecedent treatments with steroids/adrenocorticotropic hormone (ACTH). The chronic use of antiinflammatory medications such as aspirin, nonsteroidal antiinflammatory drugs (NSAIDS), or steroids may prevent or slow the onset of AD.[18] These findings are consistent with prior studies that have hinted at inverse relationships between AD and rheumatoid arthritis with the use of steroids. Some investigations have detected classic complement-mediated inflammatory changes in brains with AD. Clinical trials using antiinflammatory therapy to retard or prevent the expected progression of AD symptoms are well under way, along with other research into the possible relationship between AD and inflammatory or musculoskeletal diseases.

Research suggests a link between estrogen and AD on the basis of reports that postmenopausal women who use estrogen are less likely to develop AD than those who do not. Estrogen receptors have been shown to regulate nerve growth factor (NGF); NGF increases estrogen binding. This coregulation may control neuronal sensitivity to neurotropic factors and mediate NGF production and activity for enhanced neuronal survival.[92] Thus the low estrogen levels seen in aging or disease would prevent neurons with estrogen receptors from responding to NGF, possibly increasing their vulnerability to AD or other degenerative processes. Although little is known about these mechanisms in men, estrogen replacement has proven to be beneficial in AD therapy for women.

Evidence is also emerging that AD may be caused by heterogenous mechanisms. One form may have an early-age onset that is associated with more severe neuropathological changes, more rapid progression, dermatographical changes similar to those found in Down's syndrome, and platelet abnormalities such as increased membrane fluidity. The second type may occur in older patients and follow an indolent course. Other theories of causation of AD include the excess deposition of aluminum in the brain and the possibility of a slow viral infection. However, there is no compelling evidence that aluminum, heavy metals, or infections cause AD.

Humans are not the only species to develop AD. Aged primates develop both the clinical and neuropathological features of this disease.[19] Other aged mammals develop senile plaques and neurofibrillary tangles that resemble the human pathological condition (e.g., bears).[27]

Brain Imaging Techniques, Findings, and Research

Although it is not possible to diagnose dementia or AD with brain imaging, brain imaging *does* provide a useful adjunct to clinical evaluations. Abnormalities have been noted on computed tomography (CT) and MRI scans.[87] Cerebral atrophy, cortical sulci widening, deep white matter lesions with periventricular distribution, and ventricular enlargement changes have been observed. These changes may be seen in older

table 9.1

Most Common Regional Abnormalities in Metabolism Detected by PET in Some Dementias

DISEASE	PATTERN OF ABNORMALITY
Alzheimer's disease	Temporoparietal hypometabolism Frontal association cortex may also be hypometabolic
Multi-infarct dementia	Multiple, usually asymmetrical focal areas of hypometabolism
Parkinson's disease with dementia	Temporoparietal hypometabolism
Pick's disease	Frontal hypometabolism Basal ganglia may also be hypometabolic
Frontal lobe dementia of the non-Alzheimer's type	Frontal hypometabolism

From Foster NL: PET imaging. In Terry RD, Katzman R, Bick KL, editors: *Alzheimer disease,* Philadelphia, 1994, Lippincott-Raven.

patients without AD; alternatively, many patients with AD have normal CT and MRI scans. Thus the primary use of CT and MRI scanning is for excluding any potentially treatable causes of cognitive impairment such as a brain tumor or chronic subdural hematoma.

Longitudinal CT studies over periods of 6 to 60 months have shown that patients with AD have significantly increased rates of ventricular and sulcal enlargement compared with age-matched controls.[66] The rates of increase in lateral ventricular size are not different for mild versus moderate AD cases. A strong correlation is found between decrements on neuropsychological tests of cognition and lateral or third ventricular enlargement.[3] White matter changes in AD consistently show periventricular lucency. Cerebral amyloid angiopathy has also been associated with such changes in white matter.

MRI images are better than CT images at discriminating between AD subjects and normals. Several studies have demonstrated the effectiveness of MRIs in showing quantitative differences in cerebral atrophy between AD, depression, and control subjects.[84] The abnormal volume of temporal lobe structures has renewed special attention in the diagnosis of AD. Hippocampal formation

changes are discriminated in up to 85% of AD cases.[59] Studies show differences between patients with AD and controls by using semiquantitative measures of temporal and entorhinal cortex, hippocampal formation, and temporal horns.[40] The entorhinal cortex atrophy ratings prove to be the most discriminatory, with a sensitivity of 90% in 34 mildly affected AD patients versus 39 controls. These radiological alterations coincide with pathological studies and show consistent, severe damage to mesial temporal structures in AD (see Figure 9.2).

Positron emission tomography (PET) has provided insights about AD by allowing the degenerative process of AD to be observed as patients gradually and progressively develop symptoms.[46] These insights include the following:[46]

• AD is not a diffuse disease.
• AD is qualitatively different from normal aging.
• Presenile and senile dementia appear the same.
• AD damages both cortical and subcortical structures.
• AD severity correlates with hypometabolism.

Some of the most common regional abnormalities in metabolism detected by PET are noted in Table 9.1. The metabolic abnormalities observed with PET can be used to differentiate AD from other causes of dementia.[11] An exception may be cases of Parkinson's disease or normal-pressure hydrocephalus.

PET and single photon emission computed tomography (SPECT) demonstrate lowered parietal and temporal metabolism and blood flow in AD. Hippocampal atrophy and parietal hypometabolism with asymmetry have been observed in patients with memory complaints that are too mild to confirm a diagnosis of dementia. In contrast, elderly patients with depression show greater white matter lesions, cortical atrophy, and generalized cortical hypometabolism when compared with nondepressed elders. Thus imaging approaches may potentially identify AD at preclinical stages and assist in the selection of patients suitable for antidementia drugs while also distinguishing the differential diagnosis of treatable depression from progressive AD.

Metabolic dysfunction revealed by PET (or SPECT) is an indication of the first detectable cortical degeneration predominantly in the temporal and/or parietal area and, in more advanced cases, in the frontal brain cortex. The anatomical changes seen with CT and MRI reflect later manifestations of the disease.[3] Despite such potential utility, the NIH Consensus Development Conference on the diagnosis of dementia recommends that brain neuroimaging studies be generally optional in the diagnostic evaluation.

Clinical Applications
Clinical Findings and Course

The DSM-IV diagnostic criteria for dementia of the Alzheimer's type emphasizes the presence of memory impairment and the associated presence of at least one other symptom of cognitive decline (e.g., aphasia, apraxia, agnosia, or abnormal executive functioning).[5] The criteria also require a continuing and gradual decline in functioning, impairment in social or occupational functioning, and the exclusion of other causes of dementia (Box 9.1).[102,103]

The symptoms of dementia are understood only within the context of the functional organization of the human brain. There is compartmentalization of function within the human brain, and different brain regions perform different functions. Most dementias damage a random distribution of brain regions, which results in a random expression of clinical symptoms. No two patients with dementia have identical clinical symptoms because no two patterns of brain injury are identical. Clinicians must contend with broad categories of cognitive deficits rather than with the precise clinical measurements that are possible in disorders such as hypertension or chronic lung disease. The progressive nature of dementia produces clinical manifestations that worsen over time at variable rates and require periodic reassessment to define cognitive deficits.

Amnesia

Amnesia, the inability to remember recent or remote facts or events, is the most common symptom encountered with dementia.[29,63] The human brain has two types of memory: recent and remote. Recent memories are things or facts that have occurred within the last 15 to 30 minutes. Remote memories are facts from the distant past that are stored in the cortex. Human beings do not remember every face, event, or conversation because the memory capacity of the brain would be saturated. Information is processed and stored for brief periods of time, and the decision is made whether to store facts in long-term memory or allow erasure of information. For example, a person may remember what he or she had for breakfast this morning but cannot recall breakfast 5 years ago. Using the personal computer as an analogy, short-term memory is held on the workstation, and long-term memory is stored on hard disk.

Recent memory is processed in the human hippocampus (see Figure 9.2). This mesial temporal lobe structure is essential for placing new information into long-term storage.[10] The hippocampus begins to lose neurons at approximately 50 years of age and is selectively and severely damaged in most dementias.[34,53,58] The hippocampus is predisposed to a range of neurodegenerative (e.g., neurofibrillary degeneration, Pick's bodies), ischemic (e.g.,

box 9.1

Diagnostic Criteria for Dementia of the Alzheimer's Type

A. The development of multiple cognitive deficits manifested by both
   (1) Memory impairment (impaired ability to learn new information or to recall previously learned information)
   (2) One (or more) of the following cognitive disturbances:
       (a) Aphasia (language disturbance)
       (b) Apraxia (impaired ability to carry out motor activities despite intact motor function)
       (c) Agnosia (failure to recognize or identify objects despite intact sensory function)
       (d) Disturbance in executive functioning (i.e., planning, organizing, sequencing, abstracting)
B. The cognitive deficits in Criteria A1 and A2 each cause significant impairment in social or occupational functioning and represent a significant decline from a previous level of functioning.
C. The course is characterized by gradual onset and continuing cognitive decline.
D. The cognitive deficits in Criteria A1 and A2 are not due to any of the following:
   (1) Other central nervous system conditions that cause progressive deficits in memory and cognition (e.g., cerebrovascular disease, Parkinson's disease, Huntington's disease, subdural hematoma, normal-pressure hydrocephalus, brain tumor)
   (2) Systemic conditions that are known to cause dementia (e.g., hypothyroidism, vitamin B_{12} or folic acid deficiency, niacin deficiency, hypercalcemia, neurosyphilis, HIV infection)
   (3) Substance-induced conditions
E. The deficits do not occur exclusively during the course of a delirium.
F. The disturbance is not better accounted for by another Axis I disorder (e.g., major depressive disorder, schizophrenia).
   Code based on type of onset and predominant features:
   With Early Onset: if onset is at age 65 years or below
       290.11   With Delirium: if delirium is superimposed on the dementia
       290.12   With Delusions: if delusions are the predominant feature
       290.13   With Depressed Mood: if depressed mood (including presentations that meet full symptom criteria for a major depressive episode) is the predominant feature. A separate diagnosis of mood disorder due to a general medical condition is not given.
       290.10   Uncomplicated: if none of the above predominates in the current clinical presentation
   With Late Onset: if onset is after age 65 years
       290.3   With Delirium: if delirium is superimposed on the dementia
       290.20   With Delusions: if delusions are the predominant feature
       290.21   With Depressed Mood: if depressed mood (including presentations that meet full symptom criteria for a major depressive episode) is the predominant feature. A separate diagnosis of mood disorder due to a general medical condition is not given.
       290.0   Uncomplicated: if none of the above predominates in the current clinical presentation
   Specify if:
   With Behavioral Disturbance
   Coding note: Also code 331.0 Alzheimer's disease on Axis III.

From American Psychiatric Association: *Diagnostic and statistical manual of mental disorders,* ed 4, Washington, DC, 1994, The Association.

hypoxic injury to pyramidal neurons), and metabolic (e.g., hypoglycemic pyramidal cell loss) injuries (see Chapter 10). Deficits in recent memory are a constant feature in AD and many other types of dementia.[32,95,106] Remote memory remains intact until later in the disease, which creates a confusing paradox for health care workers. Patients may not be able to remember events that occurred 10 or 20 minutes ago, but they may recall facts from 10 or 20 *years* ago. The uninformed clinician infers that this intact remote memory should be accompanied by intact recent memory. This misunderstanding leads to the conclusion that the patient is stubborn rather than amnestic. Family caregivers often make this inaccurate conclusion. Patients often conceal memory problems by writing notes to themselves, using old memory to distract interviewers, and vehemently denying the problem. These patients live in the past because they cannot remember the present.

The hippocampal circuits that encode recent memory can be disconnected at three levels.[89] The hippocampus processes information in a sequential manner. Information comes out of the temporal lobe and synapses in the outer layer of the entorhinal cortex, where the information is relayed to the molecular layer of the dentate gyrus and synapses on dendrites of the granule cells. The transmission passes via granule cells to neurons of the CA4/CA3 region and then to neurons of the CA1/subicular region, where the information is returned to the deep layers of the entorhinal cortex and into the temporal lobe or other areas.[89] Disconnecting this chain at any point results in hippocampal dysfunction and impairment of recent memory.[58] The dentate gyrus and CA3 region are heavily innervated by both cholinergic and catecholaminergic fibers. These catecholamines are necessary for proper transmission through the human hippocampus.[14]

AD disrupts the hippocampal circuits at multiple levels, including the entorhinal cortex, CA1 subiculum, and ascending catecholaminergic or cholinergic inputs.[58] Norepinephrine and serotonin, which are essential to proper hippocampal function, are depleted in many dementias. Neurons in both the raphe (a source of serotonin) and

locus ceruleus (a source of norepinephrine) are damaged in AD and other dementias. These catecholamine levels are also lowered in depression, which may provide a possible explanation for the memory problems associated with mood disorders.[113,115]

Aphasia

Aphasia is a complicated neuropsychiatric condition beyond the scope of this chapter. It is the second most common cognitive deficit experienced by patients with dementia.[65] Language function is roughly divided into receptive and expressive components.[10] Auditory inputs are received via the tympanic membrane and eighth cranial nerve, where they are transmitted to the medial geniculate nucleus and into the primary auditory cortex (Brodmann's area 41) in the tranverse temporal gyrus. In right-handed individuals, receptive language skills are located in the left temporal lobe and inferior parietal lobe.[78,91] The auditory area in the temporal lobe can be divided into four regions: (1) the primary auditory receptive cortex, located in the transverse temporal gyrus (area 41); (2) the unimodal association cortex, located in the superior temporal gyrus (areas 22 and 52); (3) the specialized auditory association cortex in the planum temporale area (area 42); and (4) the multimodal or heteromodal association cortex, which is probably located in the temporal lobe (see Figure 9.4, *A*). AD spares the primary receptive cortex and the peripheral auditory system, which leaves the patient with intact auditory acuity.[42,48] However, the auditory association cortex that translates spoken language into meaningful words is selectively damaged by the disease process, which results in patients who can hear but cannot understand.[10] Spoken language is accompanied by other nonverbal messages, including tone of voice, body language, facial expressions, and context of the spoken word, all of which may be integrated in the heteromodal association cortex.[10]

Receptive or sensory aphasia is common in middle or advanced stages of AD.[65] Significant behavioral consequences occur when staff or caregivers do not recognize that the patient is unable to understand spoken words. A typical example of receptive aphasia is the elderly nursing home resident with AD who is asked to disrobe for a bath. The patient cannot remember that he or she is living in a nursing home and that the nursing assistant is there to help. The nursing assistant asks the patient to disrobe, put on a bathrobe, and go to the shower, where he or she will assist the patient. The patient does not understand the spoken word and cannot remember the nursing assistant; the patient smiles and nods to hide his or her deficits. The nursing assistant returns in 5 minutes to find the patient fully clothed and abruptly begins to steer the patient toward the bath area. The patient misinterprets the spoken words but does understand the nurse's look of frustration and the potential physical threat associated with having clothing removed. The patient therefore begins to fight and is described as a "behavior problem." Antipsychotic medications do not help this condition. Staff education and alternative communication skills are pivotal to avoiding this behavior.

Basic management skills for patients with dementia and impaired communication include the following:

- Ensuring that hearing aids are in place with batteries turned on
- Ensuring that staff faces hearing-impaired patients who lip read
- Ensuring that glasses are worn by visually impaired patients
- Speaking in slow, direct, simple terms
- Giving simple, one-step commands
- Using multiple visual cues
- Speaking in a calm, empathic voice
- Maintaining a smile, even with the most frustrating patient

Expressive language skills involve a complex mixture of frontal, temporal, and parietal function. The motor language area (Broca's area) is located in the posterior inferior frontal lobe and is damaged in many patients with dementia (see Figure 9.1). These individuals develop a range of expressive language problems, including difficulty finding words, naming objects, constructing sentences, and speaking with a smooth musical qual-

ity. Spoken language has two components: (1) the organized script, which is constructed in the left brain; and (2) the musical/emotional quality of speech, which is programmed in the right hemisphere.[10] Patients with AD often have difficulty finding words or use alternative words or terms to convey the message (i.e., production anomia). This phenomenon is similar to cognitively intact individuals who experience "words stuck on the tip of their tongue." Patients with more advanced AD may say the same word or phrase repetitively—a condition called *perseveration*. Some patients lose left brain function and fail to communicate but can sing or curse because their right brain function continues.[10] Staff often misinterpret the patient's ability to curse or sing as a sign that he or she can speak. Similarly, patients with intact auditory acuity are said to be stubborn and mean because they "hear fine" but act as though they do not understand. The appropriate intervention for language-impaired patients is a calm and reassuring attitude by the staff toward the patients. All clinicians must recognize the likelihood of communication deficits in patients with AD.

Apraxia

Apraxia, the third common cognitive deficit experienced by patients with dementia, is the inability to perform preprogrammed motor activities.[10,95] Retaining sufficient information to execute complex motor skills without thought requires weeks or months of learning by small children. Walking, dressing, personal hygiene, self-feeding, and a multitude of other complex skills that become automatic over time require months of training by parents. Three major groups of apraxias pose the greatest obstacles to the care of patients with AD or other dementia: activities of daily living (ADLs) function, gait apraxia, and feeding apraxia.

Any previously learned motor activity can be lost, whereas other, even more complex activities can be retained. This patchy, discrete functional loss often frustrates professional staff and caregivers, who infer that ability in one area implies global motor competence (e.g., the patient can play the piano but not dress himself or herself).

Fighting during ADLs often results from patient anxiety or fear and from staff or caregivers whose expectations exceed the intellectual ability of the patient. Appropriate interventions include dressing the patient, laying out clothing, and acting and speaking in a calm, reassuring way.

Dressing apraxias (one type of ADL dysfunction) are common in patients with AD. These patients often struggle as family or staff attempt to place garments on their body in the correct order and position. Dressing requires a complex mixture of social, memory, and motor skills. An individual must remember the location of the clothes, the season of the year, and the social context in which the clothes will be worn. Social and executive functions prevent normal individuals from wandering about while naked. Once the clothing has been chosen, the patient must place the garments on his or her body. Putting on a blouse and fitting the hands through the sleeves requires knowing where the upper extremities are located in space at all times. During dressing, the parietal lobe monitors the spatial position of the extremities to track their location and ensure that the arms slip easily through the sleeves (Figure 9.7). Buttons and shoelaces require thousands of tiny movements by joints in the fingers to insert the button or tie the shoelace. Each step of this process requires proper functioning of discrete brain regions that can be damaged by AD.

Patients with severe dementia forget how to walk (i.e., gait apraxia) (see Figure 9.7).[95] The motor cortex, which is responsible for arm and leg movement, is less severely damaged by AD than are the prefrontal and parietal cortices, which store complex motor activities such as walking.[10] Patients with advanced AD often stand in a rigid, wide-based, and unsteady gait that resembles an adult who is learning to snow ski or roller skate. These patients cannot walk, but they can climb out of bed or kick staff. Patients with AD are not paralyzed because the primary motor circuits are less severely damaged by this disease. Gait apraxia is irreversible, and individuals with this disorder may require movement restrictions to prevent falls and fractures. Patients with static brain lesions such as strokes or head trauma may relearn walk-

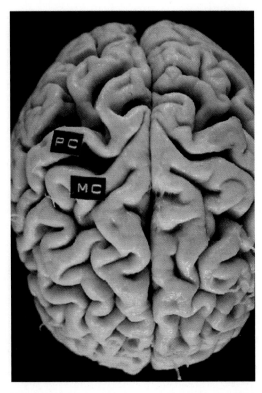

figure 9.7   Atrophy of parietal cortex *(PC)* with sparing of motor cortex *(MC)* in an Alzheimer's brain. The patient would have normal strength but forget sophisticated functions such as walking (i.e., gait apraxia). *(Courtesy Dr. Richard E. Powers, Director, University of Alabama at Birmingham Brain Resource Program.)*

ing skills through rehabilitation. However, progressive dementias such as AD rarely allow patients to relearn basic motor skills such as walking or feeding.

Feeding requires a complex mixture of social and motor skills that integrates movement of the upper extremities and the head, neck, and masticatory muscles. Children require approximately 20 years to refine basic eating skills into fine table manners. The use of fingers versus utensils, as well as table etiquette and personal hygiene during eating, are sophisticated skills that require the proper functioning of frontal and parietal cortices. Patients with AD initially lose sophisticated dining habits and revert to adolescent behavior (e.g.,

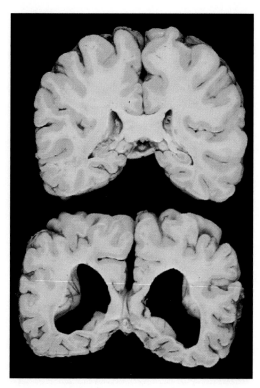

figure 9.8   Coronal sections of occipital lobe from normal *(top)* and Alzheimer's brains *(bottom)*. Significant atrophy and ventriculomegaly in the visual association regions could explain visual agnosia. *(Courtesy Dr. Richard E. Powers, Director, University of Alabama at Birmingham Brain Resource Program.)*

picking up food, spilling, taking food off other's plates). The use of eating utensils is learned during the first 5 years of life; this function is often lost in patients with AD. The final phase of feeding apraxia includes an inability to coordinate chewing and swallowing to allow proper feeding. Patients with advanced AD require special diets to prevent choking, and they eventually deteriorate to the point where they hold food in their mouth for prolonged periods of time. Aspiration pneumonia is a common occurrence in advanced dementia, with pneumonia being a common cause of death in patients with AD. Feeding tubes are of limited value because patients with severe dementia lose the ability to clear oral secretion from their mouth.

Agnosia

Agnosia is the fourth cognitive deficit manifested by patients with dementia. It is the inability to recognize preprogrammed sensory patterns or information.[10,95] Visual agnosia is fairly common in patients who begin to misidentify or not recognize family, friends, and caregivers. Visual information (e.g., faces) is encoded in the retina and transmitted via the optic nerves and lateral geniculate body to area 17 of the occipital cortex (Figure 9.8).[8,23] Patients with dementia develop selective injury to areas 18 and 19, which is the visual association cortex where visual information is processed.[64,83] Damage to occipital and parietal cortices results in patients who can see but not recognize. Patients may forget the appearance of familiar faces (including their own) and become alarmed when looking in the mirror (prosopagnosia). The appropriate intervention for such patients is to cover or remove mirrors and keep windows covered at night to prevent patients from seeing "strange faces looking in." Patients may fail to recognize other sensory inputs, including tactile, visceral, and olfactory information. Patients may see a toilet but fail to understand its meaning or use. Visceral sensory information is probably organized in the insular cortex. This region is extensively damaged in AD, and therefore patients with dementia may fail to accurately interpret internal bodily sensations (e.g., fecal versus urinary urgency).

Typical Clinical Presentation

Most patients with dementia usually experience multiple cognitive impairments. An elderly woman who resides in a nursing home and experiences angina is an excellent example. This patient has amnesia and cannot remember the identity of her staff or her location and cannot remember where her nitroglycerin tablets are located. Her receptive language deficit limits the ability of the staff to communicate with her, and her expressive deficit limits her ability to explain her symptoms to the staff. Her motor apraxia limits her ability to open a bottle or place a tablet under her tongue. Her agnosia prevents her from recognizing staff or family as helpers and may limit her ability to interpret chest pains as angina. This patient manifests her angina through agitation, yelling, or striking out. Antipsychotic medications do not help. Appropriate interventions include a physical examination to determine possible angina (e.g., diaphoresis, heart rate changes) and a trial of nitroglycerin with observations of subsequent behavior.

Diagnosis

The diagnosis of dementia begins with a careful clinical history and examination.[26,104] A mental status, neurological, and physical examination are the critical first steps in the evaluation of dementia. The clinician must examine the family history and require the caregiver to bring all medications—both prescribed and over-the-counter—consumed by the patient. Many arrive with a positive shopping-bag sign (i.e., a bag full of medicines).

Mental status examination. The basic dementia evaluation outlined in Box 9.2 identifies treatable, reversible, and arrestable causes of cognitive decline. These causes are presented in Box 9.3.[10] Depression can mimic dementia and distinguishing features. The features mentioned in Table 9.2 can be elicited with a mental status examination.[112] Numerous neuropsychological batteries[95,106] can identify cognitive loss, but the Folstein Mini-Mental State Examination[44] remains a simple, cost-efficient instrument used by primary care practitioners. This brief, easy cognitive screen can be performed in 30 minutes or less by office staff with basic training. It is valid in a broad range of patients and has good rate-rerate reliability.[44] These scores can monitor the progression of symptoms or the efficacy of treatment. Other clinical instruments such as the Psychogeriatric Dependency Rating Scale monitor behavioral or ADL function.[95,106,108]

Laboratory evaluation. Laboratory tests should include a complete blood cell count, erythrocyte sedimentation rate, electrolytes, blood glucose, blood urea, liver functions, vitamin B_{12} concen-

---

box 9.2

Comprehensive Work-up of Dementia and Delirium

Physical examination, including thorough neurological examination
Vital signs
Mental status examination
Mini-Mental State Examination (MMSE)
Review of medications and drug levels
Blood and urine screens for alcohol, drugs, and heavy metals*
Physiological work-up
    Serum electrolytes/glucose/Ca, Mg
    Liver, renal function tests
    SMA-12 or equivalent serum chemistry profile
    Urinalysis
    Complete blood cell count with differential cell type count
    Thyroid function tests (including TSH level)
    RPR (serum screen)
    FTA-ABS (if CNS disease suspected)
    Serum B_{12}
    Folate levels
    Urine corticosteroids*
    Erythrocyte sedimentation rate (Westergren)
    Antinuclear antibody (ANA)*, C_3, C_4, Anti-DS DNA*
    Arterial blood gases*
    HIV screen*†
    Urine porphobilinogens*
Chest x-ray examination
Electrocardiogram
Neurological work-up
    CT or MRI scan of head*
    SPECT‡
    Lumbar puncture*
    EEG*
Neuropsychological testing§

From Stoudemire A, Thompson TL: Recognizing and treating dementia, *Geriatrics* 36:112-120, 1981.
*If indicated by history and physical examination.
†Requires special consent and counseling.
‡May detect cerebral blood flow perfusion deficits.
§May be useful in differentiating dementia from other neuropsychiatric syndromes if this cannot be done clinically.

box 9.3
Reversible Causes of Dementia

D **Drug** toxicity
Psychoactive drugs, sedatives, hypnotics, anticholinergics, antiparkinsonian agents, antispasmodics, cardiac drugs, antihypertensives, diuretics, digoxin

E **Emotional** disorders
Involutional depression, schizophrenic decompensation

M **Metabolic** and endocrine disorders
Myxedema, hyperadrenocorticism, apathetic thyrotoxicosis, hypoglycemia, hyperosmolar states, electrolyte abnormalities, chronic obstructive pulmonary disease with hypercapnea, hypoxia, hepatic encephalopathy

E Visual and hearing disorders (**eyes and ears)**

N **Nutritional** disorders
Vitamin B_{12} and folate deficiency, other water-soluble vitamin deficiencies, iron deficiency anemia
Normal-pressure hydrocephalus

T Intracranial masses (**tumors and trauma)**
Chronic subdural hematoma, primary or metastatic neoplasms

I **Infection**
Tertiary syphilis, encephalitis, meningitis, pneumonia

A **Arteriosclerotic** complications
Strokes, transient ischemic attacks, congestive heart failure

tration, thyrotropin levels, free thyroid index, and serological tests for syphilis. CT or MRI imaging of the brain should be requested if a diagnosis is not established by history and laboratory tests. Electroencephalography, lumbar puncture, heavy metal screen, human immunodeficiency (HIV) tests, SPECT, and other specialized tests should be requested when the clinical findings suggest that they will provide useful information. As previously discussed, testing for the E4 allele for Apo-E4 does not predict which individuals will get AD and does not contribute to the routine evaluation of the patient with dementia.

Diagnostic probability. The diagnosis of AD is stratified as definite, probable, or possible according to the certainty of the available information. A diagnosis of definite AD requires that the patient exhibit a characteristic clinical syndrome and confirmatory histological evidence of AD pathology as obtained from biopsy or autopsy (see Figure 9.6). Probable AD requires that the patient meet the criteria for dementia on the basis of clinical examinations, a structured mental status examina-

tion, and neuropsychological testing; defects in at least two areas of intellectual functioning together with progressive worsening of memory; no disturbance of consciousness; and disease onset between ages 40 and 90. In addition, no systemic or other brain disorders can account for the deficits observed. An accurate diagnosis depends on a combination of inclusionary clinical features and the exclusion of other possible causes of dementia. AD should not be regarded as a purely exclusionary diagnosis. Possible AD is diagnosed when there are variations in the onset, presentation, or course of a dementing illness that has no alternate explanation; there is a systemic illness or brain disease present that is not considered to be the cause of the dementia syndrome; and there is a single, gradual progressive cognitive deficit in the absence of any other brain disorder. Focal neurological signs, sudden onset, or the early occurrence of a gait disorder or seizures make a diagnosis of AD unlikely. Neuropathological studies have demonstrated that between 65% and 90% of patients identified as having probable AD have the diagnosis confirmed at autopsy.[30,88]

table 9.2
Features That Distinguish Depression from Dementia

PRIMARY DEPRESSION	PRIMARY DEMENTIA
General	
Family usually aware of illness	Family unaware of illness
Onset dated and more acute	Insidious onset, broadly and vaguely dated
Symptoms are of short duration	Symptoms are of long duration
Rapid progression	Slow progression
Family history of affective disorder	Possible family history of AD
Personal History	
Patient with history of depression	No history of depression
Patient complains of cognitive deficits and seeks help	No complaints of cognitive deficits
Patient complains in detail	Vague complaints
Patient's complaints of cognitive deficits are emphasized	Deficit is concealed
Patient highlights his or her failures	Patient delights in his or her accomplishments
Patient makes little effort at task	Patient struggles with tasks
Patient does not try to keep up	Patient relies on notes, calendars, and similar items
Patient is in distress	Patient is unconcerned
Affective symptoms are pervasive	Affect is labile and shallow
Behavior incongruent with cognitive dysfunction	Behavior compatible with cognitive dysfunction
Examination	
No sundowning	Sundowning
Attention and concentration preserved	Faulty attention and concentration
"I don't know" answers are typical	Frequent "near-miss" answers
"Don't know" answers on orientation	Orientation tests poor
Recent and remote memory loss are similar	Recent memory loss greater than remote memory loss
Decreased memory for specific periods is common	No gaps in memory
No glabellar or snout reflexes	Glabellar and snout reflexes present
Psychological Testing	
Variable performance	Consistently poor performance
Weschler test shows no typical pattern	Great discrepancy between verbal and performance scores
Examination of Mental Status	
Absence of apraxia and agnosia	Has apraxia or agnosia
Will correct any word intrusions	Demonstrates word intrusions

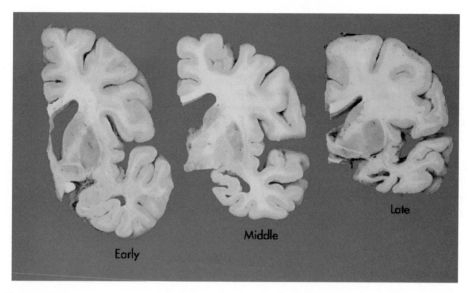

figure 9.9   Coronal brain sections from three patients with early-, middle-, and late-stage dementia. The hemispheres demonstrate mild (early), moderate (middle), and severe (late) cortical atrophy with a corresponding reduction in brain volume. Temporal lobe damage causes language impairment and auditory hallucinations. Progressive brain atrophy explains the progressive nature of AD. *(Courtesy Dr. Richard E. Powers, Director, University of Alabama at Birmingham Brain Resource Program.)*

Symptom Progression

The clinical progression of dementia can be divided into three phases: early, middle, and late (Figure 9.9) as characterized in Box 9.4. The classic dementia syndrome of AD includes impairment of learning new information, poor recall of remote material, impaired naming and verbal comprehension, deterioration in constructional and visual spatial abilities, and poor calculations, abstracting, and judgment. Amnesia is the common symptom of early dementia. Fluency of verbal output, repetition skills, and the ability to read aloud are retained until later in the disease. Motor and sensory functions are also spared throughout most of the course of the illness. In the final phases there is total abolition of intellectual function, progressive loss of ambulation and coordination, dysphagia, and incontinence. Aspiration pneumonia, sepsis associated with urinary tract infection or decubitus ulcers, or an independent age-related disease usually accounts for the pa-

tient's death. Differential diagnoses, including the detailed differential between dementia and depression in AD dementia, are included in Box 9.1 and Table 9.2.

Because AD is progressive, the patient's cognitive impairment worsens over time at variable and unpredictable rates. Patients require systematic reevaluation every 6 months to determine their level of cognition and basic functional skills. The Folstein Mini-Mental State Examination can be used as a basic assessment of cognitive function.[44] The Psychogeriatric Dependency Rating Scale can be used to monitor ADLs and behavioral symptoms in patients with dementia.[108] Language skills can be screened with simple, structured instruments. This information should be recorded in the medical record but communicated to the treatment team and caregivers. Staff must understand the nature and severity of the cognitive deficits so that they can develop appropriate individual treatment plans.

box 9.4

Cognitive Symptoms of Early, Middle, and Late Stages of Alzheimer's Disease*

Early Stage

Forgetfulness for faces, names, and conversations

Subtle decline in performing work or ADLs (trouble learning new routines, slowing of work performance, and decreased output)

Subtle personality changes (decline in social graces and withdrawal from social contacts)

Early language problems (difficulty expressing complex ideas, shortening of phraseology)

Repetitiveness

Anxiety, worry, and depression concerning the decline of these abilities

Early-Middle Stage

Pervasive memory problems (forgetting major, important items; "forgetting to remember")

Inability to work in one's customary job

Paranoia, apathy, or delusions

Need for supervision in household chores

Difficulties in naming objects

Disorientation outdoors, especially in relatively unfamiliar places

Definite decline in personal grooming

Occasional incontinence

Need for reminders to bathe and assistance in dressing

Late-Middle Stage

Frequent disorientation indoors

Need for supervision in bathroom

Very limited vocabulary and comprehension

Disorders of sleep/wakefulness cycle

Extremes of emotional reactivity

General withdrawal from all social contacts

State of "living in the past"

Purposeless hyperactivity or energy

Late Stage

Dissolution of personality

Lack of recognition

Severe language impairment

Inability to feed oneself

Incontinence

Severe motor deficits

*There is much variation in the order, intensity, and duration of symptoms among patients. Seizures, myoclonus, or gait disturbances may predominate in some subsets of patients.

box 9.5

Neuropsychiatric Characteristics of Alzheimer's Disease

Personality alterations	Anxiety
Disengagement	Psychomotor activity disturbances
Disinhibition	Agitation or combativeness
Delusions	Wandering
Persecutory	Pacing
Theft	Purposeless activity
Infidelity	Miscellaneous
Capgras syndrome	Sexual activity changes
Hallucinations	Decreased sexual interest
Auditory	Increased sexual interest
Visual	Appetite changes
Mood changes	Sleep disturbances
Depressive symptoms	Klüver-Bucy syndrome
Elevated mood	
Catastrophic reactions	
Mood lability	

From Cummings JL. Neuropsychiatric aspects of Alzheimer's disease and other dementing illnesses. In Yudofsky SC, Hales RE, editors: *The American Psychiatric Press textbook of neuropsychiatry*, ed 2, Washington, DC, 1992, American Psychiatric Press.

Clinical Consequences

The principal psychiatric consequences of AD include personality alterations, delusions, hallucinations, mood changes, agitation, anxiety, disturbances of psychomotor activity, and various miscellaneous behavioral changes, including disturbances of sleep and appetite, altered sexual behavior, and Klüver-Bucy syndrome (Box 9.5). [95,106]

Alteration of Personality

Personality changes are ubiquitous in AD, with the most common being passivity or disengagement. Patients may exhibit diminished emotional responsiveness, decreased initiative, loss of enthusiasm, diminished energy, and decreased volition. [80] Self-centered, resistive, and disinhibited behaviors may also occur. Patients may be labile and sensitive, excitable, or unreasonable. Personality changes affect essentially all AD patients; they often occur early in the course and may pre-date intellectual abnormalities. Catastrophic reactions may occur when patients exhibit massive emotional outbursts of crying and weeping. Frontal lobe damage may explain some symptoms (Figure 9.10, *A*). [33]

Psychosis

Delusions are common in AD and affect between 30% and 50% of all patients. [20] The most common delusions involve false beliefs of theft, spousal infidelity, abandonment, that the house is not one's home, persecution, and Capgras syndrome (i.e., the false belief that an individual is an imposter). [86] There is no specific delusional content that distinguishes the psychosis of AD from other psychoses. Delusions are most common in the middle phase of illness but may occur early in the clinical course and sometimes persist until late in the disease. Delusions do not correlate with the severity of the dementia or with specific aspects of intellectual dysfunction. Patients who are experiencing delusions are more behaviorally disturbed, difficult to manage, and more often show rapid decline when compared with patients without delusions. [38] Hallucinations are a less common

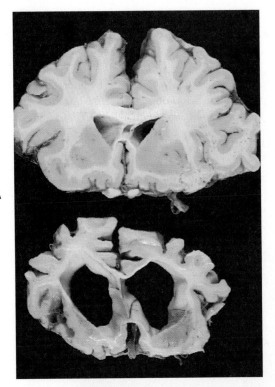

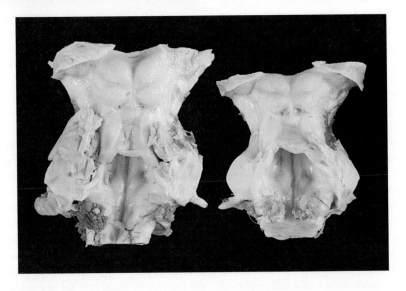

figure 9.10   Damage to frontal lobes and brainstem nuclei may explain some psychiatric symptoms in AD. **A,** Coronal sections through the frontal lobes of a normal brain *(top)* versus an Alzheimer's brain *(bottom)*, which demonstrates frontal lobe atrophy and ventriculomegaly. **B,** Brainstem of patient with end-stage AD *(right)* is significantly smaller as compared with an age-matched normal individual *(left)*. Patients with AD lose neurons from multiple brainstem nuclei, including substantia nigra (dopamine), locus ceruleus (norepinephrine), raphe (serotonin), and pedunculopontine (acetylcholine). Patients with AD do not have cranial nerve abnormalities (except olfaction) because brainstem motor and sensory nuclei are spared. *(Courtesy Dr. Richard E. Powers, Director, University of Alabama at Birmingham Brain Resource Program.)*

manifestation of AD and occur between only 9% and 27% of patients. Visual hallucinations are most common, followed by auditory or combined auditory and visual hallucinations. Typical visual hallucinations include persons from the past, intruders, animals, complex scenes, or inanimate objects.[74] Visual hallucinations may be indicative of a co-occurring delirium. Auditory hallucinations are often persecutory and usually accompany delusions. There is no precise anatomical localization for delusions,[31,115] but auditory hallucinations may be produced by damage to the temporal lobe.[78]

Mood Disorder

A variety of mood changes have been observed with AD, including depression, elation, and lability. Although few patients with AD meet the criteria for major depressive disorder, elements of depression do occur in 20% to 40% of AD patients. Tearfulness and thoughts of burden and worthlessness are often expressed. Suicide is rare but may occur. A family history of depressive disorders is quite common.[77] Anxiety has been reported in approximately 40% of patients. The most common manifestation is excessive worry and anticipatory concern regarding upcoming events.[74] Damage to brainstem nuclei may explain some depressive symptoms (Figure 9.10, B).[113]

Agitation

Agitation, a common symptom in dementia patients, is a vague clinical term indicating emotional, motor, or verbal activity not explained by the patient's needs or situation.[106] Caregivers or staff often misinterpret symptoms of cognitive impairment as agitation (e.g., repetitive question asking, struggling during ADLs, wandering about the unit, pacing). Distressed, vocal, or combative patients should be carefully evaluated before receiving sedatives. Patients with dementia become agitated for a variety of reasons, including pain, hunger, fear, boredom, fatigue, environmental chaos, and as a consequence of medications or medical problems (i.e., delirium). Staff should carefully document the time, duration, frequency, severity, and behavioral features of agitation.

Pain. Chronic, persistent pain is common in the elderly; approximately 25% of nursing home residents require some form of analgesic therapy. Extremity and joint pain, as well as visceral distress, are common. Oral pain caused by improperly fitting dentures or carious teeth causes agitation during eating. Patients with dementia and aphasia lose their ability to explain physical pain or to request pain medications. Rectal impaction and constipation are extremely uncomfortable, even for cognitively intact individuals, and may provoke agitation in patients with dementia. Ulcer pain and angina can go unrecognized in these patients. Clinicians should conduct a thorough review of physical conditions to determine whether a patient needs antacids, analgesics, laxatives, or nitrates to lessen pain and "agitation." Patients with severe dementia may not be able to accurately localize pain, and staff should not depend on patients to precisely define areas that hurt them. Patients with amnesia may forget that they experienced pain (e.g., angina) following the episode.

Hunger. Hunger can cause agitation in a patient with dementia. Physically active patients who eat part of their meals can become hungry. Patients with AD lose weight even with aggressive nutrition. Patients may develop very selective food preferences (e.g., sweets) or lose their appetite. Damage to hypothalamic or brainstem structures may explain these symptoms (see Figures 9.3 and 9.10, B). Staff should consider offering snacks to patients who become restless 1 or 2 hours following meals. Rigid diabetic calorie control is not worth the use of antipsychotic medication if the patient becomes hostile or restless. Patients with AD and diabetes may require less stringent glucose control to prevent hypoglycemic episodes and hunger. Dehydration and thirst are also important causes of agitation. Some patients forget the location of water and the operation of faucets or water fountains. Therefore patients should be prompted to take fluids every 2 hours to avoid becoming dehydrated, irritable, and constipated.

Fear. Patients with dementia can become afraid. Patients with AD cannot remember the names of their family, staff, or even themselves. This disorientation and lack of familiarity cause distress and fear. Reassurance and distraction are appropriate interventions for disoriented, fearful individuals. Verbal reassurance may have limited value in a patient with aphasia; in such cases caregivers must use nonverbal communication (e.g., smiling, gentle touch, calm voice) to assure distressed patients that all is well.

Boredom. Boredom is a major problem for patients with dementia. Recreational activities should consume as much patient time as possible. Television talk shows are not entertaining for patients with dementia and aphasia. The recreational staff can develop programs that entertain and engage patients with limited memory, communication skills, and motor skills.

Delirium. The abrupt onset of agitation is highly suggestive of delirium; a careful evaluation is required to exclude medical causes of confusion. Urinary tract infections, pneumonia, and other infections can lead to an acute mental status change. A new medication such as antihistamines, benzodiazepines, and narcotics can also cause confusion and agitation (see Chapter 12).

Akathisia. Patients may appear agitated as a consequence of neuroleptic medications. All antipsychotic medications and some medical drugs such as metoclopramide (Reglan) and cisapride (Propulsid) can cause akathisia. Akathisia is an inner sense of restlessness and motor activity caused by dopamine-blocking agents. Patients with akathisia often pace the halls, fail to sit still, and appear quite restless. Increasing the use of antipsychotic medications for this type of "agitation" will only worsen symptoms. Appropriate interventions include neuroleptic dose reductions, pro-

pranolol (Inderal), and low-dose benzodiazepines.

Environmental chaos. Environment can provoke agitation in some patients with dementia. Noisy, chaotic units cause such patients to become restless. Crowded, noisy day rooms can make patients fearful and restless. Hostile or loud roommates who disrupt sleep patterns can cause patients to become irritable.

An "agitated" patient with dementia presents a special diagnostic challenge to clinical staff. Clinicians must identify the cause of the agitation and consider behavioral interventions before using medications or restraints. Many types of agitation are made worse by sedatives and antipsychotic medications. Before administering these medications, clinicians should consider pain, hunger, fear, boredom, delirium, and medication side effects as possible causes of agitation. Patients who become agitated in response to hallucinations, delusions or depression warrant a careful trial with psychotropic medications. Patients who are depressed should be treated with antidepressant medications. Appropriate documentation for agitation includes a precise description of the frequency and severity of symptoms.

Sundowning. *Sundowning* refers to increased late afternoon or nocturnal activity by patients with AD.[33,95,106] Many patients with dementia are relatively calm in the morning and early afternoon but appear more confused and less manageable by approximately 4 or 5 PM. Psychotic symptoms may worsen, and the patient may not sleep at night. These patients often nap during the day and require less sleep than typical elders. The neuropathology of sundowning is unknown, but damage to subcortical structures may play some role in this behavior (see Figures 9.3 and 9.10). A combined pharmacological and behavioral management strategy is required to manage a patient who is experiencing sundowning. Sedating medications such as antipsychotics can be given in divided doses later in the afternoon and early evening. Sedative hypnotics are generally ineffective but can be tried. Behavioral management strategies include performing important activities such as bathing and shaving in the morning, when patients are less confused. Home safety programs, dead-bolt door locks to prevent escape, and nighttime sitters may be necessary for home management.[57] Patients with sundowning may exhaust caregivers; family support such as sitters or respite care is essential for maintaining home placement. Institutionalized elders (e.g., nursing home residents) can remain up until later hours but require supervision to prevent intrusion into other patients' rooms.

Other Behavioral Complications

New, troublesome behaviors are common in AD. Pacing and wandering are pervasive behaviors in the middle and late stages of AD. Providing self-contained spaces for wandering is a major challenge for residential facilities. Restlessness is reported in up to 60% of patients; angry outbursts occur in 50%, and assaultive behavior occurs in 20%.[32] Other behavioral changes have been described, including hypersexuality, sleep disturbance, and the Klüver-Bucy syndrome, which is characterized by hyperorality, hypermetamorphosis, emotional placidity, agnosia, and altered sexual behavior. This syndrome may occur in fragmentary form in the late stages of AD and may be associated with bilateral damage to amygdalae (see Figure 9.5).[10]

Clinical Management Implications

The management of dementia of the Alzheimer's type has four major components: (1) treating the cognitive deficit in selected patients, (2) ameliorating associated behavioral disturbances, (3) reducing the consequences of disability, and (4) addressing the needs of the caregiver (Table 9.3). In addition, patients who have a co-existing medical condition or psychiatric disorder contributing to the cognitive impairment will require treatment of that underlying disorder. Untreated or undertreated medical problems (e.g., COPD, ulcer disease) may worsen the patient's distress and confusion.

The cognitive deficit of AD improves moderately in some patients who are treated with tacrine (Cognex) or donepezil (Aricept). These drugs inhibit cholinesterase, enhance cholinergic function, and modestly produce improvement in cognition in one half to two thirds of those patients who can tolerate the drugs. Patients who respond usually improve to the level of function they had the previous year. Tacrine is potentially hepatotoxic, and liver aminotransferase (ALT) must be monitored every other week for several months as a safety precaution. Tacrine therapy also requires that the patient have a well-established diagnosis of AD, normal liver function, and a caregiver who is willing to administer the drug four times daily. Donepezil, which has been recently approved, requires no such monitoring and is not associated with hepatotoxicity. In addition, the dosage is 5 or 10 mg once daily, with clinical results similar to those seen with tacrine. Although the specific longitudinal or long-term effects of these cognitive-enhancing drugs remain to be seen, there is some indication that cognitive enhancers favorably affect the course of AD and improve noncognitive functions. Cholinominergic agents must be administered in therapeutic doses and meticulously monitored according to pharmaceutical company protocols. Families must be discouraged from expecting major improvement but encouraged to hope for sustained patient function that maintains independence and avoids nursing home care. Abrupt cessation of cholinomimetic agents may cause rapid deterioration of patient function.

Present treatment strategies focus on improving the function of surviving cholinergic neurons (see Figure 9.5). Newer medications or a combination of drugs may enhance the function of existing neurons in key transmitter systems such as the cholinergic, noradrenergic, and serotonergic systems. However, these medications do not address the fundamental problem in dementia (i.e., neuronal death). Future therapeutic strategy may include the prospective treatment of at-risk individuals with medications that either prevent the deposition of potentially toxic substances such as amyloid or directly correct the genetic factors that produce Alzheimer-type brain changes. Because multiple genes have been identified as possible

table 9.3
Treatment of Dementia

TREATMENT DOMAIN	FOCUS OF TREATMENT	INTERVENTION
Underlying disorder	Vascular dementia	Aspirin, ticlopidine
	Parkinson's disease	Selegiline, levodopa, bromocriptine, pergolide
	Depression	Antidepressants, electroconvulsive therapy
	Brain tumor	Surgery, radiation therapy, chemotherapy
	Hydrocephalus	Ventriculoperitoneal shunt
	Infections	Antibiotics
Cognitive impairment	Alzheimer's disease	Tacrine
Behavioral symptoms	Depression	Antidepressants, electroconvulsive therapy
	Psychosis	Antipsychotic agents
	Agitation	Antipsychotic agents, trazodone, carbamazepine, anxiolytics, propranolol
	Anxiety	Anxiolytics
	Insomnia	Sedative hypnotics
Consequences of disability	Seizures	Anticonvulsants
	Pneumonia	Antibiotics
	Urinary tract infection	Antibiotics
	Pressure ulcers	Preventive measures
Family	Psychotic distress	Counseling, support group, psychiatric care
	Exhaustion	Assisted home care, day care, respite care, residential care
	Financial planning, power of attorney	Legal consultation

From Cummings JL: Dementia: the failing brain, *Lancet* 345:1481-1484, 1995.

linkage sites for the disease, genetic strategies will require sophisticated, therapeutic interventions. The genetic locus for Huntington's disease (chromosome 4) has been known for more than a decade without the development of an effective preventive measure.[95] Preventive health measures such as hypertension control and smoking cessation have had limited success in the United States; AD prevention will probably follow the same course. Although molecular neurobiology is progressing rapidly, it is probable that effective prevention of AD may require 10 to 20 years for mass-scale implementation. It is anticipated that even with effective prevention, many mild-to-moderate cases will require treatment well into the twenty-first century.

Behavioral or noncognitive symptoms of AD often respond to nonpharmacological interventions such as avoiding circumstances that provoke behavioral outbursts, developing tolerant patient care environments, and teaching behavioral management strategies to family members and/or nurses. Nonpharmacological approaches are best exhausted before psychotropic drugs are used to control behaviors. When medications are used, the drug therapies should be guided by the specific diagnosis and target symptoms. Starting doses should be small, and doses should be increased slowly. The clinician should be aware of potential side effects and drug interactions, as well as of the effects of aging on metabolism. Patients with AD and other patients with dementia are especially vulnerable to the side effects of psychotropic drugs, which include sedation, confusion, and postural instability. The patient's medication regimen should be reviewed regularly; the amounts should be reduced or the drugs eliminated whenever possible.

Home-based dementia care addresses the needs of two individuals: the patient and the caregiver who provides assistance 24 hours per day, 7 days per week.[9] Care of the caregiver is an essential aspect of the total management of AD.[29,52] Family members provide most of the care that patients with AD receive, and this is a stressful undertaking. Increased rates of depression, psychotropic medication use, and stress-related illnesses are found among AD caregivers. Community resources such as assisted home care, day care, respite care, and extended residential care may reduce the burden. Participation in an Alzheimer's support group can help immensely, but some caregivers may require formal counseling or psychotherapy.[9]

Caregivers require detailed information and constructive realistic suggestions for each phase of the patient's illness.[45] They need information on the basic disease process, medications and side effects, monitoring for new medical or dental problems, organizing legal or financial issues, preparing for long-term care, and considerations for end-of-life planning. Extensive, consumer-friendly literature for family caregivers is available through most Alzheimer's support groups and through texts such as *The 36 Hour Day*.[67]

Conclusion

The four *As* of AD (actually the four *As* of dementia) are present in a range of neurodegenerative disorders. It is difficult for cognitively intact persons to understand the stress and anxiety produced by dementia. In the early phases of their disease, many patients with dementia understand they are losing cognitive functions. The stress of dementia can be likened to the emotions experienced by a person who begins a new job. The new employee cannot remember people's names, job

expectations, or even the location of the bathroom. To the patient with dementia and communication problems, dementia is like beginning a new job in a foreign country in which the patient speaks the language poorly. The patient may need to orient himself or herself to person, location, and schedule on a daily basis using a foreign language (i.e., his or her own). The cognitive disability of dementia can provoke the stress of a first day on a new job, except that patients with dementia relive this experience every day for the rest of their lives.

REFERENCES

1. Adams JH, Duchen LW, editors: *Greenfield's neuropathology,* ed 5, New York, 1992, Oxford University Press.
2. Agid Y, Javoy-Agid F, Ruberg M et al: Progressive supranuclear palsy: anatomoclinical and biochemical considerations, *Adv Neurol* 45:191-206, 1986.
3. Albert MS, Fleche G: Neuroimaging in Alzheimer's disease, *Psychiatr Clin North Am* 14:443, 1991.
4. Alzheimer A: Uber eine eigneartige Erkankung der Hirnrinde, *Alegemeine Zeitschrift fur Psychiatrie* 64:146, 1907.
5. American Psychiatric Association: *Diagnostic and statistical manual of mental disorders,* ed 4, Washington, DC, 1994, The Association.
6. Arendt T, Bigl V, Tennstedt A et al: Neuronal loss in different parts of the nucleus basalis is related to neuritic plaque formation in cortical target areas in Alzheimer's disease, *Neuroscience* 14:1, 1985.
7. Arispe N, Pollard HB, Rojas E: Giant multilevel cation channels formed by Alzheimer disease amyloid beta-protein [A beta P (1-40)] in bilayer membranes, *Proc Natl Acad Sci U S A* 90(22):10573-10577, 1993.
8. Bailey PA, Bonin GV. In Ivy AC, Kampmeier OF, Schour I et al, editors: *The isocortex of man,* Champaign, 1951, The University of Illinois Press.
9. Barrett JL, Haley W, Powers RE: Alzheimer's disease and their caregivers: medical care issues for primary care physicians, *South Med J* 89:1-90, 1996.
10. Benson DF: *The neurology of thinking,* New York, 1994, Oxford University Press.

11. Berglund M, Hagstadius S, Risberg J et al: Normalization of regional cerebral blood flow in alcoholics during the first 7 weeks of abstinence, *Acta Psychiatr Scand* 75:202-208, 1987.

12. Blessed G, Tomlinson BE, Roth M: The association between quantitative measures of dementia and of senile change in the cerebral grey matter of elderly subjects, *Br J Psychiatry* 114:797-811, 1968.

13. Boller F, Lopez OL, Moossy J: Diagnosis of dementia: clinicopathologic correlations, *Neurology* 38:76-79, 1989.

14. Braak H. In Barlow HB, Bizzi E, Florey E et al, editors: *Studies of brain function: architectonics of the human telecephalic cortex,* New York, 1980, Springer-Verlag.

15. Braak H, Braak E: Neuropathological staging of Alzheimer's-related changes, *Acta Neuropathol (Berl)* 82:239-259, 1991.

16. Braak H, Braak E, Grundke-Iqbal I et al: Occurrence of neuropil threads in the senile human brain and in Alzheimer's disease: a third location of paired helical filaments outside neurofibrillary tangles and neuritic plaques, *Neurosci Lett* 65:351-355, 1985.

17. Breitner JCS, Folstein MF: Familial Alzheimer's dementia: a prevalent disorder with specific clinical features, *Psychol Med* 14:63, 1994.

18. Breitner JC, Gau BA, Welsh KA et al: Inverse association of anti-inflammatory treatments and Alzheimer's disease: initial results of a co-twin control study, *Neurology* 44:227-232, 1994.

19. Brizzee KR, Ordy JM, Hofer H et al: Animal models for the study of senile brain disease and aging changes in the brain. In Katzman R, Terry RD, Bick KL, editors: *Alzheimer's disease: senile dementia and related disorders,* New York, 1978, Raven Press.

20. Brook P, Berrios GE: Delusions and the psychopathology of the elderly with dementia, *Acta Psychiatr Scand* 72:296-301, 1985.

21. Brun A, Englund E: A white matter disorder in dementia of the Alzheimer type: a pathoanatomical study, *Ann Neurol* 19:253-262, 1986.

22. Callaway R, Haley WE, Wadley VG: An Alzheimer's disease outreach education program for primary care physicians, *Gerontologist* 1994.

23. Celesia GA: Organization of auditory cortical areas in man, *Brain* 99(3):403-414, 1976.

24. Coleman PD, Flood DG: Neuron numbers and dendritic extent in normal aging and Alzheimer's disease, *Neurobiol Aging* 8:521-545, 1987.

25. Corder EH, Saunders AM, Strittmatter WJ et al: Gene dose of apolipoprotein E type allele and the risk of Alzheimer's disease in late-onset families (see comments), *Science* 261:828-829, 1993.

26. Corey-Bloom J, Thal LJ, Galasko D et al: Diagnosis and evaluation of dementia, *Neurology* 45:211-218, 1995.

27. Cork LC, Powers RE, Selkoe DJ et al: Neurofibrillary tangles and senile plaques in aged bears, *J Neuropathol Exp Neurol* 47:629-641, 1988.

28. Corsellis JAN: Posttraumatic dementia. In Katzman R, Terry RD, Bick KL, editors: *Alzheimer's disease and related disorders,* New York, 1978, Raven Press.

29. Council on Scientific Affairs AMA: Physicians and family caregivers: a model for partnership, *JAMA* 269:1282-1284, 1993.

30. Crystal H, Dickson D, Fuld P et al: Clinicopathologic studies in dementia: nondemented subjects with pathologically confirmed Alzheimer's disease, *Neurology* 38:1682-1687, 1988.

31. Cummings JL: Organic delusions: phenomenology, anatomical correlations, and review, *Br J Psychiatry* 146:184-197, 1985.

32. Cummings JL: Neuropsychiatric aspects of Alzheimer's disease and other dementing illnesses. In Yudofsky SC, Hales RE, editors: *The American Psychiatric Press textbook of neuropsychiatry,* ed 2, Washington, DC, 1992, American Psychiatric Press.

33. Cummings JL, Benson DF: *Dementia: a clinical approach,* ed 2, Boston, 1992, Butterworth-Heinemann.

34. Dam AM: The density of neurons in the human hippocampus, *Neuropathol Appl Neurobiol* 5:249-264, 1979.

35. Delaere P, He Y, Fayet G et al: βA4 deposits are constant in the brain of the oldest old: an immunocytochemical study of 20 French centenarians, *Neurobiol Aging* 14:191-194, 1993.

36. Dickson DE, Schmidt ML, Lee VM-Y et al: Immunoreactivity profile of hippocampal CA2/3 neurites in diffuse Lewy body disease, *Acta Neuropathol* 87:269-276, 1994.

37. Doty RL: Olfactory capacities in aging and Alzheimer's disease: psychophysical and anatomic considerations, *Ann NY Acad Sci* 640:20-27, 1991.

38. Drevets WC, Rubin EH: Psychotic symptoms and the longitudinal course of senile dementia of the Alzheimer type, *Biol Psychiatry* 25:39, 1989.

39. Eggers R, Haug H, Fischer D: Preliminary report on macroscopic age changes in the human prosencephalon: a stereologic investigation, *J Hirnforsch* 25:129-139, 1984.

40. Erkinjuntti T, Lee DH, Gao F et al: Temporal lobe atrophy on magnetic resonance imaging in the diagnosis of early Alzheimer's disease, *Arch Neurol* 50:305-310, 1993.

41. Ernst RL, Hay JW: The US economic and social costs of Alzheimer's disease revisited, *Am J Public Health* 84:1261-1264, 1994.

42. Esiri MM, Pearson RCA, Powell TPS: The cortex of the primary auditory area in Alzheimer's disease, *Brain Res* 366:385-387, 1986.

43. Flood DG, Buell SJ, Defiore CH et al: Age-related dendritic growth in dentate gyrus of human brain is followed by regression in the 'oldest old,' *Brain Res* 345:366-368, 1985.

44. Folstein MF, Folstein S, Robins P: "Mini mental state": a practical method for grading the cognitive state of patients for the clinician, *J Psych Res* 12:189-198, 1975.

45. Fortinsky RH, Hathaway TJ: Information and service needs among active and former family caregivers of persons with Alzheimer's disease, *Gerontologist* 30:604-609, 1990.

46. Foster NL: PET imaging. In Terry RD, Katzman B, Bick KL, editors: *Alzheimer disease*, New York, 1994, Raven Press.

47. Gearing M, Mirra S, Hedreen JC et al: The consortium to establish a registry for Alzheimer's disease (CERAD). X. Neuropathology confirmation of the clinical diagnosis of Alzheimer's disease, *Neurology* 45(3):461-466, 1995.

48. Giaquinto S: *Aging and the nervous system,* New York, 1988, John Wiley & Sons.

49. Glenner GG: Congophilic microangiopathy in the pathogenesis of Alzheimer's syndrome, *Med Hypotheses* 5:12-31, 1979.

50. Goldman JE, Yen S-H: Cytoskeletal protein abnormalities in neurodegenerative diseases, *Ann Neurol* 19:209-223, 1986.

51. Gottfries CG: Neurochemical aspects on aging and diseases with cognitive impairment, *J Neurosci Res* 27:541-547, 1990.

52. Haley WE, Clair JM, Saulsberry K: Family caregiver satisfaction with medical care of their demented relatives, *Gerontologist* 32:219, 1992.

53. Hanks SD, Flood DG: Region-specific stability of dendritic extent in normal human aging and regression in Alzheimer's disease. I. CA1 of hippocampus, *Brain Res* 540:63-82, 1991.

54. Haug H: Brain sizes, surfaces, and neuronal sizes of cortex cerebri: a stereological investigation of man and his variability and a comparison with some mammals (primates, whales, marsupials, insectivores, and one elephant), *Am J Anat* 180:126-142, 1987.

55. Haug H, Barmwater U, Eggers R et al: Anatomical changes in aging brain: morphometric analysis of the human prosencephalon. In Cervos-Navarro J, Sarkander HI, editors: *Brain aging: neuropathology and neuropharmacology,* New York, 1983, Raven Press.

56. Haug H, Kuhl S, Mecke E et al: The significance of morphometric procedures in the investigation of age changes in cytoarchitectonic structures of human brain, *J Hirnforsch* 25:353-374, 1984.

57. Hof PR, Morrison JH: Quantitative analysis of a vulnerable subset of pyramidal neurons in Alzheimer's disease. II. Primary and secondary visual cortex, *J Comp Neurol* 301:55-64, 1990.

58. Hyman BT, Van Hoesen GW, Damasio AR et al: Alzheimer's disease: cell-specific pathology isolates the hippocampal formation, *Science* 225:1168-1170, 1984.

59. Jack CR, Petersen RC, O'Brien PC et al: MR-based hippocampal volumetry in the diagnosis of Alzheimer's disease, *Neurology* 42:183, 1992.

60. Jellinger K: Quantitative changes in some subcortical nuclei in aging, Alzheimer's disease and Parkinson's disease, *Neurobiol Aging* 8:556-561, 1987.

61. Katzman R, Terry R, DeTeresa R et al: Clinical, pathological, and neurochemical changes in dementia: a subgroup with preserved mental status and numerous neocortical plaques, *Ann Neurol* 23:138-144, 1988.

62. Kemper T: Neuroanatomical and neuropathological changes in normal aging and dementia. In Albert ML, editor: *Clinical neurology of aging,* New York, 1984, Oxford University Press.

63. Larson EB, Reifler BV, Sumi SM et al: Diagnostic evaluation of 2000 elderly outpatients with suspected dementia, *J Gerontol* 40(5):536-543, 1985.

64. Lewis DA, Campbell MJ, Terry RD et al: Laminar and regional distributions of neurofibrillary tangles and neuritic plaques in Alzheimer's disease, *J Neurosci* 7:1799-1808, 1987.

65. Lubinski R, Orange JB, Henderson D et al: *Dementia and communciation,* San Diego, 1995, Singular Publishing.

66. Luxenberg JS, Haxby JV, Creasey H et al: Rate of ventricular enlargement in dementia of the Alzheimer type correlates with rate of neuropsychological deterioration, *Neurology* 37(7):1135-1140, 1987.

67. Mace NL, Rabins PV: *The 36-hour day,* Baltimore, 1991, Johns Hopkins University Press.

68. Mann DMA, Yates PO, Marcyniuk B: Monoaminergic neurotransmitter systems in presenile Alzheimer's disease and in senile dementia of Alzheimer type, *Clin Neuropathol* 3:199-205, 1984.

69. Masliah E, Miller A, Terry RD: The synaptic organization of the neocortex in Alzheimer's disease, *Med Hypotheses* 41:334-340, 1993.

70. Matsuyama H, Nakamura S: Senile changes in the brain in the Japanese: incidence of Alzheimer's neurofibrillary change and senile plaques. In Katzman R, Terry RD, Bick KL: *Alzheimer's disease: senile dementia and related disorders,* New York, 1978, Raven Press.

71. Maurer K, Riederer P, Beckmann S, editors: *Alzheimer's disease: epidemiology, neuropathology, neurochemistry, and clinics,* New York, 1990, Springer-Verlag.

72. McAllister TW, Powers RE: Approaches to treatment in dementing illness. In Emery OB, Oxman TE, editors: *Dementia: presentations, differential diagnosis, and nosology,* Baltimore, 1994, Johns Hopkins University Press.

73. McKhann G, Drachman D, Folstein M et al: Clinical diagnosis of Alzheimer's disease: report of the NINCDS-ADRDA work group under the auspices of Department of Health and Human Services task force on Alzheimer's disease, *Neurology* 34:939-944, 1984.

74. Mendez MF, Martin RJ, Smyth KA et al: Psychiatric symptoms associated with Alzheimer's disease, *J Neuropsychiatry Clin Neurosci* 2:28, 1990.

75. Mohs RC, Breitner JCS, Silverman JM et al: Alzheimer's disease: morbid risk among first-degree relatives approximates 50% by 90 years of age, *Arch Gen Psychiatry* 44:405, 1987.

76. O'Connor DW, Pollitt PA, Hyde JB et al: Do generational practitioners miss dementia in elderly patients? *Br Med J* 297:1107-1110, 1988.

77. Pearlson GD, Ross CA, Lohr WD et al: Association between family history of affective disorder and the depressive syndrome of Alzheimer's disease, *Am J Psychiatry* 147:452, 1990.

78. Penfield W, Perot P: The brain's record of auditory and visual experience, *Brain* 86:595-705, 1963.

79. Peng I, Binder LI, Black MM: Biochemical and immunological analyses of cytoskeletal domains of neurons, *J Cell Biol* 102:252-262, 1986.

80. Perry S, Cummings JL, Hill MA: Personality alterations in dementia of the Alzheimer type, *Arch Neurol* 45:1187, 1988.

81. Perry G, Cras P, Kawai M et al: Transformation of neurofibrillary tangles in the extracellular space, *Bull Clin Neurosci* 56:197, 1991.

82. Powers RE: The neurobiology of aging. In Coffey CE, Cummings JL, editors: *Textbook for geriatric neuropsychiatry,* Washington, DC, 1994, American Psychiatric Press.

83. Price JL, Davies PB, Morris JC et al: The distribution of tangles, plaques and related immunohistochemical markers in healthy aging and Alzheimer's disease, *Neurobiol Aging* 12:295-312, 1991.

84. Rabin PV, Pearlson GD, Aylward E et al: Cortical magnetic resonance imaging changes in elderly inpatients with major depression, *Am J Psychiatry* 148:617, 1991.

85. Rebeck GW, Reiter JS, Strickland DK et al: Apolipoprotein E in sporadic Alzheimer's disease: allelic variation and receptor interactions, *Neuron* 11:575,1993.

86. Reisberg B, Sorentien J, Salob SP et al: Behavioral symptoms in Alzheimer's disease: phenomenology and treatment, *J Clin Psychiatry* 48(suppl 5):9, 1987.

87. Riege WH, Metter EJ: Cognitive and brain imaging measures of Alzheimer's disease, *Neurobiol Aging* 9:69, 1988.

88. Risse SC, Raskind MA, Nochlin D et al: Neuropathological findings in patients with clinical diagnoses of probable Alzheimer's disease, *Am J Psychiatry* 147:168, 1990.

89. Rosene DL, Van Hoesen GW: The hippocampal formation of the primate brain: a review of some comparative aspects of cytoarchitecture and connections. In Jones EG, Peters A, editors: *Cerebral cortex,* New York, 1986, Plenum Press.

90. Schellenberg GD, Bird TD, Wijsman EJ et al: Genetic linkage evidence for a familial Alzheimer's disease locus on chromosome 14, *Science* 258:668, 1992.

91. Seldon HL: Cerebral cortex. In Jones EG, Peters A, editors: *The anatomy of speech perception: human auditory cortex,* New York, 1987, Plenum Press.

92. Sohrabji F, Miranda RC, Toran-Allerand CD: Estrogen differentially regulates estrogen and nerve growth factor mRNAs in adult sensory neurons, *Neuroscience* 14:459, 1994.

93. Strittmatter WJ, Weisgraber KH, Huang DY et al: Binding of human apolipoprotein to synthetic amyloid beta peptide: isoform-specific effects and implications for late-onset Alzheimer disease, *Proc Natl Acad Sci U S A* 90(17):8098-8102, 1993.

94. Strittmatter WJ, Weisgraber KH, Goedert M et al: Hypothesis: microtubule instability and paired helical filament formation in the Alzheimer disease brains are related to apolipoprotein E genotype (review), *Exp Neurol* 125:163, 172, 1994.

95. Strub RL, Black FW: *Behavioral disorders: a clinical approach,* Philadelphia, 1981, FA Davis.

96. Terry RD, Wisniewski HM: The ultrastructure of the neurofibrillary tangles and the senile plaque. In Wolstenholme GEW, O'Connor M, editors: *CIBA Foundation symposium on Alzheimer's disease and related conditions,* London, 1970, J&A Churchill.

97. Terry RD, Eliezer M, Hansen LA: Structural basis of the cognitive alterations in Alzheimer disease. In Terry RD, Katzman R, Bick KL, editors: *Alzheimer disease,* New York, 1994, Raven Press.

98. Tomlinson BE, Blessed G, Roth M: Observations on the brains of demented old people, *J Neurol Sci* 11:205-242, 1970.

99. Torack RM, Morris JC: The association of ventral tegmental area histopathology with adult dementia, *Arch Neurol* 45:497-501, 1988.

100. Uchihara T, Kondo H, Kosaka K et al: Selective loss of migral neurons in Alzheimer's disease: a morphometric study, *Acta Neuropathol (Berl)* 83:271-276, 1992.

101. Ulrich J: Senile plaques and neurofibrillary tangles of the Alzheimer type in nondemented individuals at presenile age, *Gerontology* 28:86-90, 1982.

102. Wallin A, Blennow K: Pathogenetic basis of multiinfarct dementia, *Alzheimer Dis Assoc Disord* 5:91-102, 1991.

103. Wallin A, Brun A, Gustafon L: Classification and nosology, *Acta Neurol Scand Suppl* 157:8-18, 1994.

104. Wallin A, Brun A, Gustafon L: Clinical methodology, *Acta Neurol Scand Suppl* 157:19-26, 1994.

105. Weinberger M, Gold DT, Divine GW et al: Expenditures in caring for patients with dementia who live at home, *Am J Public Health* 83:338-341, 1993.

106. Weiner MF: *The dementias: diagnosis, management, and research,* ed 2, Washington, DC, 1996, American Psychiatric Press.

107. Whitehouse PJ, Price DL, Clark AW et al: Alzheimer disease: evidence for selective loss of cholinergic neurons in the nucleus basalis, *Ann Neurol* 10:122-126, 1981.

108. Wilkinson IM, Graham-White J: Psychogeriatric dependency rating scale: a method of assessment for use by nurses, *Br J Psychiatr* 137:558-565, 1980.

109. Williams ME, Connolly NK: What participating physicians in North Carolina rate as their most challenging geriatric medicine concerns, *J Am Geriatr Soc* 38:1230-1234, 1990.

110. Winograd CH, Jarvik LF: Physician management of the demented patient, *J Am Geriatr Soc* 34:295-308, 1986.

111. Yamaguchi H, Hirai S, Morimatso M et al: A variety of cerebral amyloid deposits in the brains of Alzheimer's-type dementia demonstrated by beta-protein immunostaining, *Acta Neuropathol* 76:541, 1988.

112. Yesavage J: Differential diagnosis between depression and dementia, *Am J Med* 94(Suppl 5A):23S-28S, 1993.

113. Zubenko GS, Moossy J: Major depression in primary dementia, *Arch Neurol* 45:1182, 1988.

114. Zubenko GS, Huff FJ, Beyer J et al: Familial risk of dementia associated with a biologic subtype of Alzheimer's disease, *Arch Gen Psychiatry* 45:889, 1988.

115. Zubenko GS, Moossy J, Martinez J et al: Neuropathologic and neurochemical correlates of psychosis in primary dementia, *Arch Neurol* 48:619-624, 1991.

Other Dementias

Dementia is the permanent loss of multiple intellectual functions as a result of the death or dysfunction of neurons; it has multiple potential causes.[3,15,33] Alzheimer's disease (AD) is the most common cause of dementia, but many other conditions such as infections, tumors, vitamin deficiencies, intoxications, and metabolic disorders can destroy sufficient numbers of neurons to cause cognitive loss.[4,63] The five most common causes of dementia in adults are AD, vascular dementia, alcohol, diffuse Lewy body disease, and trauma.[33] Several other types of dementia receive considerable attention, including Pick's disease, normal-pressure hydrocephalus, and Creutzfeldt-Jakob disease. Comprehensive national statistics are not available on the incidence, prevalence, and causes of dementia in adults. Epidemiological studies are limited because a brain biopsy or autopsy examination is needed to confirm a diagnosis.

This chapter discusses the following three groups of dementias:

1. The most common types of dementia besides AD
2. Uncommon dementias that receive considerable attention by clinicians
3. Treatable disorders such as CNS infections and tumors

Neuropsychiatric symptoms associated with parkinsonism and other movement disorders are discussed in Chapter 13. Many other important causes of dementia such as progressive supranuclear palsy,[2] frontal lobe degeneration,[4] and Wilson's disease[26,43] are beyond the scope of this book.

This chapter focuses on cognitive loss in adults. Dementia is uncommon in children and is defined as mental retardation if the cognitive loss occurs before 18 years of age.[3] Brain trauma and infection are common causes of dementia in young adults, but most of the other dementias discussed in this chapter do not occur in the young.[16] Metabolic disorder diseases (e.g., metachromatic leukodystrophy, Krabbe's disease) occur in children and young adults but rarely in older adults.[1] A small number of uncommon dementias occur in young adults and middle-aged individuals (e.g., Wilson's disease,[26,43] Huntington's disease,[18] systemic lupus erythematosus[72]).

Vascular or Multiinfarct Dementia

There are many types or names of vascular dementia, including multiinfarct dementia (MID), mini-stroke dementia, hardening of the arteries, Binswanger's disease, and subcortical arteriosclerotic leukoencephalopathy (Table 10.1). Each type has a specific history or medical literature that lacks diagnostic precision because few patients have a single specific type of vascular disease. Most vascular dementia involves multiple types of ischemic brain injury. Before 1970 most cognitive loss in elderly patients was attributed to loss of brain tissue from multiple infarcts because most older patients with dementia have atherosclerosis and often have strokes of varying degrees and locations.[9,65] A stroke or infarct is the death or permanent dysfunction of neurons caused by insufficient oxygen and nutrients (Figure 10.1).[1] Cessation or reduction of blood flow causes most strokes. The common assumption that dementia is caused by vascular injury originated from medical folklore rather than the hard sciences. In the late 1960s Blessed, Tomlinson, and Roth[9,65] were the first to advocate that most dementia is caused by AD (see Chapter 9).

A broad range of psychopathology is produced

table 10.1
Common Types of Vascular Dementia

DISEASE TERMINOLOGY	COMMON LOCATION OF BRAIN LESION	CAUSE	CLINICAL FREQUENCY	PATHOLOGICAL FREQUENCY
Vascular dementia	Anywhere in CNS	All types of vascular or ischemic disease	Common	Common
Multiinfarct dementia	Anywhere in CNS but often cortical	Usually atherosclerotic vascular disease	Common	Common
Arteriosclerotic subcortical leukoencephalopathy	Deep white matter	Atherosclerosis or arteriolar sclerosis	Uncommon	Rare
Binswanger's disease	Deep white matter	Arteriolar sclerosis	Uncommon	Rare
Anoxic encephalopathy	Cerebral cortex and hippocampus	Hypotension or hypoxia	Uncommon	Uncommon

Common location, Typical site of brain lesion; *cause,* underlying vascular or systemic disease; *clinical frequency,* how common the disease is seen in clinical practice; *pathological frequency,* how commonly the disease is confirmed at autopsy.

by strokes, including demoralization, depression, anxiety disorders, mania, and dementia.[60] The type of stroke-induced psychopathology depends on the size, location, and age of the infarction, as well as preexisting psychiatric disorders.[62] Poststroke psychiatric disorders must be distinguished from vascular dementia.

Any type of vascular injury that kills or disconnects neurons can contribute to vascular dementia; the brains of most patients with vascular dementia demonstrate multiple types of strokes.[1,22,23] The amount of vascular damage must be substantial (e.g., greater than 100 cc), but no practical technique is available to measure the volume of infarcted brain. Ischemic injury can be subtle.[22] Animal studies demonstrate that brief periods of hypoxia (2 to 3 minutes) cause neurons to disappear without other evidence of damage. Because some anoxic neuronal injury may escape detection, measuring the extent of anoxic brain injury becomes difficult.[23]

The definition of vascular dementia does not specify the location of strokes, but strategically placed strokes (e.g., bilateral thalamus, Broca's

area) can have profound effects on cognitive function.[7] Vascular dementia is a global term for all types of vascular injury that cause cognitive loss.[68,69] Vascular dementia causes cognitive loss in 15% to 30% of patients with dementia. Although higher rates are quoted in some clinical studies, pathological reviews rarely describe vascular disease as causing more than 20% of all dementia in the elderly. There is no clear racial or socioeconomic bias, but vascular dementia is more common in individuals with hypertension.

The clinical symptoms of vascular dementia are often indistinguishable from those of AD.[63] Table 10.2 contrasts the broad range of findings in the three most common types of dementia: AD, vascular dementia, and diffuse Lewy body disease. Patients sometimes have a "stair-step" progression in which they suffer abrupt drops in levels of function. They often have neurological signs such as weakness or upgoing toes, which can be detected through a careful neurological examination. Clinical symptoms of vascular dementia sometimes fluctuate, and psychiatric symptoms are common. Patients often have preexisting cardiovascular dis-

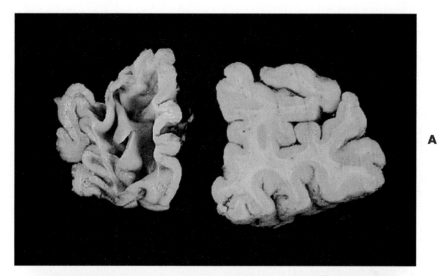

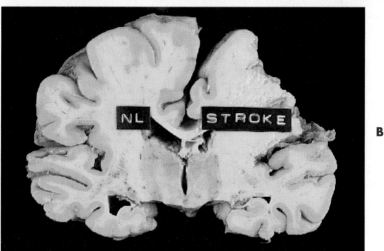

figure 10.1   Strokes in the frontal and parietal lobes caused by atherosclerosis. **A,** Extensive parenchymal loss in the left frontal lobe. **B,** Extensive infarction of the right parietal lobe caused by atherosclerotic vascular disease (see Figures 10.2 and 10.3). *(Courtesy Dr. Richard E. Powers, Director, University of Alabama at Birmingham Brain Resource Program.)*

ease, hypertension, and diabetes. Many have a past history of smoking. A detailed past medical history is therefore important to determine the risk for vascular dementia.

A simple screening instrument was developed by Hachinski[49,68,69] to assess an individual's risk for vascular dementia. The score of this brief symptom inventory correlates well with the risk for vascular dementia. Psychiatric symptoms, including hallucinations, delusions, and personality deterioration are common complications of vascular dementia. Although some authors suggest that psychiatric morbidity is more common in vascular dementia than in other cognitive disorders, these symptoms are common in all dementias.

Strokes result from three vascular factors: vessel wall abnormalities, vascular flow abnormalities, and blood constituent abnormalities. Any type of

table 10.2
Common Dementias Over Age 65

	ALZHEIMER'S DISEASE	VASCULAR DEMENTIA	DIFFUSE LEWY BODY DISEASE
Epidemiology			
Average age at onset	72	68	68
Percentage of all dementias	50%-65%	15%-20%	2%-20%
Symptoms			
Dementia	Yes	Yes	Yes
Symptom fluctuation	No	Yes	Yes
Extrapyramidal symptoms	Some	Rare	Frequent
Psychosis	Some	Some	Frequent
Dementia Treatment	Cholinomimetics	Prevention	None
Pathology	Senile plaques Neurofibrillary tangles	Ischemic brain injury (e.g., strokes, lacunes)	Lewy bodies

table 10.3
A Comparison of Atherosclerosis versus Arteriolar Sclerosis

DISEASE	LOCATION OF DAMAGE IN VESSEL	CAUSE	BRAIN PATHOLOGY	COMMON LOCATION
Atherosclerosis	Intima of large vessels	Hyperlipidemia Hypertension	Ischemia Infarction	Cortical
Arteriolar sclerosis	Media of medium and small vessels	Hypertension	Lacunar infarct, hemorrhage	Subcortical

cardiopulmonary disease, metabolic disorder, or intrinsic cerebrovascular disease that kills nerve cells may cause vascular dementia. For example, heart disease with poor perfusion, irregular heartbeats (e.g., arrhythmias), and atherosclerosis of the carotid arteries can reduce brain perfusion and destroy neurons.

Two major types of intrinsic cerebrovascular disease are common in the brains of individuals over age 50: atherosclerosis and arteriolar sclerosis (Table 10.3).[1] Atherosclerosis, or hardening of the arteries, involves damage to or fibrosis of the intima (inner layer) of the blood vessel, with deposition of cholesterol, lipid, and other debris within the vascular lining (Figures 10.2 and 10.3, *A*). Atherosclerosis is common at bifurcation points in larger diameter vessels. These damaged areas in arteries, called plaques, cause thrombosis (clots) or emboli. Debris or thrombi from plaques embolize into the cerebral arteries and occlude small vessels, which causes strokes of all degrees. Atherosclerotic vessels can also become thrombosed or occluded at the location of the plaque. Atherosclerotic occlusion of the vessel does not automatically cause stroke because collateral circulation may sustain the brain.

Arteriolar sclerosis is hypertensive damage to the muscular media (middle layer) of medium-

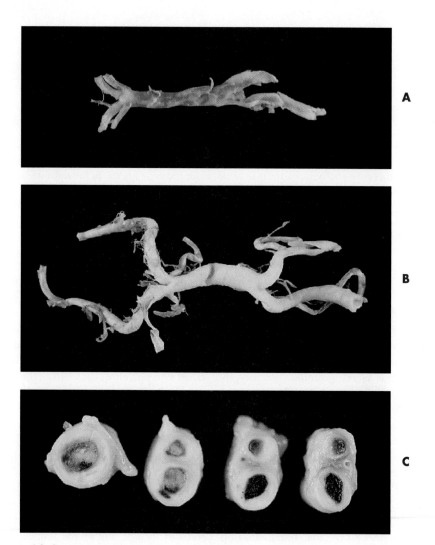

figure 10.2   Atherosclerosis in cerebral vessels. **A,** A normal basilar artery that appears translucent. The atherosclerotic vessel **(B)** has multiple yellow-white lesions along the vessel wall that are atherosclerotic plaques and a rigid appearance caused by stiffening of the wall. **C,** Cross section through the atherosclerotic blood vessel with extensive narrowing and thrombosis. The microscopic appearance is seen in Figure 10.3. *(Courtesy Dr. Richard E. Powers, Director, University of Alabama at Birmingham Brain Resource Program.)*

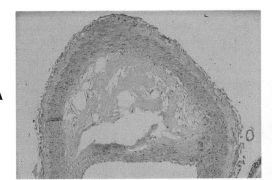
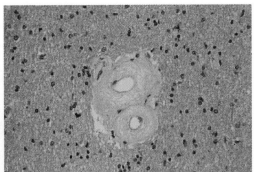

A

B

figure 10.3   Microscopic appearance of blood vessels with atherosclerosis and arteriolar sclerosis. **A,** Atherosclerosis damages the intima of this large artery. The granular material in the vessel wall represents debris that can embolize downstream in blood vessels and cause strokes. **B,** Arteriolar sclerosis damages the media and adventitia of small arteries, and this thickened small vessel can thrombose or rupture. *(Courtesy Dr. Richard E. Powers, Director, University of Alabama at Birmingham Brain Resource Program.)*

and small-caliber vessels that results in thrombosis or bleeding (Figure 10.3, *B*). The brain tissue around vessels with arteriolar sclerosis is often damaged, which may lead to slitlike strokes called lacunar infarcts (Figure 10.4).

Neurons require adequate levels of glucose and oxygen for survival.[1] Anoxic brain damage results from low blood pressure, low oxygen tension in blood, or low glucose levels. These conditions kill cortical neurons, especially those in vulnerable regions such as the hippocampus. Systemic diseases such as chronic obstructive pulmonary disease (COPD) or insulin-dependent diabetes can produce significant hypoxia or hypoglycemia.[20,27]

The diagnosis of vascular dementia is made with a careful clinical history, physical assessment, neurological examination, and brain imaging studies. There is no blood or spinal fluid test that distinguishes vascular dementia from other types of dementia such as AD. Some clinicians use the Hachinski scale to assess the risk for vascular dementia.

Both cortex and white matter can be damaged by vascular insufficiency. Brief periods (3 minutes) of hypoxia or hypotension, such as those experienced by individuals undergoing cardiopulmonary resuscitation, can kill neurons but leave the neuropil intact.[22] Neurons in selected brain regions, such as the hippocampus, are more vulnerable to anoxic damage than are neurons in other areas such as the motor strip. Patients who sustain anoxic brain damage may awaken with selective cognitive deficits such as amnesia.[52] Longer periods of hypoxia or hypoperfusion lead to strokes with necrosis and reabsorption of brain tissue, called encephalomalacia.[1] MID, the most common type of vascular dementia, results from multiple cerebral infarcts usually caused by thromboemboli (see Table 10.1).[68]

Binswanger's disease is a rare form of white matter vascular dementia and may demonstrate the stair-step progression typically seen in patients with MID.[13,21] Although this disease is often diagnosed by radiologists, it is rare in most autopsy series. Clinical symptoms are variable and can include any of the four *As* of dementia: amnesia, aphasia, apraxia, and agnosia. Psychiatric complications are common and include hallucinations, delusions, and depression. Patients with Binswanger's disease often have serious preexisting hypertension, and cigarette smoking is common.[13] There is no premortem test for Binswanger's disease. The white matter damage often appears on magnetic resonance imaging (MRI) scans; but a confirmed diagnosis requires a postmortem examination of the brain.

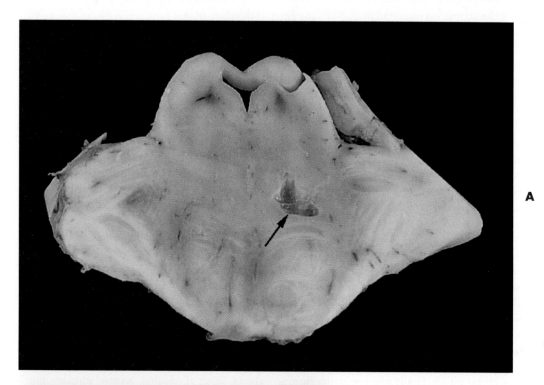

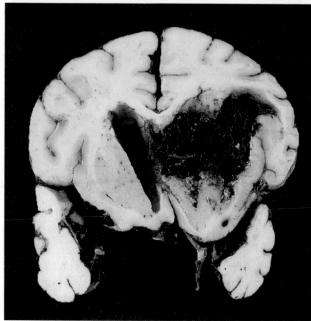

figure 10.4   Lacunar infarction (**A**) and intracerebral hemorrhage (**B**) resulting from hypertension. **A,** The pons has a small, slitlike loss of brain tissue in the middle of the basis pontis *(arrow)*. **B,** A hemorrhage into the basal ganglia extends into the lateral ventricle. *(Courtesy Dr. Richard E. Powers, Director, University of Alabama at Birmingham Brain Resource Program.)*

Dementia can be produced by primary vasculitis of the central nervous system (CNS) (i.e., inflammation of blood vessels or involvement of CNS vessels by systemic vasculitis).[47] Disorders such as lupus erythematosus often have CNS sequelae.[72] Clinicians may perform brain biopsies to identify this disease.

There is no specific treatment for vascular dementia. Anticoagulants such as aspirin may be helpful in patients with embolic disease. Controlling or correcting medical problems (e.g., controlling hypertension, stopping irregular heartbeats to improve cardiac function or blood oxygenation) may slow progression of the disease. "Vasodilator" medications such as ergots (e.g., Hydergine) are not clinically helpful.[41] The efficacy of surgically correcting extracranial cerebrovascular disease (i.e., carotid endarterectomy) is unclear. There is no known treatment for Binswanger's disease, but CNS vasculitis may respond to antiinflammatory therapy. Appropriate control of hypertension and cardiac disease may slow the progression of symptoms by slowing hypertensive damage to small blood vessels in brain white matter.[41] Although there are no specific family support groups for patients with vascular dementia, families should be encouraged to attend dementia support groups. Standard dementia behavior management techniques can be used for these patients. There is no specialty clinic or foundation for patients with vascular dementia.

Alcoholic Dementia

Alcoholic dementia accounts for between 1% and 10% of all cases of dementia in patients over age 65.[33,36] There is no genetic or racial predisposition, but men probably have higher rates than women. Alcoholic dementia usually occurs after prolonged, sustained drinking (i.e., 15 to 20 years) and may occur in patients under 65 years of age.[14,67] Patients with alcoholism often have past head trauma as a result of falls. Conditions such as subdural hematomas may worsen the symptoms of alcoholic dementia.

Alcoholic dementia is caused by the following:[36]

- The direct toxic effect of alcohol on neurons

- Alcohol-related nutritional deficiencies such as thiamine or B_{12}
- CNS effects from alcohol-induced multiorgan diseases such as cirrhosis and cardiomyopathy

Performance on neuropsychological tests is impaired in 50% to 70% of sober alcoholics, but most deficits are mild.[14] The clinical presentation of alcoholic dementia often resembles that of other dementias such as AD. Amnesia, apathy, slowness of thought process, and impaired judgment are common.[63,72] Alcohol causes multiple cognitive dysfunctions, and many patients have past episodes of other alcohol-related mental status changes.[34,63] Alcoholic blackouts, seizures, delirium tremens, and Wernicke's encephalopathy are common antecedents to dementia.[56,72] Korsakoff's psychosis is not a true dementia but includes impaired recent memory (see Chapter 8). Alcohol worsens cognitive impairment in elderly patients with other types of dementia.[32] Patients with alcoholic dementia develop both cognitive and psychiatric symptoms; behavioral manifestations may respond to the therapies previously described.

Patients with alcoholic dementia should totally abstain from all alcohol, receive adequate nutrition, and receive vitamin supplementation with thiamine, folate, and B_{12}.[14,20] The patient's dementia may be worsened by secondary health problems such as cirrhosis, pancreatitis, or hepatic encephalopathy. Cognition may improve when these serious medical problems are corrected. Good nutrition and management of health problems may result in slight improvement of alcoholic dementia over 1 to 2 years. In contrast to most patients with AD, who demonstrate a decline in Mini-Mental State Examination scores over time, patients with alcoholic dementia may show a small increase. Alcoholic dementia may not progress in patients who are abstinent.[8]

Psychotic symptoms can be treated with antipsychotic medications. Some elderly alcoholics have other major mental illnesses that require treatment (e.g., bipolar disorder).[61] Family members need to be educated about dementia and alcoholism. Patients should participate in Alcoholics Anonymous when they are intellectually capable of understanding the programs. Family members should be encouraged to attend Al

Anon. Behavioral complications can be managed with standard dementia home management programs. Patients who regain function are at a serious risk for drinking, and families must be vigilant to maintain sobriety.

Diffuse Lewy Body Disease

Diffuse Lewy body disease (DLBD) is a neurodegenerative disorder that may include dementia, abnormalities of the extrapyramidal motor system, and psychiatric symptoms.[4,50] The pathological feature of DLBD is the presence of multiple Lewy bodies in cortical or subcortical neurons. Lewy bodies are eosinophilic cytoplasmic inclusions measuring 5 to 10 μm in diameter. These masses of neurofilaments appear as circular cytoplasmic inclusions within neurons.[55] Lewy bodies in the brainstem have a central eosinophilic core that is surrounded by a clear halo (see Chapter 2); cortical Lewy bodies have only the eosinophilic core. Lewy bodies can occur in the brains of 5% of individuals over the age of 50, even in the absence of a known neurological disease. DLBD was largely unrecognized by neuropathologists until the late 1980s, but this tissue diagnosis is increasing because pathologists are searching for the inclusions and performing the necessary special stains.[38,53]

The cause of DLBD is unknown. There is no proven relationship to vascular disease, but many patients with AD also have Lewy bodies.[50] DLBD may account for 2% to 20% of all cases of dementia in elderly individuals; it is uncommon in individuals under 50 years of age. The male-to-female incidence ratio is unclear. DLBD develops earlier in life than does AD (68 years versus 72 years) and progresses more rapidly (average length of life of 5 years for DLBD versus 7 years for AD) (see Table 10.2). [42]

The typical clinical features of DLBD are dementia with fluctuating symptoms, extrapyramidal symptoms that resemble idiopathic parkinsonism, and hallucinations or delusions.[17,42] Cognition may fluctuate on a daily basis, and this fluctuation may distinguish DLBD from AD. The rapid change of symptoms can mimic the clinical feature of vascular dementia. Extrapyramidal

symptoms range from mild rigidity or bradykinesia to severe symptoms of parkinsonism. Auditory hallucinations are quite common.[50,53] The parkinsonism of DLBD results from damage to neurons in the substantia nigra. The cognitive deficits may result from global damage that includes the loss of cortical neurons or catecholamine inputs. No therapy is presently available for DLBD, but parkinsonian symptoms are improved with dopamine replacement, and psychiatric symptoms respond to psychotropic medications.[18,19]

There is no premortem diagnostic test for DLBD.[4] A definitive diagnosis requires both a brain autopsy by a pathologist who is familiar with the subtle pathological changes in this disorder and a laboratory that can perform ubiquitin immunocytochemistry.[38] The gross appearance of a brain with DLBD ranges from mild to moderate cortical atrophy that is usually less severe than in AD. Hippocampal atrophy may be present. Brainstem nuclei (i.e., the substantia nigra and locus ceruleus) are often depigmented as a result of damage to these catecholamine-producing centers.

The microscopic appearance of brains with DLBD includes multiple Lewy bodies in cortical or subcortical neurons.[53,54] These inclusions are commonly present in neurons within the temporal lobe and layers 5 or 6 of the parahippocampal cortex or cingulate cortices. Vacuolation of the neuropil, referred to as *spongiform change,* is often present, and the cortical Lewy bodies require special stains with ubiquitin antibody to accurately distinguish the number of cytoplasmic inclusions (Figure 10.5).[38] Lewy bodies are often present in subcortical neurons of the nucleus basalis of Meynert, hypothalamus, substantia nigra, locus ceruleus, and raphe. The brains of some patients (30% to 40%) with DLBD may also contain senile plaques and neurofibrillary tangles identical to those present in AD. Up to 20% of patients with AD may also have Lewy bodies present in cortical or brainstem neurons.[24] There are no specific guidelines to determine the "primary" cause of dementia in brains in which two or three pathological conditions are present.[70] The pathologist must either decide which type of injury is most intense or diagnose mixed dementia.

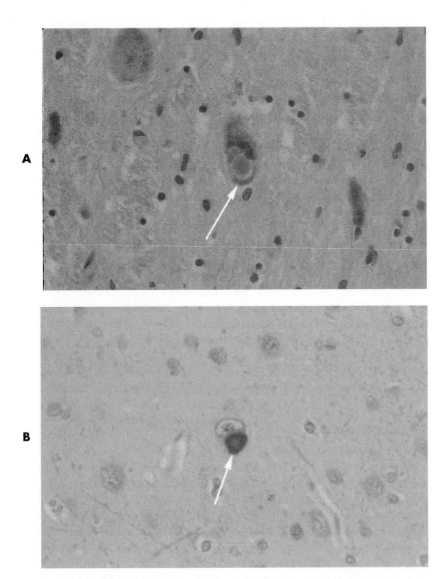

figure 10.5   Microscopic appearance of diffuse Lewy body disease. **A,** A typical Lewy body *(arrow)* within the cell of a pigmented neuron in the substantia nigra. This eosinophic inclusion has a clear halo and displaces the brown neuromelanin. **B,** A cortical Lewy body *(arrow)* stained dark brown with antibodies to ubiquitin that lacks the halo. *(Courtesy Dr. Richard E. Powers, Director, University of Alabama at Birmingham Brain Resource Program.)*

Trauma

Trauma is a common cause of neuropsychiatric disability in persons under the age of 45. Approximately 30% of all trauma fatalities result from head injury. In the United States, approximately 500,000 individuals have persistent neurological sequelae from head trauma. Up to 40% of patients with postconcussive syndrome suffer prolonged neuropsychiatric disability.[72] Patients who sustain serious head trauma may suffer from postconcussive confusion, amnesia, or dementia. Some patients never awaken but persist in a vegetative state. Head trauma also causes psychiatric sequelae that include anxiety, depression, and psychosis.[35,37]

Posttraumatic brain injury results from multiple pathogenetic mechanisms.[1] The neurological aftermath of a closed head injury includes the following: (1) direct mechanical trauma to brain parenchyma, (2) shearing of axons during massive, violent brain movement, (3) cerebral edema, (4) generalized hypoxia from other non-CNS accidental injuries (e.g., collapsed lungs, blood loss), and (5) intracranial bleeding such as subdural and subarachnoid hemorrhages or parenchymal hematomas.[16] The depth and duration of acute unconsciousness often predicts the severity of long-term brain injury and the likelihood of long-standing neuropsychiatric sequelae. Many patients with serious head trauma sustain several types of brain injury (e.g., edema, hypoxia, and bleeding). This cumulative damage results in the neuropsychiatric morbidity.

Subdural hematomas are collections of blood located beneath the dura and are caused by tearing of the bridging vein (veins that connect the brain to the sagittal sinus) (Figure 10.6). Elderly or alcoholic patients have an increased risk for developing subdural hematomas after head trauma.[14] The hematoma usually occurs over the lateral convexity; this clot may become a space-occupying mass that compresses the brain parenchyma. An untreated subdural hematoma can change from acute to chronic. Older or chronic hematomas are enclosed in membranes that resemble a sack with currant jelly in the middle. It can be absorbed over weeks or months, or it may slowly expand, with subsequent deterioration in function that causes a patient to appear demented. Subdural hematomas can be surgically drained but often recur unless the membranes are removed.[1] In contrast, epidural hematomas are located between the dura and skull and result from lacerations of the middle meningeal artery. Unless surgically drained, an epidural hemorrhage is rapidly fatal.

A subarachnoid hemorrhage involves bleeding onto the outer surface of the brain as a result of the laceration of small superficial vessels. This hemorrhage causes swelling, vasospasms, and additional brain injury. There is no effective surgical treatment.[63,72]

Direct trauma to the brain from falls or blows causes the brain tissue to collide with bony surfaces and produces a range of parenchymal lesions. Cerebral contusions (i.e., bruises) occur when the brain collides with bone (Figure 10.7). Cerebral lacerations result from the tearing of brain tissue.[1] Cerebral hematomas occur in brain parenchyma when blood vessels are torn by trauma. Massive shaking of the cranial contents can sever millions of axons as they pass through structures such as the corpus callosum, which results in diffuse axonal injury (DAI). Any brain injury can cause swelling (i.e., cerebral edema). Because the volume of the cranial vault cannot expand, the cortical surface presses against the skull as the volume of an edematous brain increases. The contents of the cranial vault can shift as the cerebrospinal fluid (CSF) is pressed out of the brain and the ventricular system is compressed (i.e., herniation). The cumulative damage of direct trauma, swelling, and herniation explains the high rates of neuropsychiatric disability that result from closed head injury.

Sixty percent of those patients with head injury make a good recovery without persistent neurological deficits. Some require extensive rehabilitation to relearn the tasks and information erased by the cortical damage. Unlike with degenerative dementias, rehabilitation is often successful in patients with brain trauma because the damage is not progressive.

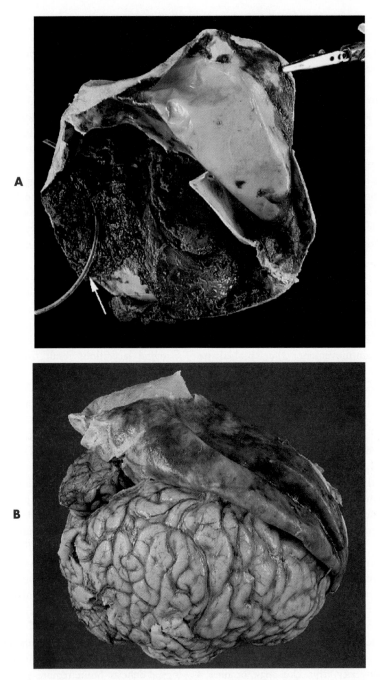

figure 10.6   Acute and chronic subdural hematomas in patients with closed head injury. **A,** An acute subdural clot is present on the underside of the dura. A catheter (*clear tube*) was surgically inserted to drain the blood (*arrow*). **B,** An older, organized subdural hematoma (i.e., chronic) with a glistening membrane on the reflected surface. *(Courtesy Dr. Richard E. Powers, Director, University of Alabama at Birmingham Brain Resource Program.)*

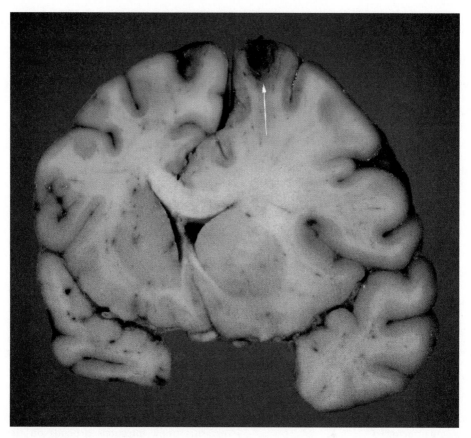

figure 10.7   Coronal brain section from an individual with head injuries following a motor vehicle accident. The V-shaped, purple-brown cortical lesion is a cerebral contusion (bruise) in the right
superior frontal gyrus (*arrow*). The brain is swollen (edema), and the right hemisphere is shifted to the
left (herniation). The blood on the outer surface is a subarachnoid hemorrhage. *(Courtesy Dr. Richard E.
Powers, Director, University of Alabama at Birmingham Brain Resource Program.)*

Infections

A variety of CNS infections cause dementia by
damaging neurons, axons, and dendrites (Table
10.4). The complications of acute bacterial infections such as edema, vascular thrombosis, and
anoxia can cause permanent cognitive decline.
Other types of meningitis (e.g., fungal, tuberculous), encephalitis, leukoencephalopathy, and
brain abscess can cause permanent cognitive loss.
The evaluation of dementia in young individuals
includes a lumbar puncture (LP) to exclude infectious etiologies. LPs are not performed in elderly

patients with "classic" AD because they are low-
yield, cost-ineffective procedures.[15,71] Clinicians
should consider CNS infection in any immunocompromised patient who has confusion or dementia (e.g., cancer patients, transplant recipients,
steroid recipients).

Syphilis was a common cause of dementia before the development of antibiotics.[51] Patients with
acquired immunodeficiency syndrome (AIDS) are
still at risk for CNS syphilis. CNS syphilis can
present with a constellation of cognitive and
neurological symptoms, including pupillary (eye)

table 10.4
Common Central Nervous System Infections That Cause Acute or Chronic Confusion*

INFECTION	TYPICAL CLINICAL COURSE	DEFINITIVE DIAGNOSTIC PROCEDURE
Bacterial meningitis	Acute	Lumbar puncture
Tuberculosis	Acute or chronic	Lumbar puncture Skin test
Fungal (e.g., cryptococcus)	Acute or chronic	Lumbar puncture
Viral (e.g., herpes)	Acute or chronic	Lumbar puncture Brain biopsy Serological tests
HIV	Chronic	Lumbar puncture Serological tests
Spirochete (e.g., syphilis)	Chronic	Lumbar puncture Serological tests
Rickettsial (e.g., Lyme disease)	Chronic	Serological tests Lumbar puncture
Prion (e.g., Creutzfeldt-Jakob)	Chronic	Brain biopsy

*The acute infection lasts for hours to days, whereas the chronic infection may persist for weeks to months. Lumbar puncture includes appropriate chemistry, cultures, and serological tests. Serological tests include the detection of antibodies against specific organisms or antigens. The definitive diagnostic procedure is the most helpful test in diagnosing the infection.

abnormalities, auditory disturbances, paresis, and sensory impairment.[39]

Tuberculous meningitis can cause confusion and dementia as a result of the meningitis or secondary vasculitis. CNS tuberculosis can present with minimal fever or other symptoms of infection.[63] Mycotic infections of the CNS can produce confusion and neurological symptoms. The most common fungal CNS infection in immunocompromised individuals is cryptococcosis, but others include blastomycosis and nocardiosis.[20]

Viral infections can cause dementia through brain damage from encephalitis, leukoencephalopathy, or the sequelae of meningitis.[5] Herpes infections of the brain can cause massive swelling and necrosis of the temporal lobe, resulting in seizures, psychiatric morbidity, and cognitive loss.[72] Many other brain infections can cause significant neuropsychiatric morbidity, including rickettsial infections (e.g., Lyme disease),[45,59,66] amebic brain infection, and CNS parasites.[1,58] The risk of significant intellectual or psychiatric

morbidity from amebic, protozoan, and other parasitic brain infections depends on the geographical location of the patient and the patient's immune status.

Appropriate antimicrobial or antiviral therapy stops the progression of dementia caused by most infections. Behavioral complications are managed as they are with all dementias (see Chapter 9).

Creutzfeldt-Jakob Disease

Creutzfeldt-Jakob (CJ) disease is a prion-mediated disorder that accounts for fewer than 1% of all cases of dementia; it produces a high level of anxiety in health care workers, undertakers, and families.[11,75] A prion is an infectious particle that is smaller than a virus. This genetic fragment resists all methods of decontamination and is almost impossible to isolate. There is no gender, racial, or socioeconomic predisposition for the infectious disease, but approximately 10% is familial. The collection of prion-mediated diseases also includes

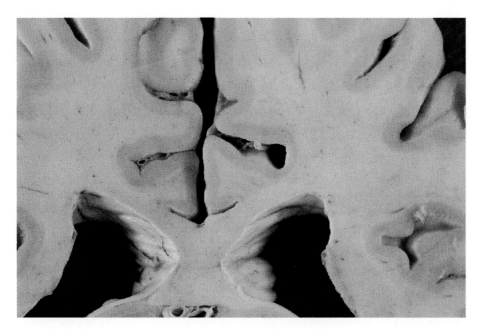

figure 10.8   The brain of a patient with Creutzfeldt-Jakob disease. The cingulate gyrus atrophy is mild despite severe spongiform degeneration (see Figure 10.9) and advanced dementia. *(Courtesy Dr. Richard E. Powers, Director, University of Alabama at Birmingham Brain Resource Program.)*

Gerstmann-Sträussler-Scheinker disease (GSS), fatal familial insomnia (FFI), and kuru.[12,25,57] A similar organism is implicated in mad cow disease and scrapie (a disease found in sheep).

Patients with CJ disease develop rapidly progressive dementia, myoclonus (jerking of arms and legs), and a characteristic electroencephalographical pattern with high voltage bursts of biphasic and triphasic slow waves. Most patients (90%) with CJ disease die within 18 months, but in rare cases a patient can survive for up to 7 years.[10,11] Some forms of CJ disease run in families (10%) and are referred to as Gerstmann-Sträussler-Scheinker syndrome. There are no specific neurological, neuropsychological, or psychiatric manifestations that confirm the clinical diagnosis of CJ disease. Brain imaging may show atrophy or a normal brain, and other blood or CSF tests are nonspecific.

The gross appearance of brains of patients with CJ disease ranges from normal to atrophic (Figure 10.8). There is no specific pattern of atrophy that distinguishes CJ disease from AD. The microscopic appearance includes cortical neuronal loss, gliosis, and spongiform degeneration, (i.e., multiple vacuoles within the neuropil) in grey matter (Figure 10.9). Amyloid plaques that contain amyloid protein derived from prion proteins may be present. The microscopic changes that occur with CJ disease are usually present in the cortex but may be found in subcortical or brainstem structures.[6,12]

CJ disease is produced by a prion that infects the brain and CNS tissues of victims. This disease can be transmitted by inoculation of brain tissues, including the brain, pituitary, and corneas.[73] The prion is not transmitted via blood products. Most cases of CJ disease occur spontaneously in the population; scientists do not know how an infected individual contracts the prion. Some health care workers have contracted the disease via neurosurgical or autopsy contamination with nervous tissues.

Antimicrobial and antiviral medications are not

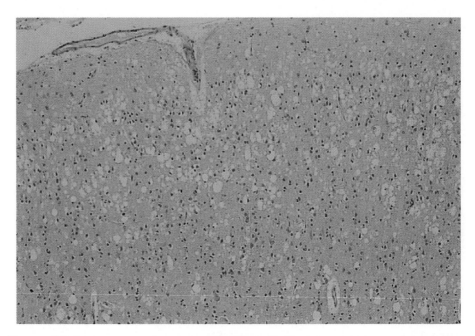

figure 10.9   Microscopic appearance of the severe spongiform change of Creutzfeldt-Jakob disease (i.e., vacuoles in the neuropil), which is undetectable in the gross specimen. *(Courtesy Dr. Richard E. Powers, Director, University of Alabama at Birmingham Brain Resource Program.)*

effective for prion-mediated diseases. Many patients develop psychiatric complications that are treated with appropriate psychotropic medications and behavioral management strategies. Surgical procedures that involve the exposure of nerve or brain tissue (e.g., cataract extractions) should be avoided. Many patients undergo a brain biopsy to exclude treatable causes of rapidly progressive dementia such as infection or vasculitis. These brain biopsies and other neurosurgical procedures should be performed with great care. Although tissue confirmation of CJ disease allows the family to make appropriate plans, most neurosurgeons are hesitant to perform a biopsy on patients who are known to have CJ disease.

Because undertakers may be hesitant to embalm patients with CJ disease, families should make advanced arrangements to identify a funeral director who is willing to provide such services. There is no evidence of person-to-person transmission of this disease other than exposure to nervous system tissue. Laboratory and histology personnel who handle brain tissue should use special precautions for these cases. Autopsy brain removal must be performed with great care because bone saws can aerosolize brain tissues. Formalin fixation does not inactivate the prion; special fixatives must be used. Formalin-fixed, paraffin-embedded blocks remain infectious. Patients who may have CJ disease should not donate blood. Because standard methods used to sterilize surgical instruments do not kill the prion, special, extraordinary measures should be used to ensure that surgical instruments are adequately sterilized following a brain biopsy or autopsy. There is no evidence that nursing personnel are at increased risk for developing CJ disease, but standard universal precautions should be used.

Pick's Disease

Pick's disease is a rare neurodegenerative disorder of unknown cause that is diagnosed in fewer than 2% of autopsy series on patients with de-

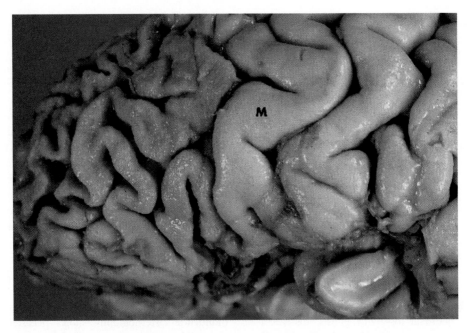

figure 10.10   Pick's disease involving the frontal lobe with marked atrophy of the prefrontal region *(left)* and sparing of the motor strip *(M) (right)*. Other lobes were of normal volume. *(Courtesy Dr.*
Richard E. Powers, Director, University of Alabama at Birmingham Brain Resource Program.)

mentia.[4] There is no race or gender bias for the
disease, and affected individuals usually manifest
symptoms between ages 50 and 70.[4] Patients with
Pick's disease commonly have language problems
and neuropsychiatric symptoms, including hallucinations, delusions, and personality changes.
Compared with AD, the initial symptoms of
Pick's disease often include personality change,
hyperorality, disinhibition, roaming, and speech
disturbances.[44] Focal neurological signs are usually
absent, with sparing of motor and sensory function. Brain imaging demonstrates selective lobular
atrophy that suggests Pick's disease more often
than AD.[44,72] Pick's disease is progressive, and the
life expectancy is similar to that of AD (3 to 20
years, with an average life expectancy of 5 to 7
years). There is no premortem diagnostic test for
Pick's disease; a brain biopsy or autopsy confirmation is required. There is no known genetic component to Pick's disease nor any evidence for toxic
causes. Cytoskeletal abnormalities differ from

those seen in AD and occur in the neurons of
damaged lobes. The pathological diagnosis is confirmed by identifying Pick's bodies within individual nerve cells.[1]

There is no treatment for Pick's disease. Psychiatric symptoms can be managed with standard
psychotropic medications. Behavior manifestations are managed using strategies identical to
those used to manage AD (see Chapter 9). Patients with Pick's disease do not develop parkinsonism.

Pick's disease is also called lobar atrophy because individuals with this disease manifest symmetrical, severe bilateral atrophy of single lobes
(Figure 10.10). Isolated bilateral temporal or
frontal atrophy is most common, but selective atrophy of the parietal or occipital lobes is also possible. This cortical atrophy is most severe in the
association cortex, with relative sparing of the primary motor or sensory cortex.[1,48]

The microscopic alterations of Pick's disease are

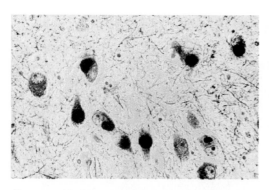

figure 10.11   Microscopic appearance of Pick bodies (i.e., circular silver-stained neuronal inclusions diagnostic of Pick's disease). *(Courtesy Dr. Richard E. Powers, Director, University of Alabama at Birmingham Brain Resource Program.)*

usually limited to the atrophic lobes and include severe neuronal loss with gliosis, distended or bloated neurons, and Pick's bodies (circular, silver-stained cytoplastic inclusions within neurons) (Figure 10.11).[28] Damaged neurons and Pick's bodies contain abnormal collections of tau, neurofilaments, and other cytoskeletal components.[29] Brains with Pick's disease do not contain large numbers of senile plaques, neurofibrillary tangles, or amyloid deposits.

No specific foundation or information centers are available for individuals with Pick's disease. However, family caregivers should receive support and education about dementia. They can also benefit from Alzheimer's or dementia support groups because their patients will develop problems similar to those experienced by patients with AD or vascular dementia.

Normal-Pressure Hydrocephalus

Normal-pressure hydrocephalus (NPH) accounts for approximately 1% of all dementia and receives this contradictory name because the patients have both a relatively "normal" CSF pressure and evidence of hydrocephalus.[4] In fact, the CSF pressure is not completely normal! There is no racial, gender, or socioeconomic bias for developing NPH.[72]

Patients with NPH usually manifest gait problems, urinary incontinence, and dementia.[31] The clinical symptoms of dementia can resemble those of AD or vascular dementia, and many patients manifest apathy, irritability, or social disinhibition (i.e., frontal lobe signs). These patients have a wide, unsteady gait with feet that shuffle along the floor; this type of gait is sometimes referred to as a magnetic gait, as though the feet are stuck to the floor with magnets. Urinary incontinence occurs early in the disease, and dementia usually follows later. Patients also develop psychiatric symptoms. The typical symptoms of increased intracranial pressure (e.g., headache, vomiting) are usually absent.

The diagnosis of NPH is suggested by a characteristic computerized axial tomography (CAT) or magnetic resonance imaging (MRI) scan, which demonstrates very large ventricles. Radionuclide cisternography shows persistent radionuclide in ventricles after 24 hours and persistence in cisterns or over convexities after 48 hours. The diagnosis of NPH can be confirmed when the neurosurgeon monitors the pressure in a patient's brain and documents periods of elevated pressure waves (i.e., B waves) for 2 hours during the 2 days of monitoring.

Although the cause of NPH is unknown, there is slowing of the flow of spinal fluid through the ventricular system, which results in periodic elevation of CSF pressure. The ventricular system is usually patent, and obstruction may occur at the level of the arachnoidal granulations (see Chapter 1). Patients often have a past history of head trauma or CNS infection that may precipitate fibrosis of arachnoidal granulations or stenosis of narrow points in the flow of CSF (e.g., cerebral aqueduct). Some patients demonstrate significant improvements when large quantities of CSF (e.g, 50 ml) are withdrawn from the arachnoidal space via the spinal canal.[74]

The autopsy examination of brains from patients with NPH shows dilation of the lateral, third, and fourth ventricles, with widening of the cerebral aqueduct.[1] The microscopic appearance is unremarkable (Figure 10.12).

Patients with NPH undergo ventriculoperi-

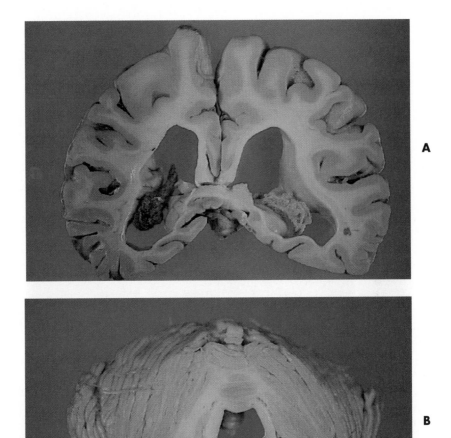

figure 10.12   Brain alterations typical of normal-pressure hydrocephalus. **A,** Massive enlargement of the occipital horn of the lateral ventricles. **B,** Dilation of the fourth ventricle. Microscopic examination of this NPH brain was unremarkable, and no obstruction to the flow of CSF was identified. *(Courtesy Dr. Richard E. Powers, Director, University of Alabama at Birmingham Brain Resource Program.)*

toneal shunt placement to drain spinal fluid out of the brain and relieve pressure (Figure 10.13). In this procedure, which is used in many diseases besides NPH, a burrhole is drilled through the skull and a catheter is threaded through brain tissue into the lateral ventricle. This fenestrated tube is connected to a reservoir that sits outside the burrhole and under the scalp. The reservoir empties into a tube that is tunneled under the scalp, neck, chest, and abdomen, where this catheter drains into the peritoneal space. The CSF is drained from the ventricle through the reservoir and out

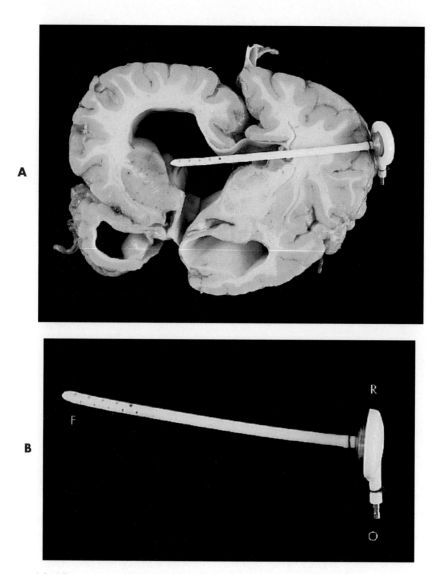

figure 10.13   Demonstration of shunting, a common neurosurgical procedure used in many neurological diseases. **A,** This coronal brain section from a child with hydrocephalus demonstrates an intraventricular shunt with the catheter in the lateral ventricle and a reservoir (the circular white bladder) that would sit outside the burrhole through the skull. **B,** The shunt includes a fenestrated drainage tube *(F)* that sits in the ventricle, a reservoir *(R)*, and the metal fitting that secures the outflow catheter *(O)*. *(Courtesy Dr. Richard E. Powers, Director, University of Alabama at Birmingham Brain Resource Program.)*

into the peritoneal space, where it is reabsorbed like all other fluids. Infection does not occur because the flow is one-way and the peritoneum is sterile. The drainage from this shunting procedure may arrest the progression of dementia and improve bladder control or gait. However, the existing dementia is often irreversible. Older patients (an average age of 75 years) show less improvement than younger patients following shunt insertion. The decision to insert a shunt is made on a case-by-case basis.[72]

Psychotic symptoms produced by NPH can be treated with standard psychopharmacology. The standard behavioral management strategies used with patients with AD are useful for NPH (see Chapter 9). Families should be referred to dementia support groups, and standard dementia education should be recommended. No regional or national association exists for patients with NPH.

Other Types of Dementia

A range of other diseases cause cognitive loss in adults.[4,72] Chronic intoxication with heavy metals such as lead or mercury can cause dementia. Chronic lead ingestion by children results in mental retardation. Chronic exposure to other toxic substances such as hydrocarbons also increases the risk for cognitive loss. For example, painters have higher rates of neuropsychological deficits than other groups.[46] The microscopic neuropathology of chronic heavy metal and hydrocarbon intoxication is nonspecific and can involve gliosis, blood vessel changes, and other conditions.

Specific endocrine disorders can cause cognitive impairment. Hypothyroidism, chronic hypoglycemia, and hypercalcemia can produce dementia, psychiatric symptoms such as depression or psychosis, and confusion.[72] There is no specific neuropathological abnormality for thyroid or parathyroid disease, but hypoglycemia can cause neuronal loss that resembles hypoxia in the hippocampus and other brain areas.[1]

Vitamin deficiencies such as B_{12} or folate can cause several neurological problems, including peripheral neuropathy, spinal cord degeneration, and dementia. Vitamin deficiencies occur in a range of medical problems, including pernicious anemia and bowel disease. Blood levels for vitamins are easily determined, and dementia may improve with vitamin replacement therapy. Vitamin deficiency dementia lacks a specific gross or microscopic neuropathological condition, except in cases of thiamine deficiency; the brains of individuals with this type of deficiency manifest alterations of Wernicke's encephalopathy.

Strategically placed brain tumors cause a range of neuropsychiatric symptoms, including psychosis, seizures, confusion, and dementia.[72] Intrinsic brain tumors such as gliomas grow very slowly and efface exisiting brain structures. A glioma is a growth of malignant astrocytic or oligodendroglial cells. This slow, insidious tumor can lead to a subtle cognitive decline that mimics dementia. Limbic gliomas are tumors that grow through the limbic system; they often present with neuropsychiatric symptoms.[40]

A broad range of neurological diseases produce neuropsychiatric symptoms, including dementia. To develop a differential diagnosis, the clinician must consider the patient's age, speed of symptom progression, neurological signs, preexisting medical conditions, sequence of neuropsychological morbidity, and psychiatric comorbidity. Basic tests such as brain imaging, heavy metal screens, and vitamin panels can exclude many diagnoses. In many instances the clinician must usually await the autopsy to establish a definitive diagnosis.

REFERENCES

1. Adams JH, Duchen LW, editors: *Greenfield's neuropathology*, ed 5, New York, 1992, Oxford University Press.
2. Agid Y, Javoy-Agid F, Ruberg M et al: Progressive supranuclear palsy: anatomoclinical and biochemical considerations, *Adv Neurol* 45:191-206, 1986.
3. American Psychiatric Association: *Diagnostic and statistical manual of mental disorders,* ed 4, Washington, DC, 1994, The Association.
4. Barba GD, Boller F: Non-Alzheimer degenerative dementias, *Curr Opin Neurol* 7:305-309, 1994.
5. Barnes DW, Whitley RJ: CNS diseases associated with varicella zoster virus and herpes simplex virus infections: pathogenesis and current therapy, *Neurol Clin* 4(1):265-283, 1986.

6. Bell JE, Ironside JW: Neuropathology of spongiform encephalopathies in humans, *Br Med Bull* 49:738-777, 1993.

7. Benson DF: *The neurology of thinking,* New York, 1994, Oxford University Press.

8. Berglund M, Hagstadius S, Risberg J et al: Normalization of regional cerebral blood flow in alcoholics during the first 7 weeks of abstinence, *Acta Psychiatr Scand* 75:202-208, 1987.

9. Blessed G, Tomlinson BE, Roth M: The association between quantitative measures of dementia and of senile change in the cerebral grey matter of elderly subjects, *Br J Psychiatry* 114:797-811, 1968.

10. Brown P, Rodgers-Johnson P, Cathala F et al: Creutzfeldt-Jakob disease of long duration: clinicopathological characteristics, transmissibility and differential diagnosis, *Ann Neurol* 16:295-304, 1984.

11. Brown P, Cathala F, Castaigne P et al: Creutzfeldt-Jakob disease: clinical analysis of a consecutive series of 230 neuropathologically verified cases, *Ann Neurol* 20:597-602, 1986.

12. Budka H, Aguzzi A, Brown P et al: Neuropathological diagnostic criteria for Creutzfeldt-Jakob disease and other human spongiform encephalopathies (prion diseases), *Brain Pathol* 5:459-466, 1995.

13. Caplan LR, Schoene WC: Clinical features of subcortical arteriosclerotic encephalopathy (Binswanger disease), *Neurology* 12:1206-1215, 1978.

14. Charness ME, Sim RP, Greenberg DA: Ethanol and the nervous system, *N Engl J Med* 321:442-453, 1989.

15. Corey-Bloom J, Thal LJ, Galasko D et al: Diagnosis and evaluation of dementia, *Neurology* 45:211-218, 1995.

16. Corsellis JAN: Posttraumatic dementia. In Katzman R, Terry RD, Bick KL: *Alzheimer's disease and related disorders,* New York, 1978, Raven Press.

17. Crystal HA, Dickson DW, Lizardi JE et al: Antemortem diagnosis of diffuse Lewy body disease, *Neurology* 40:1523-1528, 1990.

18. Cummings JL: Neuropsychiatric aspects of Alzheimer's disease and other dementing illnesses. In Yudofsky SC, Hales RE, editors: *The American Psychiatric Press textbook of neuropsychiatry,* ed 2, 26:605, 1992.

19. Cummings JL, Benson DF: *Dementia: a clinical approach,* ed 2, Boston, 1992, Butterworth-Heinemann.

20. Evans JG, Williams TF, editors: *Oxford textbook of geriatric medicine,* New York, 1992, Oxford University Press.

21. Fredriksson K, Brun A, Gustafson L: Pure subcortical arteriosclerotic encephalopathy (Binswanger's disease): a clinicopathological study, *Cerebrovasc Dis* 2:82-86, 1992.

22. Garcia JH: The evolution of brain infarcts: a review, *J Neuropathol Exp Neurol* 51:387-393, 1992.

23. Garcia JH, Brown GG: Vascular dementia: neuropathologic alterations and metabolic brain changes, *J Neurol Sci* 109:121-131, 1992.

24. Gibb WRG, Mountjoy CQ, Mann DMA et al: A pathological study of the association between Lewy body disease and Alzheimer's disease, *J Neurol Neurosurg Psychiatry* 52:701-708, 1989.

25. Goldfarb LG, Brown P: The transmissible encephalopathies, *Ann Rev Med* 46:57-65, 1995.

26. Grimm G, Prayer L, Oder W et al: Comparison of functional and structural brain disturbances in Wilson's disease, *Neurology* 41:272-276, 1991.

27. Hazzard WR, Andres R, Bierman EL et al, editors: *Principles of geriatric medicine and gerontology,* ed 2, New York, 1990, McGraw-Hill.

28. Hof PR, Bouras C, Peri DP et al: Quantitative neuropathologic analysis of Pick's disease cases: cortical distribution of Pick bodies and coexistence with Alzheimer's disease, *Acta Neuropathol* 87:115-124, 1994.

29. Izumiyama Y, Ikeda K, Oyanagi S: Extracellular or ghost Pick bodies and their lack of tau immunoreactivity: a histological, immunohistochemical and electron microscopic study, *Acta Neuropathol* 87:277-283, 1994.

30. Jack CR, Petersen RC, O'Brien PC et al: MR-based hippocampal volumetry in the diagnosis of Alzheimer's disease, *Neurology* 42:183-188, 1992.

31. Katzman R: Normal pressure hydrocephalus. In Katzman R, Terry RD, Bick KL, editors: *Alzheimer's disease: senile dementia and related disorders,* ed 7, New York, 1978, Raven Press.

32. King MB: Alcohol abuse and dementia, *Int J Geriatr Psych* 1:31-36, 1986.

33. Larson EB, Reifler BV, Sumi SM et al: Diagnostic evaluation of 2000 elderly outpatients with suspected dementia, *J Gerontol* 40(5):536-543, 1985.

34. Lee K, Moller L, Hardt F et al: Alcohol-induced brain damage and liver damage in young males, *Lancet* 2(8146):759-761, 1979.

35. Lewin W, Marshall TF, Roberts AH: Long-term outcome after severe head injury, *Br Med J* 2:1533-1538, 1979.

36. Lieber CS: Medical disorders of alcoholism. In Flier JS, Underhill LH, editors: Seminars in medicine of the Beth Israel Hospital, *N Engl J Med* 333:1058-1063, 1995.

37. Lishman WA: Brain damage in relation to psychiatric disability after head injury, *Br J Psychiatry* 114:373-410, 1968.

38. Lowe J, Mayer RJ, Landon M: Ubiquitin in neurodegenerative diseases, *Brain Pathol* 3:55-65, 1993.

39. Luxon L, Lees AJ, Greenwood RJ: Neurosyphilis today, *Lancet,* 1(8107):90-93, 1979.

40. Malamud N: Psychiatric disorder with intracranial tumors of the limbic system, *Arch Neurol* 17:113-123, 1967.

41. McAllister TW, Powers RE: Approaches to treatment in dementing illness. In Emery OB, Oxman TE, editors: *Dementia: presentations, differential diagnosis, and nosology,* Baltimore, 1994, The Johns Hopkins University Press.

42. McKeith IG, Fairbairn AF, Perry RH et al: The clinical diagnosis and misdiagnosis of the senile dementia of Lewy body type (SDLT), *Br J Psychiatry* 165:324-332, 1994.

43. Medalia A, Isaacs-Glaberman K, Scheinberg IH: Neuropsychological impairment in Wilson's disease, *Arch Neurol* 45:502-504, 1988.

44. Mendez MF, Selwood A, Mastri AR: Pick's disease versus Alzheimer's disease: a comparison of clinical characteristics, *Neurology* 43:289-292, 1993.

45. Meurers B, Kohlhepp W, Gold R et al: Histopathological findings in the central and peripheral nervous systems in neuroborreliosis: a report of three cases, *J Neurol* 237:113-116, 1990.

46. Mikkelsen S, Jorgensen M, Browne E et al: Mixed solvent and organic brain damage: a study of painters, *Acta Neurol Scand Suppl* 78(118):1-143, 1988.

47. Moore PM, Cupps TR: Neurological complications of vasculitis, *Ann Neurol* 14:155-167, 1983.

48. Munoz-Garcia D, Ludwin SK: Classical and generalized variants of Pick's disease: a clinicopathological, ultrastructural, and immunocytochemical comparative, *Ann Neurol* 6:467-480, 1984.

49. Olga V, Emery B, Oxman TE, editors: *Dementia presentations, differential diagnosis, and nosology,* Baltimore, 1994, The Johns Hopkins University Press.

50. Olichney JM, Galasko D, Corey-Bloom J et al: The spectrum of disease with diffuse Lewy body. In Weiner WJ, Lang AE: *Behavioral neurology of movement disorders: advances in neurology,* ed 65, New York, 1995, Raven Press.

51. Pachner AR: Spirochetal diseases of the CNS, *Neurol Clin* 4(1):207-222, 1986.

52. Penfield W, Mathieson G: Memory: autopsy findings and comments on the role of hippocampus in experimental recall, *Arch Neurol* 31:145-154, 1974.

53. Perry RH, Irving D, Blessed G et al: Senile dementia of Lewy body type: a clinically and neurologically distinct form of Lewy body dementia in the elderly, *J Neurol Sci* 95:119-139, 1990.

54. Perry EK, McKeith I, Thompson P et al: Topography, extent, and clinical relevance of neurochemical deficits in dementia of Lewy body type, Parkinson's disease, and Alzheimer's disease, *Ann NY Acad Sci* 640:197-202, 1991.

55. Pollanen MS, Dickson W, Bergeron C: Pathology and biology of the Lewy body, *J Neuropathol Exp Neurol* 52:183-191, 1993.

56. Price J, Kerr R, Hicks M: The Wernicke-Korsakoff syndrome: a reappraisal in Queensland with special reference to prevention, *Med J Aust* 147:561-570, 1987.

57. Prusiner SB, DeArmond SJ: Prion diseases and neurodegeneration, *Ann Rev Neurosci* 17:311-339, 1994.

58. Reik L: Disorders that mimic CNS infections, *Neurol Clin* 4(1):223-247, 1986.

59. Reik L, Burgdorfer W et al: Neurologic abnormalities in Lyme disease without erythema chronicum migrans, *Am J Med* 81:73-78, 1990.

60. Robinson RG, Bolduc PL, Price TR: Two-year longitudinal study of poststroke disorders: diagnosis and outcome at one and two years, *Stroke* 18:837-843, 1987.

61. Saunders PA, Copeland JRM, Dewey ME et al: Heavy drinking as a risk factor for depression and dementia in elderly men; findings from the Liverpool Longitudinal Community Study, *Br J Psych* 159:213-216, 1991.

62. Starkstein SE, Robinson RG, Price TR: Comparison of patients with and without poststroke major depression matched for size and location of lesion, *Arch Gen Psych* 45:247-252, 1988.

63. Strub RL, Black FW: *Behavioral disorders: a clinical approach*, Philadelphia, 1981, FA Davis.

64. Terry RD, Eliezer M, Hansen LA: Structural basis of the cognitive alterations in Alzheimer disease. In Terry RD, Katzman R, Bick KL, editors: *Alzheimer disease*, New York, 1994, Raven Press.

65. Tomlinson BE, Blessed G, Roth M: Observations on the brains of demented old people, *J Neurol Sci* 11:205-242, 1970.

66. Vallat JM, Hugon J, Lubeau M et al: Tick-bite meningoradiculoneuritis: clinical, electrophysiologic, and histologic findings in 10 cases, *Neurology* 37:749-753, 1987.

67. Victor M, Banker BQ: Alcohol and dementia. In Katzman R, Terry RD, Bick KL: *Alzheimer's disease: senile dementia and related disorders*, New York, 1978, Raven Press.

68. Wallin A, Blennow K: Pathogenetic basis of vascular dementia. In *Alzheimer's disease and associated disorders*, New York, 1991, Raven Press.

69. Wallin A, Blennow K: Heterogeneity of vascular dementia: mechanisms and subgroups, *J Geriatr Psych Neurol* 6:177-188, 1993.

70. Wallin A, Brun A, Gustafson L: Classification and nosology, *Acta Neurol Scand Suppl* 157:8-18, 1994.

71. Wallin A, Brun A, Gustafon L: Clinical methodology, *Acta Neurol Scand Suppl* 157:19-26, 1994.

72. Weiner MF: *The dementias: diagnosis, management, and research*, ed 2, Washington, DC, 1996, American Psychiatric Press.

73. Weller RO, Steart V, Powell-Jackson JD: Pathology of Creutzfeldt-Jakob disease associated with pituitary-driven human growth hormone administration, *Neuropathol Appl Neurobiol* 12:117-129, 1986.

74. Wikkelso C, Anderson H, Blomstrand C et al: Normal pressure hydrocephalus: predictive value of the cerebrospinal fluid tap–test, *Acta Neurol Scand* 73:566-573, 1986.

75. Will RG, Matthews WB: A retrospective study of Creutzfeldt-Jakob disease in England and Wales 1970-1979 I. Clinical features, *J Neurol Neurosurg Psych* 47:134-140, 1984.

AIDS Dementia and Other AIDS-Related Neuropsychiatric Disorders

Infectious diseases of the central nervous system (CNS) often produce neurological or psychiatric morbidity. Human immunodeficiency virus (HIV)–related neuropsychiatric syndromes occur in approximately one third of adults and one half of children with acquired immunodeficiency syndrome (AIDS).[18] Four broad categories of neuropsychiatric problems arise from HIV infection:[2]

- Psychological distress related to a fatal illness
- Neuropsychiatric complications of the primary HIV brain infection
- Neuropsychiatric complications of secondary opportunistic brain infections or secondary brain tumors
- Nervous system complications from medical therapies

The frail physical health of patients with AIDS complicates the interpretation and management of their neuropsychiatric problems.

Epidemiology and Demographics

AIDS is a costly national and international problem. The National Foundation for Brain Research estimates the cost of AIDS in the United States to be approximately $66.5 billion per year when both personal costs and mortality costs are combined.[22] This spending level represents an enormous portion of the American health care dollar. The rate of AIDS dementia has fallen with

antiviral therapy, but neuropsychiatric complications continue to pose major problems with patient management (Box 11.1).[26,29] All health care professionals who treat patients with AIDS must become familiar with the neuropsychiatric complications.

AIDS is caused by the Lentivirus subfamily of the human retrovirus, which attacks the human immune system. AIDS is distinguished from HIV infection by the presence of opportunistic infections (e.g., *Pneumocystis carinii*), AIDS-related malignancies (e.g., Kaposi's sarcoma), or a significant depression of the CD4/CD8 lymphocyte ratio. Patients with AIDS often develop a range of fluctuating physical complaints, including fatigue, weight loss, anorexia, and malaise. The patient's suppressed immune system allows unusual fungal, viral, and bacterial infections to occur in the brain, which causes a multitude of neuropsychiatric symptoms.

It is estimated that 22 million people are infected with HIV worldwide, with 10,000 new cases occurring daily.[26] Furthermore, 6.8 million people have developed AIDS, and another 1 million deaths have been documented since 1981.[26] In the United States, approximately 1.5 million people are infected with HIV. This total includes between 107,000 and 150,000 women.[31] The incidence of HIV infection among white men is declining, but as much as 3% of the black male population

box 11.1 ▰▰▰▰▰▰

Neuropsychiatric Disorders Associated with HIV Infection and AIDS

Adjustment disorders: can include depressed or anxious mood

Affective disorders: depression, mania, suicidal ideation

Anxiety disorders: generalized anxiety disorder, panic attacks

Organic mental disorders: AIDS dementia complex, tumor-associated diseases such as cerebral lymphoma

Delirium: related to infection, medication, or multiorgan failure

Personality disorders: borderline or antisocial

Substance abuse disorders: polysubstance abuse, intravenous drug usage

Other: hypochondriasis, obsessive-compulsive disorder, bereavement

between ages 30 and 44 is affected.[29] These differences among racial and ethnic groups may be more reflective of socioeconomic variables.[26]

Three broad groups of patients contract HIV infections: neonates, children and adolescents, and adults. A small but growing number of elderly patients are now contracting the disease. Approximately 10% of the AIDS cases reported in the United States in 1995 involved individuals over 50 years of age, and 30% of this cohort was 60 years of age or older.[8,28]

The clinical manifestations and neuropsychiatric complications of HIV infection and AIDS vary by group. The typical neonate develops HIV from its HIV-positive mother; the transmission rate ranges from 21% to 27%.[33] The neurodevelopmental implications of congenital HIV infections are unknown. Most infants do not survive into late adolescence or adulthood to demonstrate the effect of the virus on intellectual development. However, a few infants born seropositive do become seronegative within approximately 1 year. Neurological manifestations are common in children with AIDS. A progressive encephalopathy

occurs in which children lose motor milestones.[33] However, the long-term developmental and psychiatric effect on children is unknown. A small number of children contract the virus via sexual contact or drug usage. Adolescents are also vulnerable to HIV infection and AIDS as a result of high-risk behaviors (i.e., unprotected sex and intravenous [IV] drug use).

HIV is not transmitted via casual contact; it is transmitted via blood products or bodily fluids (e.g., semen).[26] Specific adult high-risk groups include IV drug users, prostitutes, promiscuous homosexual men, and individuals with hemophilia. HIV infection is highly preventable but requires the alteration of highly driven behaviors (e.g., discontinuing IV drug usage, using safe sexual practices). HIV transmission via the stored blood transfusion supply is rare, but patients who receive large volumes of blood products, such as those with hemophilia, remain at risk. Health care workers assume slightly higher risks for developing HIV through exposure to blood or bodily fluids.[8]

Psychobiological Considerations

HIV infection is detected by the host's production of antibodies against the virus. Following infection, the human body requires 2 to 6 months to produce detectable levels of antibodies. This latency period allows small numbers of unsuspecting donors who have been infected with HIV to give blood that is negative for antibodies. Two tests screen for these antibodies: the Enzyme-Linked ImmunoSorbent Assay (ELISA) method, which is less specific but more cost-effective; and the Western blot method, which is highly specific and expensive.[9] Some false-positives and false-negatives occur with the ELISA/enzyme immunoassay (EIA) method and require the Western blot for confirmation.[9] HIV testing should always include patient counseling and strict confidentiality. Individuals who are HIV-seropositive should be educated on ways to prevent transmission and on their responsibility to inform others of the infection (e.g., spouses, health care workers).

Individuals infected with HIV do not develop AIDS until 5 to 7 years after the primary infection. The initial viral infection resembles a flulike syndrome. The virus infects the immune system and other organs. It enters the human brain through the bloodstream by crossing the blood-brain barrier. Significant brain infection probably does not occur during the initial asymptomatic stages and may be delayed until the development of AIDS.[25] The CNS infection has three general stages[18]:

1. Entry into CNS macrophages
2. Invasion and replication within brain macrophages
3. Production of neurotoxic substances by CNS macrophages and astrocytes, which causes neuronal damage or death

The initial stage of CNS infection includes the virus crossing the blood-brain barrier and entering the microenvironment of the brain. The timing of and mechanism for HIV infection of the CNS is unknown. In the second stage of CNS infection, the HIV attaches to the brain macrophage by using the gp120 proteoglycans that bind to macrophage receptors (Figure 11.1). The macrophage internalizes this complex, and the cell begins to produce low levels of neurotoxins that are released into the extracellular environment. Following ingestion by the macrophage, the virus inserts itself into the macrophage genome and begins to replicate. This process produces large quantities of various neurotoxic substances that stimulate adjacent astrocytes to elaborate additional substances, including cytokines, tumor necrosis factor, and interleukins.[18,25] Each chemical has a profound effect on the microenvironment of the brain. The astrocyte plays a dual role by attempting to control the environment while also producing substances that increase damage.

There is no direct evidence that HIV infects the neuron.[18] Patients both with and without dementia have the virus in their CNS tissue, and the viral load does not predict the risk for developing dementia.[11] Neuronal damage may be caused by an excitotoxic effect produced by alterations of

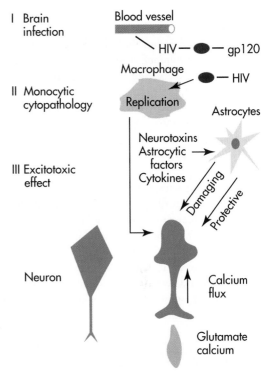

figure 11.1   The basic molecular mechanisms by which HIV infection damages the brain. Although neuronal dysfunction explains the clinical symptoms of AIDS, the pathogenetic mechanisms involve macrophages and astrocytes. Neuronal dysfunction may be caused by the disruption of brain microenvironment rather than by direct viral infection of neurons. *(Courtesy Dr. Richard E. Powers, Director, University of Alabama at Birmingham Brain Resource Program.)*

neuronal calcium metabolism and overactivation of *N*-methyl-D-aspartate (NMDA) receptors.[18] The end result is neuronal death or diminished neuronal function as a result of decreased numbers of dendrites. The complicated cascade of events causes proliferation of macrophages, activation of astrocytes, and neuronal loss or dendritic regression. Pharmacological attempts to block the viral brain damage are hampered by this complicated cascade of cellular events.

Some research focuses on preventing viral entry into the target cell or replication of the virus within the CNS.[12] Other research focuses on blocking the excitotoxic effects that mediate neuronal damage.[18] Drugs that block calcium channels (e.g., nimodipine), medications that antagonize the NMDA receptor (e.g., memantine), and drugs that stabilize the postsynaptic NMDA receptor (e.g., nitroglycerin) are three potential methods of protecting the brain from HIV damage caused by substances released from macrophages and astrocytes.

HIV infection also damages white matter via unknown mechanisms. It is unknown whether HIV infects the oligodendrocyte, but multiple theories attempt to explain the white matter pallor that commonly occurs in the brains of patients with AIDS. Some scientists theorize that HIV infection triggers an autoimmune phenomenon similar to multiple sclerosis,[32] whereas others hypothesize that soluble cytotoxic substances damage the oligodendrocytes.[18]

Clinical Applications

Clinical Findings and Course

Patients with AIDS experience a range of psychiatric complications as a result of the primary HIV brain infection.[6,10,19,20] Many patients complain of depressive symptoms typical of endogenous depression and difficulties with concentration. The mechanism of AIDS-induced depression is unknown, but depressive symptoms are common in other chronically medically ill patients. Depression can be confused with dementia, but depressive symptoms are improved with antidepressants. Patients with AIDS may also develop manic symptoms and anxiety disorders. The standard medications for depression, anxiety, and mania are effective in patients with HIV-related neuropsychiatric complications.

AIDS Dementia Complex

AIDS dementia complex is a term that describes a variable mixture of cognitive, motor, and behavioral abnormalities in patients with AIDS.[18] Approximately 60% of those individuals infected with HIV who develop AIDS will also develop dementia.[25] Dementia may be the presenting symptom in some HIV-infected individuals.[27] Approximately 90% of AIDS fatalities demonstrate neuropathological alterations in the brain at autopsy; this observation suggests that more patients may develop symptoms as improved medical therapy lengthens the duration of survival.[15,24,25,32] These abnormalities are distinct from the opportunistic CNS infections that result from immunosuppression.

The clinical course of AIDS dementia can be divided into three stages: early, middle, and late.[25] The speed of progression, symptom constellation, and terminal end points vary from patient to patient. Early symptoms include difficulties with concentration, memory, and conceptualization. As the dementia progresses, patients can develop apraxia, hyperreflexia, dysarthria, and frontal lobe dysfunction. Patients with late-stage dementia may demonstrate apathy, withdrawal, and unresponsiveness. Neurodiagnostic testing for AIDS dementia does not confirm or exclude the diagnosis. Structural brain imaging (computed axial tomography [CAT] or magnetic resonance imaging [MRI] scans), electrophysiological studies (electroencephalograms [EEGs]), and functional brain imaging (single photon emission computed tomography [SPECT] and positron emission tomography [PET] scans) consistently show nonspecific abnormalities in patients with clinically diagnosed AIDS dementia.[2,16] Premortem clinical studies can exclude other diseases such as meningitis but cannot confirm the AIDS dementia complex. Other infectious diseases common to patients with AIDS, including cryptococcosis and progressive multifocal leukoencephalopathy (PML), can produce dementia-like symptoms. These diseases must be excluded before the diagnosis of primary AIDS dementia can be made. Many cases of dementia result from a combination of primary HIV brain infection and secondary AIDS-related CNS disease.[16,17,24]

The variable pathological findings in the brains of patients with AIDS dementia fail to correlate with the severity of dementia. Brains from individuals with AIDS dementia complex manifest variable degrees of cortical atrophy and ventricu-

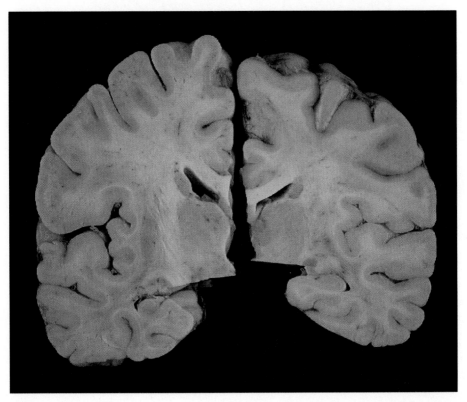

figure 11.2   The gross appearance of AIDS dementia. Comparison of a coronal section through cerebral hemispheres from a normal patient *(left)* and a patient with AIDS *(right)*. Although the AIDS brain is smaller and atrophic, there is no specific distinguishing lesion. *(Courtesy Dr. Richard E. Powers, Director, University of Alabama at Birmingham Brain Resource Program.)*

lomegaly (Figure 11.2).[16] No specific brain region is consistently damaged by the virus.

The microscopic findings in the brains of patients with AIDS and dementia are usually non-specific, and the histopathological alterations of cortex are variable. Some cases demonstrate almost no abnormal microscopic findings, whereas other brains have extensive gliosis, microglial nodules, and a proliferation of individual glial cells (Figure 11.3). Immunoperoxidase preparations with anti-HIV antibodies stain macrophages and microglial cells and indicate the presence of HIV within these cells.[15,23,24,34] Quantitative measures of cerebral cortex show variable reductions in the numbers of neurons and simplification of dendritic arborization.[25] Massive, region-specific neu-

ronal loss is not consistently identified. The microscopic appearance of white matter damage includes pallor and thinning. Microglial cells, astrocytes, and multinucleated giant cells are often present without massive white matter necrosis or inflammation. Basal ganglia, brainstem, and cerebellar histopathology are equally nonspecific. Biochemical and neurochemical studies fail to demonstrate specific abnormalities in the brain tissue of patients with AIDS dementia complex. The white matter of the spinal cord can develop a vacuolar myelopathy, which is a peculiar degeneration of the lateral and posterior columns with marked vacuolation. Some patients with AIDS also develop a peripheral neuropathy with either motor or sensory symptoms.

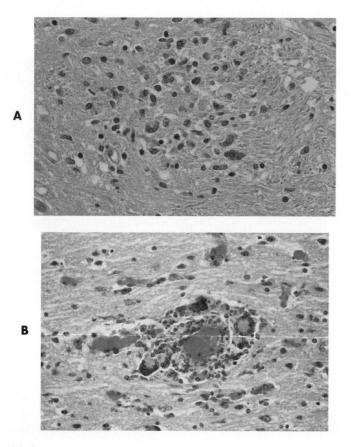

figure 11.3   The typical microscopic features of AIDS encephalopathy include microglial nodules **(A)** and perivascular inflammation in white matter **(B)**. *(Courtesy Dr. Richard E. Powers, Director, University of Alabama at Birmingham Brain Resource Program.)*

Secondary Opportunistic Brain Infections

Patients with AIDS are predisposed to fungal, bacterial, viral, and other infections of the brain and spinal cord (Table 11.1). These infections can present with symptoms that range from confusion to coma. The four common types of secondary brain infections in patients with AIDS are meningitis, cerebritis, brain abscess, and leukoencephalopathy. Meningitis is an infection of the leptomeninges of the brain, whereas cerebritis is the direct infection of brain tissue. A brain abscess is a circumscribed focus of parenchymal brain infection with associated inflammation, edema, and necrosis. Brain abscesses can persist for weeks or months and can develop a "capsule" composed of astrocytes, fibroblasts, and inflammatory cells. Leukoencephalopathy involves damage to white matter with the loss of myelinated axons.

Bacterial infections. Bacterial infections can cause meningitis, cerebritis, or brain abscess. Bloodborne bacteria can seed the brain, or bacteria can extend directly from sinus infections.[4] The microscopic examination of brains with meningitis shows inflammatory cells in the arachnoidal spaces; this purulent exudate follows blood vessels into the brain parenchyma. Cultures of the cerebrospinal fluid (CSF) of patients with bacterial meningitis often grow the caustive organism. Appropriate antimicrobial therapy on the basis of CSF culture and sensitivity eliminates this infection.

CNS tuberculosis occurs in patients with AIDS, who often present with confusion and lethargy. The spinal fluid studies and cultures often assist with this diagnosis.[15,21,32] The CSF of these patients commonly displays elevated numbers of lymphocytes, high protein, and positive

table 11.1
Common CNS Infections Associated with HIV

CLASS	COMMON ORGANISMS	RESPONSE TO ANTIMICROBIAL THERAPY
Bacterial	Gram +	Excellent
	Gram −	Excellent
Fungal	*Cryptococcus*	Fair
	Aspergillus	Fair
Viral	HIV	Poor
	CMV	Fair
	Herpes	Good
	PML	Poor
Protozoan	*Toxoplasma*	Good

Excellent, Most patients recover with proper therapy; *Good,* therapy helps most patients; *Fair,* some patients improve with therapy; *Poor,* most patients will die even with therapy.

mycobacterial cultures. Appropriate antituberculosis antimicrobial therapy will eradicate the infection.

Fungal (mycotic) infections. Immunocompetent individuals rarely develop mycotic brain infections, but mycotic infections occur commonly in patients with AIDS. *Cryptococcus* organisms are a common cause of meningitis (6% to 25%) and may cause confusion or dementia-like syndromes.[15,21,32] *Aspergillus* organisms and fungi that cause mucormycosis produce brain abscess and brain hemorrhage by proliferating within blood vessels, thrombosing the vessels, and infarcting the brain. *P. carinii* is a common pulmonary pathogen but almost never involves the CNS.[15,24]

Viral infections. Viral brain infections are common in patients with AIDS and can damage any part of the nervous system. Although many patients with AIDS develop generalized cytomegalovirus infections (CMV), brain involvement is less common. CMV and herpes simplex virus (7% to 10%) can infect brain tissue, leading to seizures, confusion, coma, or other neurological problems.[16,23,24] Herpes encephalitis often involves the temporal lobes, causing seizures and altered

consciousness. The infected brain shows inflammation, necrosis, and viral inclusions called Cowdry type A inclusion bodies within neurons or astrocytes.[1] Immunocytochemical preparations of brain tissue stained with antibodies that recognize the herpes simplex virus will label both neurons and astrocytes and indicate the presence of the herpes virus. Standard antiviral therapies are effective in stopping the infection following an accurate diagnosis.

The JC papovavirus attacks oligodendrocytes in white matter, which causes PML. This disease can produce confusion, lethargy, and weakness. The gross appearance of PML includes punched-out necrotic white matter lesions that appear well circumscribed. The white matter is selectively involved, and the cortex is usually spared. The microscopic appearance of these lesions shows a loss of myelinated axons, macrophages, inflammation, and viral inclusions in oligodendrocytes. No therapy is effective in patients with PML. CMV encephalitis or retinitis occurs in AIDS; this disabling infection may respond to antiviral therapy.[5]

Parasitic infections. *Toxoplasma gondii* brain infections occur in 8% to 20% of all patients with AIDS.[23] These organisms are protozoan with a life cycle outside of humans and often produce brain abscess. Appropriate antimicrobial therapy eradicates the *Toxoplasma* organism.[2]

Patients with AIDS can contract a variety of other CNS infections, including syphilis and unusual parasitic infections such as amebic abscess. Every patient with AIDS and confusion requires a careful evaluation to exclude CNS infections.[21]

Secondary Brain Tumors

Kaposi's sarcoma is commonly associated with AIDS but rarely occurs in the CNS. However, patients with AIDS may develop B-cell lymphomas of the brain.[30] These CNS tumors are unusual in healthy subjects but occur in the brains of 1% to 8% of individuals with AIDS.[16,17,24] These tumors can occur in any CNS location and commonly occur as a mass lesion. This monotonous proliferation of malignant lymphocytes often produces neuropsychiatric symptoms.

Other CNS Complications

Patients with AIDS have complicated medical problems resulting from numerous infections, multiorgan dysfunction, and the prescription of numerous toxic medications. Medical delirium occurs in 1% to 3% of these patients. Patients with AIDS develop multiple nutritional deficiencies (e.g., B_{12} deficiency) that cause or worsen neuropsychiatric deficits. Many anti-AIDS drugs have powerful CNS effects. For example, zidovudine (AZT) can cause mania, and antiviral agents can cause confusion or depression. Hepatic or renal failure can produce metabolic encephalopathy. This combination of organ failure and toxic medications predisposes patients with AIDS to delirium.[3,7] AIDS wasting syndrome involves the slow or rapid loss of weight. This multifactorial process may be associated with infection and can be confused with depression.[4]

Clinical Consequences

The psychological effect of HIV infection and AIDS resembles that of any terminal illness. Patients often react with shock or disbelief followed by anger and frustration when informed that they are infected with the virus. Many individuals withdraw from their social circle and begin to exhibit mourning behaviors. Seropositive individuals may develop anxiety disorders, including panic attacks, generalized anxiety disorders, hypochondriasis, and obsessive-compulsive disorder.[20] These conditions usually result from disease-related stress and not from intrinsic brain infection. Reactive depressions most often present as sadness accompanied by tearfulness, expressions of worthlessness, hopelessness, and helplessness. Not surprisingly, many patients (17%) manifest adjustment disorders.

Data on the psychological effect of this disease are confounded by observations that some groups of patients who are HIV-positive suffer high rates of preexisting psychopathology. Individuals at high risk for developing AIDS often have preexisting substance abuse, antisocial personality disorder, and other psychiatric illnesses.[20] Patients with chronic mental illness have a significantly increased rate of HIV infection as compared with the general population.[20] Patients with serious mental illness have higher rates of substance abuse, high-risk behaviors, and socioeconomic factors such as poverty and homelessness, all of which increase the risk for infection.

Clinical Management Implications

The medical management of HIV infection and AIDS is well described in several recent textbooks and is not reviewed here.[2] New immunological and antiretroviral drug therapy holds promise for slowing or stopping the progression of infection. The following section focuses on clinical management of the neuropsychiatric features of the disease.

Clinical Management of the Psychological Impact of AIDS

As previously stated, individuals with AIDS react to their diagnosis as most people do to news of a terminal illness. Anxiety reactions can be treated with benzodiazepines. However, some caution should be exercised because of the high instance of substance abuse among this population. Anecdotal reports indicate that stress management techniques such as progressive relaxation have proven beneficial for some patients.

Manipulative behaviors may appear with this population. These behaviors often anger caregivers and complicate treatment unless recognized and confronted. As a rule, structure and limit setting are useful when dealing with manipulative patients. Power struggles between patients and caregivers or the treatment team are nontherapeutic. Staff should validate the patient's suffering and enable the patient to articulate needs.

Clinical Management of Neuropsychiatric Complications of AIDS

As mentioned earlier, many patients complain of depressive symptoms that are typical of endogenous depression or of anxiety consistent with DSM-IV criteria. Standard medications for depression or anxiety are effective for AIDS-related neuropsychiatric disorders and are thoroughly reviewed in *Psychotropic Drugs,* second edition.[13] The secondary amine nortriptyline is particularly beneficial if depressive symptoms include insomnia, weight loss, anxiety, or gastrointestinal disturbances. Patients exhibiting hypersomnia, weight gain, and expressed suicidal ideation may benefit from the more "activating" selective serotonin reuptake inhibitors (SSRIs).[20] Lithium is the drug of choice for mania that occurs early in the disease process (at serum levels of 1 mEq/L), but it is poorly tolerated in later stages of the disease.[20] In such instances small doses of a high-potency neuroleptic such as haloperidol or fluphenazine may be effective.

Clinical Management of AIDS Dementia Complex

Some evidence suggests that high-dose AZT administration may slow the progression of HIV dementia, and formal treatment trials are under way.[20] The symptomatic treatment of cognitive deficits is similar to the management of other dementias (see Chapter 9).[31]

Intellectual and cognitive dysfunction. Patients with AIDS dementia complex experience impaired concentration, memory deterioration, impaired abstracting ability, slowing of mental and psychomotor capabilities, delirium and, at a late stage, akinetic mutism. These dysfunctions are manifested as difficulty in following directions, forgetfulness, concrete thinking, verbal and physical slowness, confusion, disorientation, immobility, and an inability to speak. Several strategies that compensate for the cognitive losses associated with AIDS dementia complex have been developed for professional and related caregivers and include the following:
1. Limit communication to simple and straightforward ideas and tasks.
2. Use written or verbal cues to facilitate recall.
3. Limit options to a few concrete choices, and structure routine into the patient's life.
4. Allow time for the patient with slowed verbal and psychomotor skills to react.
5. Provide reorientation and memory aids for the patient with delirium who is confused.

Sensorimotor dysfunction. Patients with AIDS dementia complex also commonly experience sensorimotor dysfunction. In these individuals, motor incoordination and increased muscle tone lead to gait disturbances, clumsiness, intention tremors, ataxia, slurred speech, deterioration of handwriting, weakness, fatigue, and bladder/bowel incontinence. Appropriate clinical management includes environmental manipulation such as accident-proofing living quarters, clearly labeling potential hazards (e.g., hot water faucet), and assessing for signs of urinary tract infections.

Personality and behavioral disturbances. Patients with AIDS dementia complex may also develop impaired impulse control that manifests as agitation, combativeness, or angry outbursts. Caregivers can reduce external stimulation of these behaviors by identifying and removing sources of agitation and by redirecting patient behavior instead of attempting to control it.

Summary

Neurological dysfunction in patients with AIDS results from numerous causes. Psychological responses, neuropsychiatric complications of primary HIV infection, secondary opportunistic infections, malignancies, and disease-related toxic-metabolic states can cause significant neuropsychiatric morbidity. Management of the neurologically impaired patient with AIDS includes treatment of CNS infections, management of psychiatric symptoms, resolution of toxic-metabolic problems, and psychological supports for these individuals, who are confronting a fatal disease.

REFERENCES
1. Adams JH, Duchen LW, editors: *Greenfield's neuropathology*, ed 5, New York, 1992, Oxford University Press.
2. Bennett JC, Plum F, editors: *Cecil's textbook of medicine*, Philadelphia, 1996, WB Saunders.
3. Chaisson RE, Barditch-Crovo P: Adverse reactions to therapy for HIV infection, *Emerg Med Clin North Am* 13(1):133-146, 1995.
4. Currier JS, Feinberg J: Bacterial infections in HIV disease. In Volderding P, Jacobson MA, editors: *AIDS Clinical Review 1995/1996* 1:131, 1996.
5. Dunn JP, Jabs DA: Cytomegalovirus retinitis in AIDS: natural history, diagnosis, and treatment. In Volderding P, Jacobson MA, editors: *AIDS Clinical Review 1995/1996* 1:99, 1996.

6. Faulstich ME: Psychiatric aspects of AIDS, *Am J Psychiatry* 144:551-556, 1987.

7. Galetto G, Morrow CT: Noninfectious manifestations of human immunodeficiency virus infection, *Emerg Med Clin North Am* 13(1):105-131, 1995.

8. Gordon SM, Thompson S: The changing epidemiology of human immunodeficiency virus infection in older persons, *J Am Geriatr Soc* 43(1):7-9, 1995.

9. Hansen KN: HIV testing, *Emerg Med Clin North Am* 13(1):43-59, 1995.

10. Janicak PG: Psychopharmacotherapy in the HIV-infected patient, *Psychiatric Ann* 25:609-613, 1995.

11. Johnson RT, Glass JD, McArthur JC et al: Quantitation of human immunodeficiency virus in brains of demented and nondemented patients with acquired immunodeficiency syndrome, *Ann Neurol* 39:392-395, 1996.

12. Johnson VA: New developments in antiretroviral drug therapy for HIV-1 infections. In Volderding P, Jacobson MA, editors: *AIDS Clinical Review 1995/1996* (1):305, 1996.

13. Keltner NL, Folks DG: *Psychotropic drugs,* ed 2, St Louis, 1997, Mosby.

14. Kotler DP, Grunfeld C: Pathophysiology and treatment of the AIDS wasting syndrome. In Volderding P, Jacobson MA, editors: *AIDS Clinical Review 1995/1996* (1):229, 1996.

15. Lang W, Miklossy J, Deruaz JP et al: Neuropathology of the acquired immune deficiency syndrome (AIDS): a report of 135 consecutive autopsy cases from Switzerland, *Acta Neuropathol* 77:379-390, 1989.

16. Levy RM, Bredesen DE: Central nervous system dysfunction in acquired immunodeficiency syndrome. In Rosenblum ML, Levy RM, Bredesen DE, editors: *AIDS and the nervous system,* New York, 1988, Raven Press.

17. Levy RM, Janssen RS, Bush TJ et al: Neuroepidemiology of acquired immunodeficiency syndrome. In Rosenblum ML, Levy RM, Bredesen DE, editors: *AIDS and the nervous system,* New York, 1988, Raven Press.

18 Lipton SA, Gendelman E: Dementia associated with acquired immunodeficiency syndrome. In Flier JS, Underhill LH, editors: *Seminars of the Beth Israel Hospital, N Engl J Med* 332:934-940, 1996.

19. Lyketsos CG, Federman EB: Psychiatric disorders and HIV infection: impact on one another, *Epidem Rev* 17:152-164, 1995.

20. Lyketsos CG, Fishman M, Treisman G: Psychiatric issues and emergencies in HIV infection, *Emerg Med Clin North Am* 13(1):163-177, 1995.

21. Marco CA: Presentations and emergency department evaluation of HIV infection, *Emerg Med Clin North Am* 13(1):61-71, 1995.

22. National Foundation for Brain Research: *The cost of disorders of the brain,* Washington, DC, 1992, The Foundation.

23. Navia BA, Cho E-S, Petito CK et al: The AIDS dementia complex. II. Neuropathology, *Ann Neurol* 19:525-535, 1986.

24. Petito CK, Cho E-S, Lemann W et al: Neuropathology of acquired immunodeficiency syndrome (AIDS): an autopsy review, *J Neuropath Exp Neurol* 45:635-646, 1986.

25. Portegies P: AIDS dementia complex: a review, *J Acquir Immune Defic Syndr* 7(suppl 2):S38-S49, 1994.

26. Quinn TC: The epidemiology of the acquired immunodeficiency syndrome in the 1990s, *Emerg Med Clin North Am* 13(1):1-25, 1995.

27. Rabins PV: Dementia as a symptom of HIV disease, *Lancet* 347:769-770, 1996.

28. Riley MW: AIDS and older people: the overlooked segment of the population. In Riley MW, Ory MG, Zablotsky D, editors: *AIDS in an aging society: what we need to know,* New York, 1989, Springer.

29. Rosenberg PS: Scope of the AIDS epidemic in the United States, *Science* 270:1372-1375, 1995.

30. So YT, Beckstead JH, Davis R: Primary central nervous system lymphoma in acquired immune deficiency syndrome: a clinical and pathological study, *Ann Neurol* 20:566-572, 1986.

31. Terwilliger EF: Biology of HIV-1 and treatment strategies, *Emerg Med Clin North Am* 13(1):27-42, 1995.

32. Vinters HV, Anders KH: *Neuropathology of AIDS,* Boca Raton, Fla, 1990, CRC Press.

33. Walker AR: HIV infections in children, *Emerg Med Clin North Am* 13(1):147-162, 1995.

34. Wiley CA, Achim C: Human immunodeficiency virus encephalitis is the pathological correlate of dementia in acquired immunodeficiency syndrome, *Ann Neurol* 36:673-676, 1994.

Delirium

Delirium is a reversible confusional state with rapid onset and fluctuating symptoms.[1] Unlike with dementia, the symptoms of delirium appear over hours or days and may include alterations in the level of consciousness. The manifestations of delirium may include cognitive impairment, psychiatric symptoms, and autonomic changes.

Delirium is the most common psychiatric syndrome found in the general medical hospital setting. The mortality and morbidity associated with delirium may surpass all other psychiatric disorders. Only dementia, when followed for several years, has a higher mortality rate.[21] Patients who have other disorders of cognitive impairment, including dementia, are significantly vulnerable to the development of delirium and do so with greater frequency. Delirium is an ignored and underresearched phenomenon, and therefore little is known about the epidemiology. Figure 12.1 represents a conceptual overview of delirium. A wide variety of different physiological insults and general medical conditions can produce delirium. As discussed in Chapter 8, it can also be a consequence of substance intoxication or withdrawal. Multifactorial etiologies often account for the high incidence of the syndrome and for the evolution of many equivalent diagnostic terms.

Epidemiology and Demographics

Systematic research of delirium is, for the most part, lacking.[21] Because many cases of delirium probably go undetected, estimates of the prevalence of delirium are probably quite low. Among medical inpatients the prevalence of delirium is between 11% and 16%; in the acute hospitalized elderly patient, the prevalence rises to between 24% and 65%.[13] Many elderly patients admitted to the hospital for a general medical condition develop delirium during their hospitalization. In nursing home settings, patients with dementia have frequent intercurrent bouts of delirium; these episodes may not be noticed by staff because baseline levels of confusion or disorientation pre-exist. The only clue in many cases may be an increase in irritability or a sudden change in the patient's sleep-wake cycle.

The frequency of delirium varies with the type of brain insult and the predisposition of the individual involved. Anthony, LeResche, and Niaz et al[2] found that 34% of cases seen on a psychiatric consultative service had cognitive impairment on the day of admission. Cameron, Thomas, and Mulvihill et al[3] found that 13.5% of 133 consecutive patients admitted to an acute medical ward were delirious; an additional 3.3% became delirious during hospitalization. Approximately 30% of patients in a surgical intensive care unit (ICU) or cardiac ICU and 40% to 50% of those recovering from surgery for hip fractures will have an episode of delirium. An estimated 20% of patients with severe burns and 30% of patients with acquired immunodeficiency syndrome (AIDS) have episodes of delirium while hospitalized. Individuals with chronic cognitive impairment, impaired vision or hearing, sleep deprivation, sensory deprivation, or bone fractures on admission to the hospital are also at increased risk for delirium.[21] The causes of postoperative delirium include the stress of surgery, postoperative pain, insomnia, pain medication, electrolyte imbalances, infection, fever, and blood loss.

Delirium is certainly more common in the elderly as a consequence of underlying subclinical brain damage, increased vulnerability to hypoxia,

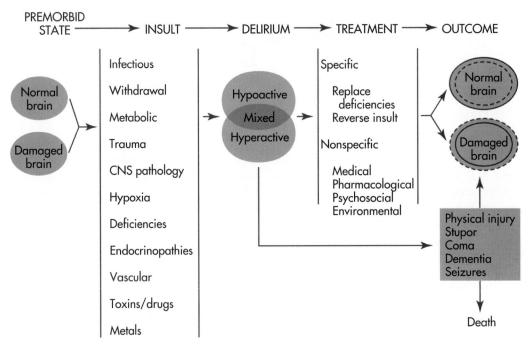

figure 12.1   A conceptual view of delirium. *(From Yudofsky SC, Hales RE, editors:* The American Psychiatric Press textbook of neuropsychiatry, *ed 2, Washington, DC, 1992, American Psychiatric Press.)*

and increased susceptibility to adverse drug reactions. Advanced age is a major risk factor for the development of delirium. Approximately 30% to 40% of hospitalized patients over the age of 65 have an episode of delirium. Other predisposing factors for the development of delirium are young age, preexisting brain damage, a history of delirium, alcohol dependence, diabetes, cancer, sensory impairment, and malnutrition. The presence of delirium is a poor prognostic sign. The 3-month mortality rate of patients who have an episode of delirium is estimated to be between 23% and 33%. The 1-year mortality rate for patients who have an episode of delirium may be as high as 50%.[20]

Psychobiological Considerations

Beyond electroencephalographic findings, the neurophysiology of delirium has received little study. There are no structural brain alterations that cause delirium. Most forms of delirium have shown decreased global metabolic brain activity, which is manifested as diffuse generalized slowing on the electroencephalogram (EEG). Hyperactive delirious states such as those associated with alcohol or sedative withdrawal often show increased "fast" activity on the EEG. However, a normal EEG does not rule out delirium per se.

In most cases of delirium, the close working relationship between subcortical and cortical structures is obviously disrupted. The reversible cortical dysfuntion may result from disruption of ascending cholinergic, serotonergic, and histaminergic inputs.

Specifically, disruption of cholinergic input to the cortex from the pons and ventral medial thalamus may underlie most delirious states. Acetylcholine is hypothesized to be the major neurotransmitter involved in delirium; the major neuroanatomical site affected is the reticular formation.[19]

Several studies have reported a variety of factors that produce delirium, with the common cause being decreased acetylcholine activity in the brain.

One of the more common causes of delirium from prescribed medications results from direct anticholinergic effects. In addition to anticholinergic agents themselves, tricyclic antidepressants and low-potency neuroleptics have significant anticholinergic effects. Therefore it is not surprising that these agents are also associated with drug-induced delirium.

Other neurotransmitters possibly implicated in some cases of delirium include serotonin, glutamate, and histamine. Histaminergic neurons may be involved in some cases observed in patients who have been oversedated with antihistamines. The disruption of histaminic input from the hypothalamus to the cortex may lead to some confusional states.

The reticular formation of the brainstem is the principal area regulating attention and arousal. The major pathway implicated in delirium is the dorsal tegmental pathway, which projects from the mesencephalic reticular formation to the tectum and thalamus.[19] More recent research of delirium has focused on basal ganglia structures such as the caudate and putamen, which are usually associated with abnormal movements. The basal ganglia may be quite important in maintaining or sustaining levels of conscious awareness. Therefore structural changes in the basal ganglia may also predispose an individual to delirium.[4,5]

Clinical Applications
Clinical Findings and Course

The diagnostic features of delirium are noted in Box 12.1. The primary symptom of delirium is impairment of consciousness together with global cognitive impairment. Abnormalities of mood, perception, and motor behavior are commonly observed; tremors, asterixis, nystagmus, incoordination, and urinary incontinence are common neuropsychiatric symptoms. Classically, delirium has a sudden onset within hours or days, with a brief fluctuating course. Improvement is rapid when the causative factor is identified and eliminated.

The prodromal features of delirium include

---

box 12.1

Diagnostic Criteria for Delirium Due to a General Medical Condition

A. Disturbance of consciousness (i.e., reduced clarity of awareness of the environment) with reduced ability to focus, sustain, or shift attention

B. A change in cognition (e.g., memory deficit, disorientation, language disturbance) or the development of a perceptual disturbance that is not better accounted for by a preexisting, established, or evolving dementia

C. Disturbance that develops over a short period of time (usually hours to days) and tends to fluctuate during the course of the day

D. Evidence from the history, physical examination, or laboratory findings that the disturbance is caused by the direct physiological consequences of a general medical condition

Modified from American Psychiatric Association: *Diagnostic and statistical manual of mental disorders,* ed 4, Washington, DC, 1994, The Association.

---

symptoms such as restlessness, anxiety, irritability, or sleep disruption. The clinical features are outlined in Box 12.2; these symptoms vary significantly over time.[1] Many patients have a mixed clinical picture that fluctuates between hypoactive and hyperactive states.[16] This variability and fluctuation is characteristic of delirium and leads to diagnostic confusion.

As previously discussed, the reticular activating system of the brainstem may be hypoactive in some cases of delirium, which causes the patient to appear apathetic, somnolent, and quietly confused. Other cases probably involve brainstem activation, in which the patient is agitated and hypervigilant and exhibits psychomotor hyperactivity.

The patient with a hypoactive type of delirium is less apt to be diagnosed as delirious and is often labeled as depressed, uncooperative, or personality

box 12.2
Clinical Features of Delirium

Prodrome (restlessness, anxiety, sleep distur-
   bance, irritability)
Rapidly fluctuating course
Decreased attention (easily distractible)
Altered arousal and psychomotor abnormality
Disturbance of sleep-wake cycle
Impaired memory (cannot register new infor-
   mation)
Disorganized thinking and speech
Disorientation (time, place, and [very rare]
   person)
Altered perceptions (misperceptions, illusions,
   delusions [poorly formed], and hallucina-
   tions)
Neurological abnormalities
   Dysphagia
   Constructional apraxia
   Dysnomic aphasia
   Motor abnormalities (tremors, asterixis, my-
      oclonus, and reflex and tone changes)
   EEG abnormalities (almost always global
      slowing)
Other features (sadness, anger, euphoria, or
   other affects)

From Wise MC, Brandt GT: Delirium. In Yudofsky SC,
Hales RM, editors: *The American Psychiatric Press textbook of
psychiatry,* ed 2, Washington, DC, 1992, American Psychiatric Press.

disordered. The diagnosis of clinical depression in
an apathetic and quietly confused patient can lead
to inappropriate treatments with antidepressants.
Misdiagnosis further increases morbidity and
mortality as a result of failure to treat the underlying causes of the delirium, and additional insult
may result from the side effects of antidepressant
medications.

The sleep-wake cycle of a patient with delirium
is often reversed. The patient may be somnolent
during the day and active during the night when
the nursing staff is sparse. This sleep-wake disturbance is not only symptomatic of delirium but
also exacerbates the confusion that results from
sleep deprivation. Resolution of a normal diurnal

sleep cycle is an important component of treatment.

A patient with delirium has difficulty sustaining attention and is easily distracted by incidental
activities in the environment. This inability to
sustain attention undoubtedly plays a key role in
memory and orientation difficulties. A patient
with delirium experiences severe impairments in
registering events into memory. Whether a result
of attentional deficits, perceptual disturbances, or
malfunction of the hippocampus, the patient fails
tests of immediate and recent memory. After recovery from delirium, some patients are amnestic
for the entire period; others have islands of memory for events that occurred during the episode.
Whether these islands of memory correspond to
lucid intervals is unknown.[21]

Except for lucid intervals, the patient with
delirium is usually disoriented to time and is often
disoriented to place; however, he or she is rarely if
ever disoriented to person. It is not unusual for a
patient with delirium to feel that he or she is in a
familiar place while also nodding agreement that
he or she is being monitored in a surgical intensive
care unit. The extent of the patient's disorientation fluctuates with the severity of the delirium.

The thought patterns of a patient with delirium
are disorganized, and reasoning is defective. As the
severity of the delirium increases, spontaneous
speech becomes incoherent and rambling and
shifts from topic to topic.

Virtually all patients with delirium have misperceptions. These patients often experience illusions, delusions, or hallucinations. They may in-
corporate misperceptions into a loosely knit
delusional system, which can result in paranoid
thoughts. Visual hallucinations are quite common
and may involve either simple visual distortions or
complex scenes. Visual hallucinations occur more
often than do auditory hallucinations; tactile hallucinations are the least common.

Delirium may be associated with motor system abnormalities, including tremors, myoclonus,
asterixis, muscle tone changes, or alterations in reflexes. The tremor associated with delirium, particularly toxic-metabolic delirium, is absent at rest
but is apparent during movement. Myoclonus and

asterixis (so-called "liver flap") may occur in many toxic and metabolic conditions. Other clinical features of delirium include emotional lability and intense responses to the mental confusion that is present. Emotional responses vary and include anxiety, panic, fear, anger, rage, sadness, apathy, and euphoria.

The diagnosis of delirium is made by the combination of clinical observations and formal changes in the patient's mental status. Recording these observations over time is of paramount importance. Such checking is especially helpful in pinpointing the fluctuation in a patient's mental status over a 24-hour period. Family members may also be helpful in documenting mental status changes and in relating any previous history of drug or alcohol dependence.

Repeated testing of mental status not only strengthens the diagnosis of delirium but also adds to the documentation that assists others in recognizing the presence of a confusional state. To test mental status, the patient may be asked to draw a clock face. This exercise and other constructional tasks have been shown to be sensitive tests of the degree of confusion present. Naming objects and writing sentences are other sensitive items in assessing delirium. Writing exercises may demonstrate motor impairment, misspellings, and linguistic errors. Dysgraphia in delirium tends to be more severe than that found with Alzheimer's disease and other dementias.

Clinical Consequences

Although no direct studies of morbidity in delirium exist, research indicates that hospitalizations are prolonged because of the condition. Gustafson, Berggren and Brannstrom et al[7] found that delirium seemed to be the best predictor of outcome in patients who presented with femoral neck fractures. Patients with a hip fracture and delirium had longer hospital stays than those who were not delirious and were more likely to require walking aids, extensive rehabilitation, or nursing home placement, or to be bedridden or die.

Other common problems that result from delirium include disruptive behaviors such as the removal of nasogastric tubes, intravenous lines, arterial lines, nasopharyngeal tubes, and intraaortic balloon pumps. Inouye, van Dyck, and Alessi et al[9] reported that the risk of complications such as decubitus ulcers and aspiration pneumonia are six times greater for patients who are delirious compared with patients who are not. Levkoff, Besdine, and Wetle[12] project a 1 to 2 billion dollar savings each year if the hospital stay of each patient with delirium could be reduced by just one day!

Clinicians underestimate the mortality rates associated with delirium. Three months after diagnosis, the mortality rate for delirium is fourteen times greater than the mortality rate for affective disorders. A patient diagnosed with delirium during a hospital admission has a 5.5 times greater hospital mortality rate than a patient diagnosed with dementia. Furthermore, an elderly patient who develops delirium in the hospital has a 22% to 76% chance of dying during that hospitalization.[21] In another study of 77 patients who received a diagnosis of delirium on a consultation service, 19 died within 6 months.[18]

Clinical Management Implications

The cardinal rule in the evaluation of patients with delirium is to detect and correct the underlying disturbance(s) that are contributing to the patient's condition. Lipowski[14] has documented the most common physical illnesses associated with delirium, including congestive heart failure, pneumonia, urinary tract infections, cancer, uremia, malnutrition, hypokalemia, dehydration, hyponatremia, and cerebrovascular accidents. Systemic illnesses that result in brain dysfunction are more commonly the cause of delirium than are primary CNS disorders. Intoxications with medications, especially psychotropic agents and drugs that have sedative or anticholinergic effects, are among the most common causes of delirium in older patients (Box 12.3). Alcoholics, particularly those with a history of heavy drinking, are at significant risk for withdrawal delirium (see Chapter 8). Other drugs that involve a significant potential for withdrawal include barbiturates, sedative-hypnotics, and benzodiazepines; these drugs must

box 12.3
Drugs That Can Cause Delirium

Antibiotics
Acyclovir (antiviral)
Amphotericin B (antifungal)
Cephalexin (Keflex)
Chloroquine (antimalarial)
Metronidazole (Flagyl)

Anticholinergics
Antihistamines
Chlorpheniramine (Ornade and
   Teldrin)
Antiparkinson drugs
Antispasmodics
Atropine/homatropine
Belladonna alkaloids
Benztropine (Cogentin)
Biperiden (Akineton)
Diphenhydramine (Benadryl)
Phenothiazines (especially
   thioridazine)
Promethazine (Phenergan)
Scopolamine
Tricyclic antidepressants
   (especially amitriptyline)
Trihexyphenidyl (Artane)

Anticonvulsants
Phenobarbital
Phenytoin (Dilantin)
Sodium valproate (Depakene)

Antiinflammatory
Adrenocorticotropic hormone
Corticosteroids
Ibuprofen (Motrin and Advil)
Indomethacin (Indocin)
Naproxen (Naprosyn)
Phenylbutazone (Butazolidin)

Antineoplastic
5-Fluorouracil

Antiparkinson
Amantadine (Symmetrel)
Carbidopa-levodopa (Sinemet)
Levodopa (Larodopa)

Antituberculous
Isoniazid
Rifampin

Analgesic
Opiates
Salicylates
Synthetic narcotics

Cardiac
β-Blockers
Clonidine (Catapres)
Digoxin (Lanoxin)
Disopyramide (Norpace)
Lidocaine (Xylocaine)
Methyldopa (Aldomet)
Mexiletine
Quinidine (Quinaglute)
Procainamide (Pronestyl)
Propranolol (Inderal)

Drug withdrawal
Alcohol
Barbiturates
Benzodiazepines

Sedative-hypnotic
Barbiturates (Miltown and
   Equanil)
Benzodiazepines
Glutethimide (Doriden)

Sympathomimetic
Amphetamines
Phenylephrine
Phenylpropanolamine

Miscellaneous
Aminophylline
Bromides
Chlorpropamide (Diabinese)
Cimetidine (Tagamet)
Disulfiram (Antabuse)
Lithium
Metrizamide (Amipaque)
Podophyllin by absorption
Propylthiouracil
Quinacrine
Theophylline
Timolol (optic)

Over-the-counter
Compōz
Excedrin P.M.
Sleep-Eze
Sominex

From Wise MC, Brandt GT: Delirium. In Yudofsky SC, Hales RM, editors: *The American Psychiatric Press textbook of psychiatry,* ed 2, Washington, DC, 1992, American Psychiatric Press.

be assiduously evaluated and the appropriate detoxification regimen instituted.

The differentiation between dementia and delirium is quite important (Table 12.1).[15] However, dementia and delirium often co-exist and may be superimposed on one another. In general, the differential diagnosis of delirium is both extensive and straightforward. It is important to re-

alize that delirium may have multiple causes; each potential contributor needs to be pursued and reversed independently.

Other nonspecific causes of delirium, such as ICU psychosis, may result from isolation or trauma. ICU psychosis and postcardiotomy delirium have been well described in the literature and are best characterized as deliria with psychotic

table 12.1
Differential Diagnosis of Delirium and Dementia

FEATURE	DELIRIUM	DEMENTIA
Onset	Acute, often at night	Insidious
Course	Fluctuating, with lucid intervals, during day; worse at night	Stable over course of day
Duration	Hours to weeks	Months or years
Awareness	Reduced	Clear
Alertness	Abnormally low or high	Usually normal
Attention	Lacks direction and selectivity; distractibility; fluctuates over course of day	Relatively unaffected
Orientation	Usually impaired for time; tendency to mistake unfamiliar for familiar place and persons	Often impaired
Memory	Immediate and recent memory impairments	Recent and remote memory impairments
Thinking	Disorganized	Impoverished
Perception	Illusions and hallucinations (usually visual) are common	Often absent
Speech	Incoherent, hesitant, slow or rapid	Difficulty in finding words
Sleep-wake cycle	Always disrupted	Fragmented sleep
Physical illness or drug toxicity	Either or both present	Often absent, especially in Alzheimer's disease

From Lipowski ZJ: Delirium (acute confusional states), *JAMA* 258:1789-1792, 1987.

components. Delirious states in the ICU are usually multifactorial and may arise from the inherent stresses of the ICU itself, particularly the sleep-depriving effects. Many patients in the ICU setting are gravely ill, medically compromised, and receiving multiple medications. In addition, sleep deprivation and the loss of the normal diurnal light-dark rhythm (in units without windows) may be biologically disrupting. Delirium after cardiac surgery classically occurs 3 or 4 days postoperatively. Contributing factors include increased age, total time spent on the cardiopulmonary bypass pump, intraoperative hypotension, severity of illness, sleep deprivation, and sensory monotony.[8]

The clinical evaluation of a patient with delirium must follow a systematic process of elimination (Box 12.4). Thorough evaluation of the patient's mental and physical status in addition to a mental status examination, laboratory testing, and use of the EEG improves the diagnostic accuracy.[17] The Mini-Mental State Examination provides a useful serial screening tool for the evaluation and follow-up of a patient's clinical course (Box 12.5).[6] The laboratory evaluation can be conceptualized as having two levels. The basic battery is ordered in virtually every patient (Box 12.4). Other tests are considered when the specific cause is not apparent, even after information concerning the patient's mental and physical status is combined with the basic laboratory battery.

The use of the EEG in the evaluation of delirium has special significance. Although an EEG may be normal in dementia, it is almost always abnormal in delirium; this difference makes the EEG a very sensitive test in this clinical situation.

box 12.4
Neuropsychiatric Evaluation of the Patient

Mental status

Interview (assess level of consciousness, psychomotor activity, appearance, affect, mood, intellect, and thought processes)

Performing tests (memory, concentration, reasoning, motor and constructional apraxia, dysgraphia, and dysnomia)

Physical status

Brief neurological examination (reflexes, limb strength, Babinski's sign, cranial nerves, meningeal signs, and gait)

Review past and present vital signs (pulse, temperature, blood pressure, and respiration rate)

Review chart (labs, abnormal behavior and when it began, medical diagnoses, VDRL)

Review medication records (correlate abnormal behavior with starting or stopping medications)

Laboratory examination (basic)

Blood chemistries (electrolytes, glucose, calcium, albumin, blood urea nitrogen, ammonia (NH_4^+, and liver functions)

Blood count (hematocrit, white count and differential, mean corpuscular volume, sedimentation rate)

Drug levels (Need toxic screen? Medication blood levels?)

Arterial blood gases

Urinalysis

Electrocardiogram

Chest x-ray study

Laboratory (based on clinical judgment)

EEG (Seizures? Focal lesion?)

Computed tomography (normal-pressure hydrocephalus, stroke, and space-occupying lesion)

Additional blood chemistries (heavy metals, thiamine and folate levels, thyroid battery, LE prep, antinuclear antibodies, and urinary porphobilinogen)

Lumbar puncture (if indication of infection)

From Wise MC, Brandt GT: Delirium. In Yudofsky SC, Hales RM, editors: *The American Psychiatric Press textbook of psychiatry,* ed 2, Washington, DC, 1992, American Psychiatric Press.
VDRL, Venereal Disease Research Laboratory; *LE prep,* lupus erythematosus preparation.

A correlation exists between electrophysiological abnormalities and disturbance of consciousness. EEG changes are reversible to the extent that the clinical delirium is reversible. Spectral EEG analysis that measures the quantity of alpha, beta, theta, and delta background activity has further delineated the correlation between EEG slowing and cognitive deterioration.[11] The EEG abnormality may not always be characterized by slowing but may be low-amplitude fast activity; this type of activity is seen with alcohol withdrawal and sedative-hypnotic withdrawal delirium. The EEG abnormalities that accompany delirium may persist long after the clinical manifestations of the brain syndrome remit.

A two-tiered differential diagnostic system for delirium has been suggested by Wise and Brandt.[21] The first level of diagnosis represents the mnemonic "WHHHHIMP" (Table 12.2). These items are critical in determining the cause of delirium on an *emergent basis.* The second level of diagnosis involves other physiological insults and medical conditions that may cause delirium and uses the mnemonic "I Watch Death" (Table 12.3). These clinical diagnostic items are useful as the clinician considers the entire differential diagnosis

box 12.5
Mini-Mental State Examination

Patient _____
Examiner _____
Date _____

Mini-Mental State Examination

Maximum Score	Score	
		Orientation
5	( )	What is the (year) (season) (date) (day) (month)?
5	( )	Where are we: (state) (county) (town) (hospital) (floor)?
		Registration
3	( )	Name 3 objects: 1 second to say each. Then ask the patient all 3 after you have said them. Give 1 point for each correct answer. Then repeat them until he or she learns all 3. Count trials and record.
		Trials _____
		Attention and Calculation
5	( )	Serial 7s. 1 point for each correct. Stop after 5 answers. Alternatively spell "world" backwards.
		Recall
3	( )	Ask for the 3 objects repeated above. Give 1 point for each correct.
		Language

9	( )	Name a pencil and watch (2 points)
		Repeat the following "no ifs, ands, or buts." (1 point)
		Follow a 3-stage command:
		"Take a paper in your right hand, fold it in half, and put in on the floor" (3 points)
		Read and obey the following:
		    Close your eyes (1 point)
		    Write a sentence (1 point)
		    Copy design (1 point)

Total score _____

ASSESS level of consciousness along a continuum

Alert	Drowsy	Stupor	Coma

From Folstein MF, Folstein SE, McHugh PR: Mini-mental state: a practical method for grading the cognitive state of patients for the clinician, *J Psychiatr Res* 12:189-198, 1975.

table 12.2
Differential Diagnosis for Delirium: Emergent Items (WHHHHIMP)

DIAGNOSES	CLINICAL QUESTIONS
Wernicke's encephalopathy or withdrawal	Ataxia?
	Ophthalmoplegia?
	Alcohol or drug history?
	Increased mean corpuscular volume (MCV)?
	Increased sympathetic activity (e.g., increased pulse, increased blood pressure (BP), or sweating)?
	Hyperreflexia?
Hypertensive encephalopathy	Increased BP?
	Papilledema?
Hypoglycemia	History of insulin-dependent diabetes mellitus?
	Decreased glucose?
Hypoperfusion of central nervous system, arrhythmia	Decreased BP?
	Decreased cardiac output (e.g., myocardial infarct, cardiac failure)
	Decreased hematocrit?
Hypoxia	Arterial blood gases (decreased PO_2)?
	History of pulmonary disease?
Intracranial bleeding or infection	History of unconsciousness?
	Focal neurological signs?
Meningitis or encephalitis	Meningeal signs?
	Increased white blood cell count?
	Increased temperature?
	Viral prodrome?
Poisons or medications	Should toxic screen be ordered?
	Signs of toxicity (e.g., pupillary abnormality, nystagmus, or ataxia)?
	Is the patient on a drug that can cause delirium?

From Wise MC, Brandt GT: Delirium. In Yudofsky SC, Hales RM, editors: *The American Psychiatric Press textbook of psychiatry*, ed 2, Washington, DC, 1992, American Psychiatric Press.

of delirium. They also illustrate the seriousness of delirium and the potential morbidity and mortality that result from "acute brain failure."

As previously stated, the treatment of delirium involves the direct treatment of the underlying cause. Certain environmental and pharmacological strategies may facilitate the patient's course until the underlying cause can be identified. Environmental strategies include placing the patient in a room with a window. A family member or 24-hour sitter is placed at the patient's bedside to facilitate orientation and daily functioning. Calendars, clocks, familiar photographs, radio or television (during the waking hours), and other attempts to connect the patient to the outside world and provide moderate sensory stimulation can be used. Nightlights and other types of additional sensory input are useful for many patients. Psychological support both during and after the delirium is also important.

The pharmacological management of delirium generally includes the management of agitated and psychotic behavior. High-potency antipsychotic agents such as haloperidol (or risperidone) are drugs of choice because they have minimal effects on the blood pressure or physiological status

table 12.3
Differential Diagnosis for Delirium: Critical Items (I WATCH DEATH)

DISEASE CATEGORY	DIAGNOSIS
Infections	Encephalitis, meningitis, abscesses, and syphilis
Withdrawal	Alcohol, barbiturates, and sedative-hypnotics
Acute metabolic	Acidosis, alkalosis, electrolyte disturbance, hepatic failure, and renal failure
Trauma	Heat stroke, postoperative, and severe burns
CNS pathology	Hemorrhage, NPH, seizures, stroke, tumors, and vasculitis
Hypoxia	Anemia, carbon monoxide poisoning, hypotension, and pulmonary or cardiac failure
Deficiencies	Vitamin B_{12}, niacin, thiamine, and hypovitaminosis
Endocrinopathies	Hyperadrenocortisol or hypoadrenocortisol and hyperglycemia or hypoglycemia
Acute vascular	Hypertensive encephalopathy or shock
Toxins or drugs	Medications (Box 12.3), pesticides, and solvents
Heavy metals	Lead, manganese, and mercury

From Wise MG, Brandt GT: Delirium. In Yudofsky SC, Hales RM, editors: *The American Psychiatric Press textbook of psychiatry,* ed 2, Washington, DC, 1992, American Psychiatric Press.

of the patient. They also tend to be less sedating and have few anticholinergic side effects. In contrast, low-potency neuroleptics such as thioridazine or chlorpromazine can cause hypotension and have significant anticholinergic effects.

The prototypical drug used for the stabilization of delirium is haloperidol because it can be given orally, intramuscularly, or intravenously. A typical starting dose is 1 to 2 mg every 1 to 2 hours until the patient is stabilized. Once the patient is stabilized, haloperidol may be given in supplemental or maintenance doses every 4 hours as needed. The need for continuous medication should be evaluated every 24 hours, with the doses decreased and discontinued as rapidly as possible when the patient's mental status is normalized.

Some clinicians advocate the use of high-potency, short-acting benzodiazepines such as lorazepam. Lorazepam may be given in 1- to 2-mg doses orally, sublingually, or intramuscularly every hour until the patient is calm and slightly drowsy. However, it may cause anterograde amnesia when given in this manner and may exacerbate the patient's delirium as a result of disinhibited behavior. Because many patients with delirium are elderly or seriously medically ill, medication dosages are reduced according to the age and physical state of the patient.

Anticholinergic delirium can be treated with the cholinergic agonist physostigmine salicylate, 1 to 2 mg given slowly intravenously or intramuscularly, with repeated doses at no less than 15-minute intervals. Contraindications for using a cholinergic agonist include a history of heart disease, asthma, diabetes, peptic ulcer disease, or the possibility of bladder or bowel obstruction.[15]

In most instances, the resolution of delirium is accompanied by discontinuation of the psychotropic agent. Patients who are treated with neuroleptics must be carefully monitored for extrapyramidal side effects, neuroleptic-induced catatonia, and neuroleptic-induced neuroleptic malignant syndrome, which can occur as an adverse effect of neuroleptic treatment. A detailed discussion of the pharmacological strategies in this patient population, including the use of intravenous haloperidol and lorazepam in ICU settings, is discussed in the companion text, *Psychotropic Drugs*, second edition.[10]

REFERENCES

1. American Psychiatric Association: *Diagnostic and statistical manual of mental disorders,* ed 4, Washington, DC, 1994, The Association.
2. Anthony JC, LeResche L, Niaz U et al: Limits of the mini-mental state as a screening test for dementia and delirium among hospital patients, *Psychol Med* 12:397-408, 1982.
3. Cameron DJ, Thomas RI, Mulvihill M et al: Delirium: a test of the *Diagnostic and Statistical Manual III* criteria on medical inpatients, *J Am Geriatr Soc* 35:1007-1010, 1987.
4. Figiel GS, Hassen MA, Zorumski C et al: ECT-induced delirium in depressed patients with Parkinson's disease, *J Neuropsychiatry Clin Neurosci* 3(4):405-411, 1991.
5. Figiel GS, Krishnan KR, Breitner JC et al: Radiologic correlates of antidepressant-induced delirium: the possible significance of basal ganglia lesions, *J Neuropsychiatry Clin Neurosci* 1(2):188-190, 1989.
6. Folstein MF, Folstein SE, McHugh PR: Mini mental state: a practical method for grading the cognitive state of patients for the clinician, *J Psychiatr Res* 12:189-198, 1975.
7. Gustafson Y, Berggren D, Brannstrom B et al: Acute confusional states in elderly patients treated for femoral neck fracture, *J Am Geriatr Soc* 36:525-530, 1988.
8. Heller SS, Kornfeld DS, Frank KA et al: Postcardiotomy delirium and cardiac output, *Am J Psychiatry* 136:337-339, 1979.
9. Inouye SK, van Dyck CH, Alessi CA et al: Clarifying confusion: the confusion assessment method, *Ann Intern Med* 113:941-948, 1990.
10. Keltner N, Folks DG, editors: *Psychotropic drugs,* ed 2, St Louis, Mosby, 1997.
11. Koponen H, Partanen J, Paakkonen A et al: EEG spectral analysis in delirium, *J Neurol Neurosurg Psychiatry* 52:980-985, 1989.
12. Levkoff SE, Besdine RW, Wetle T: Acute confusional states (delirium) in the hospitalized elderly, *Ann Rev Gerontol Geriatr* 6:1-26, 1986.
13. Levkoff SE, Cleary PD, Liptzin B et al: Epidemiology of delirium: an overview of research issues and findings, *Int Psychogeriatr* 3(2):149-167, 1991.
14. Lipowski ZJ: Transient cognitive disorders (delirium, acute confusional states) in the elderly, *Am J Psychiatry* 140:1426-1436, 1983.
15. Lipowski ZJ: Delirium (acute confusional state), *JAMA* 258:1789-1792, 1987.
16. Lipowski ZJ: Delirium: acute confusional states, New York, 1990, Oxford University Press. In Yudofsky SC, Hales RE, editors: *The American Psychiatric Press textbook of neuropsychiatry,* ed 2, Washington, DC, 1992, American Psychiatric Press.
17. Nelson A, Fogel B, Faust D et al: Bedside cognitive screening instruments: a critical assessment, *J Nerv Ment Dis* 174:73-83, 1986.
18. Trzepacz P, Teague G, Lipowski Z: Delirium and other organic mental disorders in a general hospital, *Gen Hosp Psychiatry* 7:101-106, 1985.
19. Trzepacz PT, Sclabassi RJ, Van Thiel DH: Delirium: a subcortical phenomenon? *J Neuropsychiatry Clin Neurosci* 1(3):283-290, 1989.
20. Tune L, Rosse C: Delirium. In Coffey CE, Cummings JL, editors: *American Psychiatric Press Textbook of geriatric neuropsychiatry,* Washington, DC, 1994, American Psychiatric Press.
21. Wise MG, Brandt GT: Delirium. In Yudofsky SC, Hales RE, editors: *The American Psychiatric Press textbook of neuropsychiatry,* ed 2, Washington, DC, 1992, American Psychiatric Press.

chapter thirteen

Disorders of Movement

"Unaided by previous inquiries immediately directed to this disease, and not having had the advantage, in a single case, of that light which anatomical examination yields, opinions and not facts can only be offered." Dr. James Parkinson, 1817 (p. 33)

Conscious, intentional movement is initiated and sustained by the pyramidal motor system. Unconscious, unintentional motor activities associated with muscle tone and posture are sustained by the extrapyramidal motor system. Weakness (paresis) and paralysis (plegia) result from damage to the pyramidal motor system. Abnormalities of tone and posture result from malfunction of the extrapyramidal system. Brainstem nuclei project to many areas; thus brainstem neurotransmitter deficiencies related to movement disorders also precipitate cognitive, affective, and autonomic disruption. Beyond the specifics of the movement disorder, assessment should always address neuropsychiatric complications (e.g., dementia, depression) and autonomic disturbances (e.g., orthostasis, tachycardia).

The pyramidal system, or corticospinal tract, begins in the motor area of the cortex and is responsible for voluntary movement (see Chapter 1). The extrapyramidal system provides an unconscious stabilizing infrastructure that supports the voluntary movements of the pyramidal system. Movement disorders occur when motor activity is freed from extrapyramidal influences, both inhibitory and excitatory.

The extrapyramidal system includes brainstem

nuclei, subcortical nuclei (basal ganglia and thalamus), and motor cortex. The basal ganglia are a group of subcortical nuclei that lie beneath the outer rim of grey matter (see Chapter 1). The basal ganglia are composed of three major nuclei: the caudate nucleus, the putamen, and the globus pallidus (comprising both globus pallidus externa [GPe] and globus pallidus interna [GPi]). Other authors include the substantia nigra and subthalamic nuclei as part of this system because contributions from all of these nuclei are required for normal movement. Some confusion has occurred because other terms are sometimes used to identify these nuclei. Figure 13.1 provides a view of the basal ganglia, which lie deep within the brain and are visible only when the brain is cut (e.g., during postmortem examination) or during imaging. These nuclei are rich in both afferent and efferent projections; these projections give rise to two major "movement loops" that provide the basis for stabilizing and supporting movement and posture.

Preparation for movement, inhibition of movement, and execution of movement are three of the several known functions of the basal ganglia.[8,39] Other important functions include the facilitation of reward actions (e.g., cocaine affects the uptake

239

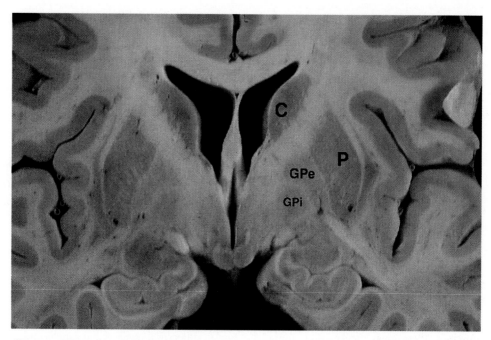

figure 13.1 Appearance of the basal ganglia in a coronal section of brain from the level of the mamillary bodies. The caudate nucleus *(C)* protrudes into the lateral ventricle, and the globus pallidus/putamen *(P)* sits beneath the internal capsule. Two segments of the globus pallidus, the globus pallidus externa *(GPe)* and globus pallidus interna *(GPi)*, are readily apparent. *(Courtesy Dr. Richard E. Powers, Director, University of Alabama at Birmingham Brain Resource Program.)*

and release of catecholamines in the basal ganglia) and the promotion of motor learning and planning.[8,22] Because basal ganglia projections reach the prefrontal, premotor, and motor cortices, dysfunctions associated with basal ganglia abnormalities have demonstrated that these nuclei are part of the extrapyramidal system.

Overview of Movement Disorders

Movement disorders are common, particularly among the elderly. These disorders have their anatomical origins in the extrapyramidal system and are caused by dysfunction of the brainstem nuclei and basal ganglia.[21] Movement disorders are broadly divided into hypokinetic, hyperkinetic, and dystonic disorders. **Hypokinetic** disorders are characterized by difficulty in initiating

movement, slowing down of movement, inability to move, and rigidity. Parkinson's disease is the prototypical hypokinetic disorder. **Hyperkinetic** disorders are characterized by excessive, involuntary movements and include choreas, ballismus, and dyskinesias. **Dystonic** disorders are characterized by the assumption of abnormal fixed positions. Many movement disorders are accompanied by neuropsychiatric symptoms, including depression, dementia, or psychosis that results from dysfunction of the brainstem or subcortical systems.

Specific Movement Disorder Categories

There are many movement disorder diagnoses (Box 13.1); the representative disorders are discussed in this book and include hypokinetic dis-

box 13.1
Movement Disorders

Choreoacanthocytosis: A rare progressive chorea-type movement disorder. Neuropathological examination reveals diffuse atrophy of the striatum with severe loss of small neurons.

Diffuse Lewy body disease: This disorder presents as parkinsonism with or without dementia or as dementia with or without parkinsonism. This disease overlaps with parkinsonism and Alzheimer's disease. Neuropathological examination reveals widespread distribution of Lewy bodies in the cortex, brainstem, hippocampus, and parahippocampal gyrus.

Gilles de la Tourette's syndrome: Characterized by progressively violent jerks of the face, shoulder, and extremities, typically beginning in childhood. No pathological abnormalities have been documented.

Hallervorden-Spatz disease: This rare autosomal recessive disorder presents with choreoathetosis, dystonia, tremors, rigidity, and dementia, with onset across the lifespan. Neuropathological examination reveals a loss of myelin in the globus pallidus and substantia nigra reticulata, increased accumulation of iron and glial pigments in the globus pallidus, and axonal swelling.

Hemiballismus: Characterized by wild, wide-ranging irregular limb movements. Pathological changes are typically found in the contralateral subthalamic nucleus.

Hereditary striatal necrosis: Rare autosomal dominant or recessive slowly progressive disorder in children with mental retardation. Characterized by rigidity, ataxia, and dysphagia. Neuropathological examination reveals bilateral necrosis of the neostriatum.

Meige's syndrome: Characterized by an orofacial dystonia. Neuropathological examination reveals patchy neuronal loss in the basal ganglia, substantia nigra, midbrain, and cerebellum.

Pallidonigral degenerations: This group of rare disorders presents with choreoathetosis, athetosis, rigid-akinetic, and hyperkinetic syndromes. Degeneration occurs in the globus pallidus and substantia nigra pathways.

Progressive supranuclear palsy: This movement disorder is sometimes referred to as parkinsonism-plus syndrome. Additional characteristic symptoms include ophthalmoplegia, dystonia, rigid akinesia, and dementia. Neuropathological examination reveals widespread neurofibrillary tangles (which differ immunochemically from Alzheimer's tangles) and widespread neuronal loss.

Shy-Drager syndrome: This disorder presents with multisystem degeneration caused by neuron loss in the basal ganglia, substantia nigra, cerebellar cortex, inferior olives, locus ceruleus, and other sites. In addition to the disorder of movement are autonomic dysfunctions such as orthostatic hypotension.

Wilson's disease: Referred to as hepatocerebral degeneration, pathological changes occur in both the liver and the brain. Specifically, spongy changes occur in the cortex, basal ganglia, dentate nucleus, and white matter.

Modified from Jellinger KA, Lantos PL, Mehraein P: Pathological assessment of movement disorders: requirements for documentation in brain banks, *J Neural Transm* 39(suppl):173-184, 1993.

orders such as Parkinson's disease and drug-induced parkinsonism, hyperkinetic disorders such as choreas and dyskinesias, and dystonias. These disorders have been selected for discussion because they are representative of the three over-arching movement disorder categories and because they are relevant for the day-to-day practice of many psychiatric clinicians.

Parkinson's Disease and Drug-Induced Parkinsonism

Parkinsonism is a general term used to describe a movement disorder that is characterized by slowness of movement (bradykinesia), failure to move (akinesia), rigidity, and tremors. Parkinson's disease (i.e., idiopathic parkinsonism) and drug-induced parkinsonism are caused by decreased bioavailability of dopamine. This disorder may respond to treatment approaches that increase dopamine availability (Parkinson's disease) or decrease acetylcholine (both disorders). Many other disorders such as progressive supranuclear palsy, olivopontocerebellar atrophy, and striatonigral degeneration can present with parkinsonism.

Choreas

Chorea (Greek for *dance*) is a hyperkinetic disorder that manifests as abrupt movements of the limbs and facial muscles. The term was first used by Sydenham[26] to describe involuntary movements in rheumatic disease, but it has since been used to describe a family of similar-appearing disorders. Sydenham was reminded of dancelike movements when he observed rapid movements of the trunk, head, face, and limbs. These movements also interrupt and interfere with normal movement.[2] They are potentiated by dopaminergic drugs and suppressed by dopamine antagonists. Huntington's disease is a common chorea and is discussed in this chapter.

Dyskinesias

Dyskinesias are characterized by involuntary movements similar to those observed in patients with chorea. Prominent dyskinesias include tardive dyskinesia, which is a late-appearing dyskinesia associated with the use of antipsychotic medications; and levodopa-induced dyskinesias, which result from an excessive reversal of dopamine deficiency. Other hyperkinetic disorders such as hemiballismus are less common.

Dystonias

Dystonias are characterized by involuntary abnormal posturing, muscle spasms, and tremors. Dystonic reactions can occur in any part of the body but are most noticeable and troublesome when they occur in the face and neck areas. Dystonias are related to a decrease in dopamine.

Overview of Basal Ganglia Function

The function of the basal ganglia is complex.[2, 26, 33, 42, 47] Attempts to reduce these complexities to diagrammatic representations are important; however, if oversimplified they minimize the aforementioned complexities, and if too detailed they pose the risk of incomprehensibility. In an attempt to balance these competing tendencies, Figure 13.2 provides a schematic of the basic pathways involved in movement.

As previously noted, the basal ganglia contain two major movement loops. These loops involve the path shown in the box below.

The basal ganglia (with the acetylcholine interneurons) receive from the cortex excitatory input that is mediated by the neurotransmitter glutamate. The thalamus receives from the basal ganglia inhibitory input that is mediated by the neurotransmitter γ-aminobutryic acid (GABA). The loop is completed when the cortex receives from the thalamus excitatory input that is mediated by the neurotransmitter glutamate. Basal ganglia activity is further affected by dopamine input from the substantia nigra (specifically, the substantia nigra pars compacta [SNpc]).

The circuits through the basal ganglia are not well understood, but it is known that input is received in the putamen from both the cortex and the substantia nigra and that output comes from the GPi. Circuitry between the putamen and GPi can be divided into two pathways: a *direct pathway* and an *indirect pathway*. The direct pathway *supports cortically initiated movement*; the indirect pathway *inhibits thalamic excitation* of the cortical premotor areas. The direct pathway is excited by

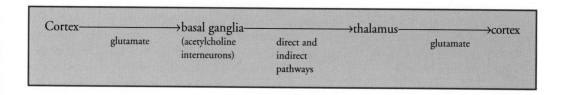

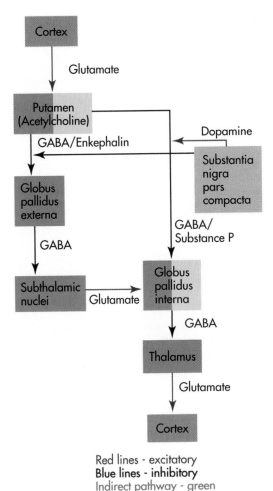

Red lines - excitatory
Blue lines - inhibitory
Indirect pathway - green
Direct pathway - yellow
GABA=gamma aminobutyric acid

Basal ganglia with direct and indirect pathways.

The putamen receives input from both the cortex and substantia nigra pars compacta. The direct pathway (putamen → globus pallidus interna → thalamus) is basically excitatory. The indirect pathway (putamen → globus pallidus externa → subthalamic nuclei → globus pallidus interna → thalamus) is basically inhibitory.

figure 13.2 The direct and indirect pathways of the basal ganglia.

SNpc dopamine projections, whereas the indirect pathway is inhibited.

The direct pathway supports cortically initiated movement. Because both tracts within the direct pathway are inhibitory, movement occurs when these inhibitory paths are themselves inhibited (similar to two negatives resulting in a positive), which results in thalamic liberation from striatal control. This disinhibition is caused by excitatory input from the cortex and SNpc, which in turn interferes with the "normal" inhibitory influence of the basal ganglia on the thalamus. The thalamus, through thalamocortical pathways, then facilitates movement by stimulating prefrontal, premotor, and motor cortices.[55] (See the box on p. 244.)

The indirect pathway inhibits thalamic excitation of the cortex. In the indirect pathway cortical input is excitatory, which enhances the inhibitory function of the putamen (mediated by SNpc dopamine) on the GPe. This inhibition in turn diminishes the inhibitory influence of the GPe on the subthalamic nuclei, which send excitatory input to the GPi and increase the ability of the GPi to inhibit the thalamus. It should be noted that the only transmitter difference between the direct and indirect pathways occurs in the putamen. The direct pathway is mediated by GABA and substance P, whereas the indirect pathway is mediated by GABA and enkephalin. This difference becomes significant in the discussion of Huntington's disease later in this chapter. (See the box on p. 244.)

Summary of Basal Ganglia Function

The SNpc, through its dopamine projections, excites the direct pathway and inhibits the indirect pathway. That is, the direct pathway selects and facilitates movement by allowing the thalamus to excite prefrontal, premotor, and motor cortices. The indirect pathway inhibits movement by inhibiting thalamic input to the prefrontal, premotor, and motor cortices. Dopamine from the SNpc, antagonized by acetylcholine interneurons in the putamen, both facilitates and inhibits movement and does so by balancing the competing influences of the direct and indirect pathways of the basal ganglia. Hallett's[26] suggestion that

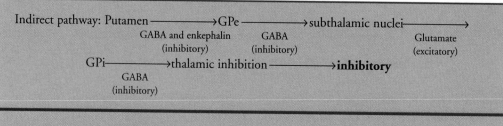

Direct pathway: Putamen ————→ GPi ————→ thalamic liberation ————→ **excitatory**
                        GABA and substance P   GABA
                        (inhibitory)   (inhibitory)

Direct pathway in summary: Liberates thalamus to *excite* cortex for movement. Overactivity causes too much movement; underactivity causes difficulty initiating movement.

Indirect pathway: Putamen ————→ GPe ————→ subthalamic nuclei ————→
                        GABA and enkephalin   GABA   Glutamate
                        (inhibitory)   (inhibitory)   (excitatory)
          GPi ————→ thalamic inhibition ————→ **inhibitory**
              GABA
              (inhibitory)

Indirect pathway in summary: Inhibition of thalamus inhibits movement. Overactivity increases inhibitory effect; underactivity decreases inhibitory effect.

types of movement disorders can be theoretically linked to changes in the activity level of the two pathways is a reasonable model for understanding these disorders. For example:

1. Disturbances that increase the function of the direct pathway (e.g., too much dopamine) "overliberate" the thalamus and may lead to overactivity (e.g., dystonia, dyskinesia, tics).
2. Disturbances that decrease the function of the direct pathway (e.g., too little dopamine) "underliberate" the thalamus and may lead to slowing of voluntary movements (e.g., bradykinesia, parkinsonism).
3. Disturbances that increase the function of the indirect pathway (e.g., too little dopamine) may lead to lack of movement or rigidity (e.g., parkinsonism).
4. Disturbances that decrease the function of the indirect pathway (e.g., too much dopamine) decrease the inhibitory influence on the thalamus, which can no longer filter out unwanted

movements; involuntary movement (e.g., chorea, dyskinesia) results.

 Parkinson's Disease

Parkinson's disease (PD) is a progressive, chronic, and degenerative disease of unknown cause (idiopathic) that involves the basal ganglia and SNpc. It was described in 1817 by Dr. James Parkinson in *An Essay of the Shaking Palsy*, which is based on his encounters with six individuals in London.[45] By the end of the century, "shaking palsy" was replaced with its Latin equivalent *paralysis agitans* as the diagnostic term for what is now called Parkinson's disease. It is interesting that few descriptions of what might be interpreted as PD appear in the literature before Parkinson's time. In a review of the history of PD, Duvoisin[15] observes that notables such as Galen, da Vinci, and Rembrandt may have been familiar with individuals with parkinsonian symptoms, but such

box 13.2
Dr. Parkinson's Progressive Symptoms of Parkinson's Disease

1. Slight weakness and tremor develop in one limb.
2. Tremor spreads to opposite side within 12 months.
3. Posture becomes less erect in a few more months.
4. Lower extremity trembling and unilateral fatigue develop. "Hitherto the patient will have experienced little inconvenience . . ."(p. 4).
5. Difficulty with hand movements and walking that require considerable will power. "At this period the patient experiences much inconvenience . . ." (p. 5).
6. Reading, writing, and the use of eating utensils become very difficult.
7. Patient leans forward when walking and ". . . adopt[s] unwillingly a running pace" (p. 7).
8. Sleep becomes disturbed and chronic constipation develops.
9. Walking becomes very difficult and patient cannot walk ". . . unless assisted by an attendant who walking backwards before him prevents his falling . . ." (p. 8).
10. The patient becomes bedridden with "the chin . . . almost immoveably bent down upon the sternum" (p. 9).
11. Finally, "the urine and feces are passed involuntarily; and at the last, constant sleepiness, with slight delirium, and other marks of extreme exhaustion, announce the wished-for release" (p. 9).

Modified from Parkinson J: *An essay on the shaking palsy,* London, 1817, Whittingham & Rowland.

musings are speculative. As the quote at the beginning of the chapter indicates, Parkinson himself lamented the lack of information on which he could build.[45] The limited historical documentation of this relatively common neurodegenerative disorder has led some scientists to search for environmental toxins that might account for the emergence of PD over the last 200 years, which is roughly the time period of the industrial age.

PD presents with a triad of symptoms: tremors, rigidity, and bradykinesia. It is one neurodegenerative disease in which the symptoms can be successfully managed; however, over time the disease eventually prevails, and motor impairment causes disability.[1] Box 13.2 lists the sequence of symptoms observed and recorded by Dr. Parkinson.

Epidemiology and Demographics

PD is rare before the age of 30 but correlates positively with age after that point. Approximately 10% of the patients with PD report an onset before age 40; 30% of the cases occur before age 50;

40% occur during the 50s; and the remainder develop after age 60.[28] Possible explanations for this age continuum include the increased neuronal vulnerability associated with aging. Indeed, some clinicians suggest that everyone would develop PD if they lived long enough. The prevalence of the disease does not seem to vary between genders, but racial differences may occur; whites seem to be more likely to develop PD than blacks. The incidence of PD is thought to be approximately 20 new cases per 100,000 population in the United States, with a prevalence rate that is between 70 and 190 per 100,000 and continues to increase until the ninth decade.[36,47,52] Approximately 2% of the population over age 65 suffers from PD.[40] A virtual epidemic of parkinsonism could develop early in the next century as a significant proportion of the U.S. population approaches that retirement milestone.

The role of genetics in PD is not clear and may be minimal, but risk factors continue to be explored, including the synergistic effects of certain environmental factors when superimposed on a genetic predisposition for the disease. The only currently accepted risk factor is age: as people age they have a greater risk of developing PD.[30]

Psychobiological Considerations
Macroscopic Brain Alterations

In the absence of other neurological disease, the uncut brain of a person with PD is unremarkable on postmortem examination. However, a midbrain section reveals degenerative changes that are visible to the naked eye. Diminution in color of two pigmented brainstem nuclei may be seen. The darkly pigmented cells of the substantia nigra are abnormally pale, whereas changes in coloration of the smaller locus ceruleus may or may not be apparent. Developmentally, melanization is a slowly evolving process, with pigmentation occurring in the SNpc between 20 and 30 years of age.[18] The pigmented cells of the SNpc synthesize dopamine, and the pigmented cells of the locus ceruleus synthesize norepinephrine. The loss of dopamine-generating cells is the single most critical factor in PD; the loss of norepinephrine-generating cells is somewhat less significant. Other neuronal systems that experience loss include the serotonergic cells in the raphe nuclei and the cholinergic cells in the nucleus basalis of Meynert. Figure 3.2 contrasts the midbrain of a person with PD with a person without PD. This figure illustrates the changes in pigmented brainstem nuclei.

Eighty percent of brain dopamine is located in the basal ganglia, which accounts for only 0.5% of the weight of the brain.[33] The rate of SNpc cell loss in nonaffected persons is approximately 0.5% per year; this rate is doubled to approximately 1% per year (approximately 10 neurons per day) in those with PD.[49] In some cases of PD, the total loss of pigmented cells in the SNpc can approach 90%.[1] A certain threshold of cell loss must occur before symptoms are noticeable: 50% to 60% of the cells in the SNpc[18] and 70% to 80% of the dopaminergic neurons that project to the putamen.[1] The concept of "threshold" is consistent with other body diseases in which extensive organ deterioration occurs before symptoms are expressed. The fact that a person with up to 50% SNpc loss can presumably continue to function without (or with minimal) motor dysfunction results from increased activity of the remaining dopamine-generating cells and an increased sensitivity of the postsynaptic dopamine receptors.[1]

Microscopic Brain Alterations
Neuronal Cell Loss and Lewy Bodies

The loss of pigmented cells in the substantia nigra can be confirmed microscopically and is associated with the cellular inclusion of Lewy bodies and pale bodies (see Figure 2.4, C). The presence of neuronal cell loss and Lewy bodies confirms the diagnosis of PD.[1] Lewy bodies are round, eosinophilic cytoplasmic inclusions with an unstained halo.[51] They always indicate neuronal degeneration but can be found before significant cell loss is apparent.[28] In fact, as much as 10% of the general population 80 years of age and older may have a few midbrain Lewy bodies without symptoms of PD.[28] These individuals, if they live long enough, may be expected to develop PD once the neuronal loss threshold is reached.

Lewy bodies are not found exclusively in the substantia nigra; they can also be found in the locus ceruleus, nucleus basalis of Meynert, and cerebral cortex. Lewy bodies are not found in the substantia nigra with certain parkinsonism-related syndromes such as striatonigral degeneration (SND) and progressive supranuclear palsy (PSP), but they are found in corticobasal ganglionic degeneration (CBGD), diffuse Lewy body disease (DLBD), and other rare disorders.[18] These findings underscore the need for continual refinement of neurological and neuropathological knowledge.

The Role of Free Radicals in Neurodegeneration

Heavy metals, including iron, are known to contribute to neuronal degeneration. Iron has a loosely bound electron that can be donated to the oxidative process; most oxidation in the human body is iron dependent.[30] The highest concentrations of iron in the brain are found in the globus pallidus, substantia nigra, and red nucleus.[43] Furthermore, brain iron levels in PD have been found to be double or triple those found in unaffected individuals.[16] It is thought that the iron-mediated oxidation process leads to the development of cytotoxic free radicals that destroy neurons, particularly neurons located in structures with high iron concentrations.

Oxidation typically requires a coenzyme such as nicotinamide-adenine dinucleotide (NAD) to transfer the electrons. A breakdown in the electron transfer mechanism has also been linked to cellular degeneration. For example, monoamine oxidase catalyzes the oxidation of dopamine to hydrogen peroxide. A deficient electron transfer system or the absence of sufficient glutathione (a detoxifying enzyme) promotes rapid conversion of hydrogen peroxide to the hydroxyl free radical that leads to lipid peroxidation. The free radical hypothesis supports the observations of heroin users in the early 1980s. Seven of these individuals intravenously injected a synthetic form of heroin that contained the toxic contaminant MPTP (1-methyl-4-phenyl-1,2,3,6-tetrahydropyridine). All seven individuals developed classic symptoms of PD. The cytotoxic effect of MPTP can be partially explained by its degradation to free radicals; its role in turning off cellular respiration is also known to contribute to cell death.[30,47] As Burkhardt and Weber[9] have noted, a self-perpetuating cycle develops in which free radicals damage enzyme complexes; this damage generates more free radicals, which damage more enzyme complexes.

Neurophysiological Brain Alterations

PD results from reductions in dopamine synthesis in the SNpc and from reductions in dopamine receptors in the putamen. A balance between dopamine from the midbrain and acetylcholine in the putamen is required for normal movement. Dopamine serves as an inhibitory influence on the basal ganglia pathways; acetylcholine serves as an excitatory influence on these pathways. When an imbalance occurs (i.e., dopamine depletion), movement disorders such as PD develop. Dopamine depletion and the resulting imbalance between dopamine and acetylcholine can occur in three ways:

1. Degeneration of dopamine-producing cells of the SNpc as exists in PD
2. Chemical depletion of neuronal dopamine (e.g., with reserpine)
3. Dopamine blockade at the postsynaptic receptor (e.g., with antipsychotic drugs)

Box 13.3 provides a representation of the imbalance between the excitatory neurotransmitter acetylcholine and the inhibitory neurotransmitter dopamine. It should be noted that acetylcholine appears to play a secondary role because drugs that increase acetylcholine (e.g., choline or physostigmine) do not precipitate parkinsonism.[6] However, cholinergics *can* increase rigidity in patients with PD.

Using the model proposed by Hallett[26] (see Figure 13.2), diminution of the dopaminergic inhibitory influence on the indirect pathway results in overactivity of this pathway, which leads to greater inhibition of thalamic activity. Accordingly, difficulty in movement and/or rigidity would be expected to occur. Decreased dopamine excitatory influence on the direct pathway results in an underactive pathway, which also suppresses thalamic expression and makes voluntary movement sluggish or bradykinetic.

Brain Imaging Techniques, Findings, and Research

Brain imaging techniques are useful in the study of PD because they allow the clinician to rule out less common but possible causes of parkinsonism-like symptoms. Magnetic resonance imaging (MRI) is of particular value because it can image iron and the level of iron accumulation in the substantia nigra and basal ganglia.[43] Width reductions in the substantia nigra have been determined by MRI. Future brain imaging research may focus on measuring iron levels in nonaffected individuals with hopes of developing therapies to block the neurodegeneration caused by iron-related oxidation processes. Positron emission tomography (PET) enables in vivo study of dopamine receptor pharmacology and neuronal activity.[25]

box 13.3
Imbalance Between Dopamine and Acetylcholine Causing Parkinson's Disease

1. A neurochemical model of Parkinson's disease.

> **Dopamine** is depleted because of loss of dopamine-generating cells in SNpc

> **Acetylcholine** bioavailability is out of balance with dopamine

2. A relative balance should be restored after treatment with dopaminergics to increase dopamine, anticholinergics to decrease acetylcholine, or both.

> **Dopamine** is increased by dopaminergic agents such as levodopa, amantadine, bromocriptine, and selegiline

> **Acetylcholine** is reduced by anticholinergic drugs such as benztropine, biperiden, and trihexyphenidyl

Clinical Applications
Clinical Findings and Course

The three primary symptoms of PD are tremors, bradykinesia, and rigidity.

Tremors

Tremors are the most common symptom of PD (approximately 75% of cases) and are probably the most annoying but the least debilitating of the primary symptoms and the most responsive to treatment. Tremors are usually detected in the arm or hand and often manifest as a "pill-rolling" motion. Stress can exacerbate tremors, and relaxation may improve them. Parkinsonian tremors occur at rest and are distinguished from tremors associated with other diseases (e.g., alcoholism), which appear with movement. Parkinsonian tremors are related to extrapyramidal system dysfunction, whereas intention tremors result from cerebellar lesions. Parkinsonian tremors respond to both anticholinergic and dopaminergic drugs.

Tremors are far from limited to PD. Other sources of tremors include other movement disorders, drug side effects (e.g., monoamine oxidase inhibitors [MAOIs], lithium, caffeine, valproate), familial or essential tremors, and anxiety. In contrast to parkinsonian tremors, familial tremors occur during voluntary movement. The decision to treat familial tremors, which may include stereotactic thalamotomy, is directly related to the level of disability. Because voluntary movement is affected, everyday tasks such as writing can become profoundly compromised. Alcohol often subdues this type of tremor. Cerebellar tremors also appear with intentional or voluntary movement. Lesions may be related to stroke, injury, or alcoholism.

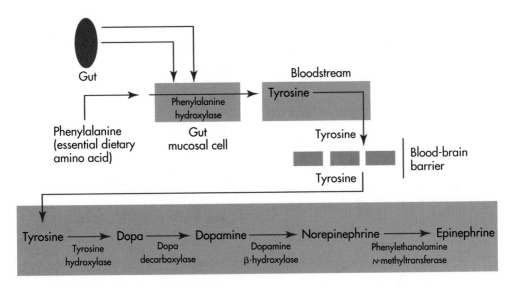

figure 13.3 The normal synthesis of catecholamines.

Bradykinesia

Bradykinesia, perhaps the most debilitating symptom of PD, is defined as a generalized slowing down of motor activity. (Akinesia is the absence of movement.) Bradykinesia makes it difficult for a person to overcome inertia; there is difficulty initiating movement, difficulty changing the speed of movement, and difficulty stopping movement. Although the ability to engage in simple motor tasks is preserved to some degree, more complex movements are significantly impaired. Dopaminergic agents usually improve bradykinesia.

Rigidity

Rigidity also makes movement difficult and can take the form of either lead-pipe or cogwheel rigidity. Lead-pipe rigidity is characterized by resistance through the entire range of motion. Cogwheel rigidity is rachetlike, with intermittent relaxing and stiffening of a muscle. Rigidity is increased by cholinergic drugs such as physostigmine and is improved by anticholingerics such as trihexyphenidyl (Artane).[4]

Other Symptoms

Other important symptoms of PD include postural difficulties; a gait disorder characterized by shuffling steps, festination, and freezing; and orthostatic hypotension. These problems contribute to the many fall-related injuries seen in this population. Postural disturbances are the least amenable to treatment and are probably related to nondopaminergic lesions "downstream" from the dopaminergic nerve terminals. Sleep difficulties, including frequent awakenings and an inability to fall asleep or stay asleep, are also prominent. An average weight loss of 10 to 30 pounds occurs in many patients. This weight loss can be attributed to dysphagia, the increased caloric demand of tremors and involuntary movements, or perhaps a hypothalamic response to the altered brain biochemistry.

Dementia develops in 15% to 20% of patients with PD; depression develops in approximately 40%.[12, 51] Depression can be partially explained by decreased dopamine, which is a precursor to norepinephrine. Figure 13.3 depicts catecholamine synthesis. Cummings[12] suggests that the development of depression in PD approximates the following model:

1. Neuronal loss in the brainstem nuclei leads to
2. Biochemical depletion of mesocortical and prefrontal neurons, which leads to
3. Decreased reward mediation, environmental dependency, and inadequate stress response, which leads to
4. Apathy, worthlessness, hopelessness, helplessness, and dysphoria.

Course

Box 13.2 outlines the course of PD as observed by Dr. Parkinson. A contemporary five-stage classification system has been developed by Hoehn and Yahr:[28]

- Stage 0: no visible disease
- Stage 1: only one side of the body is affected
- Stage 2: both sides are affected, but balance is not impaired
- Stage 3: mild balance impairment
- Stage 4: moderate balance impairment
- Stage 5: severe impairment leading to complete immobility

The progression of PD is typically slow and occurs over a period of at least 25 years. However, the problems associated with functional disabilities do affect the quality of life and can lead to physical and social withdrawal.

Clinical Consequences

A number of clinical consequences are related to the cumulative effects of the primary symptoms on specific muscles or muscle groups:

- *Facial muscles.* Masked facies, leading to the appearance of inappropriate affect in social situations
- *Eye muscles.* Blepharospasm, with difficulty opening or closing eyelids
- *Intercostal muscles.* Difficulty breathing, leading to vulnerability to respiratory disease
- *Muscles of mastication.* Difficulty chewing
- *Pharyngeal muscles.* Difficulty swallowing (dysphagia is a late symptom), leading to drooling (sialorrhea), choking

- *Vocal cord muscles.* Difficulty speaking, with a fading of volume, leading to social and interpersonal difficulties
- *Muscles of the trunk.* Difficulty with balance and posture, leading to falls
- *Bladder muscles.* Difficulty initiating urine stream, leading to urinary hesitation, retention, incontinence, and infections
- *Bowel muscles.* Difficulty initiating bowel movement, leading to constipation, impactions, and incontinence

Clinical Management Implications
Psychosocial/Behavioral Implications

Successful management of PD requires the skills and resources of many types of professionals from medicine, nursing, occupational therapy, and physical therapy. Although a great emphasis is placed on drug therapy and the fine tuning of that therapy, patients most often desire to be treated with respect, understanding, and an implied desire to help. Treatment is compromised to the degree that these needs and the needs for education and participation in treatment are not met. When practical resources from other disciplines are not used, the patient's best interests are not being considered.

Psychopharmacology

PD is associated with a dramatic decrease of dopamine levels in the basal ganglia. Although it may seem obvious to give patients dopamine, dopamine does not cross the blood-brain barrier and cannot be effective. Treatment of PD is primarily based on restoring the balance between dopamine and acetylcholine. Therefore two major categories of antiparkinson drugs have been used over the years: drugs that increase dopamine (dopaminergics) and drugs that decrease acetylcholine (anticholinergics). Dopaminergic drugs can be categorized as dopamine precursors, dopamine releasers, dopamine agonists, and dopamine metabolism blockers. Table 13.1 provides a list of dosages for selected antiparkinson drugs.

table 13.1
Antiparkinson Drugs

DRUG	STARTING ADULT DOSAGE
Dopaminergics	
Amantadine (Symmetrel)	100 mg bid
Bromocriptine (Parlodel)	1.25 mg bid
Carbidopa-levodopa (Sinemet)	1 Sinemet 25/100 mg tablet tid or 1 Sinemet 10/100 mg tablet tid or qid
Levodopa (Dopar, Larodopa)	0.5-1 g/day in divided doses
Pergolide (Permax)	0.05 mg/day
Selegiline (Eldepryl)	5 mg at breakfast and lunch
Anticholinergics	
Benztropine (Cogentin)	0.5-1 mg, hs
Biperiden (Akineton)	2 mg tid or qid
Ethopropazine (Parsidol)	50 mg qd or bid
Trihexyphenidyl (Artane)	1-2 mg/day

Phenylalanine ⟶ tyrosine ⟶ L-dopa ⟶ dopamine ⟶ norepinephrine

     phenylalanine   tyrosine   dopa   dopamine

     hydroxylase   hydroxylase   decarboxylase   β-hydroxylase

Dopamine precursors: levodopa, carbidopa-levodopa.

The sequence of dopamine synthesis is shown in the box above.

Levodopa (L-dopa) is a precursor to dopamine and crosses the blood-brain barrier. It was given to patients with PD with remarkable initial success; however, the disease soon reappeared. Some attempts at increasing the dosage of levodopa led to severe peripheral side effects. Side effects develop because, when given alone, 90% of levodopa is converted to dopamine by the enzyme dopa decarboxylase *before* it crosses the blood-brain barrier. The modest but temporary success experienced with levodopa has driven scientists to develop a drug that more completely penetrates the blood-brain barrier. A drug that effectively delivers levodopa to the brain has been synthesized by adding carbidopa, a dopa decarboxylase inhibitor, to levodopa in a combination called Sinemet.

Levodopa is the most effective antiparkinson drug. It can be given initially in mild cases and typically peaks in effectiveness within 5 years. To take advantage of this "honeymoon" period, some clinicians wait to prescribe levodopa until the disease is more advanced. Two phenomena associated with PD affect progress: the "wearing-off" phenomenon and the "off-on" phenomenon. The wearing-off phenomenon is characterized by an exacerbation of symptoms after the last dose of the day. Multiple smaller doses may help this problem. The on-off phenomenon is characterized by dramatic changes in impairment, from walking to confinement to a bed, all in the course of a few minutes.

Dopamine releaser: amantadine. Amantadine (Symmetrel) is typically used early in PD, is slightly less effective than levodopa, and is slightly more effective than anticholinergics. It causes the release of the dopamine that is still available in dopaminergic neurons; it also inhibits the reuptake of dopamine. Amantadine is effective in up to 50% of patients. The particularly bothersome side effects of amantadine include delusions, hallucinations, and confusion.

Dopamine agonists: bromocriptine, pergolide. Bromocriptine (Parlodel) and pergolide (Permax) bypass the SNpc and directly stimulate the dopaminergic postsynaptic receptors, which produces a dopamine-like effect. Bromocriptine is used most effectively in mild-to-moderate PD either alone or adjunctively with carbidopa-levodopa. Pergolide is 10 to 1000 times more potent than bromocriptine, is longer acting, and is more effective in the advanced stages of PD.

Dopamine metabolism inhibitor: selegiline. Selegiline (Eldepryl) is a monoamine oxidase-B inhibitor and can be given alone or adjunctively with levodopa in all stages of PD. The significance of this drug is twofold. First, by blocking dopamine metabolism, greater levels of dopamine are available for basal ganglia function. Second, selegiline interferes with the role of monoamine oxidase-B in the oxidation process that produces cytotoxic free radicals. This interference with the oxidation process appears to have a preventive capability. Therefore the greatest treatment potential for selegiline is in the early stages of the disease, when greater numbers of dopaminergic neurons are viable. Tetrud and Langston[53] found that selegiline slowed the progression of PD by 40% to 83%, which delays the need for levodopa. By delaying the need for levodopa, patients reserve the therapeutic but time-limited effects of levodopa and avoid or postpone the complications of long-term, high-dose levels of levodopa.

Anticholinergics: benztropine, biperiden, trihexyphenidyl. Another approach to restoring the balance between dopamine and acetylcholine is to use anticholinergics (e.g., benztropine [Cogentin], biperiden [Akineton], trihexyphenidyl [Artane]) to block the excitatory effect of acetylcholine. Such drugs have been used to treat PD for more than 100 years.[4,46] They are useful not only during the early stages of PD but also in treating drug-induced parkinsonism.[4] Anticholinergics are most effective in treating rigidity, are somewhat less effective in reducing tremors, and are least effective for bradykinesia and gait disturbances. Side effects, drug interactions, and other significant parameters of these drugs can be reviewed in the companion text, *Psychotropic Drugs*, second edition.[34a] However, it should be noted that by blocking acetylcholine, anticholinergics may cause cognitive symptoms that mimic or aggravate dementia.

Other antiparkinson drugs: diphenhydramine, ethopropazine. Diphenhydramine (Benadryl) is an antihistamine with anticholinergic properties. Ethopropazine (Parsidol) is a phenothiazine. Phenothiazines are a class of drugs that typically block dopamine and intensify the symptoms of PD. Ethopropazine is an effective antiparkinson drug, particularly for tremors, but it is rarely used.

Antioxidants. If oxidation processes lead to dopaminergic neuron degeneration, it follows that dietary supplements such as antioxidant vitamins may play a protective role in preventing PD. Tanner[52] suggests that geographical areas with lower rates of PD may not necessarily have fewer environmental toxins as commonly thought but may have a richer and more consistent source of antioxidants. Burkhardt and Weber[9] suggest that a lifelong diet abundant in antioxidants protects against developing PD. However, later supplementation with antioxidant vitamins may be too little and too late to alter the progression of the disease.

Symptoms resistant to drug therapy. Several parkinsonian symptoms are fairly resistant to drug therapy and include imbalance and postural instability, bladder dysfunction, constipation, pain related to the disease, speech difficulties, sexual dysfunction, and psychological problems.[11]

box 13.4

Model for Drug-Induced Parkinsonism

Clinical Manifestation	Theoretical Understanding	Intervention	Possible Effect of Intervention
1. Positive symptoms of schizophrenia	2. Increased bioavailability of dopamine	3. Antipsychotic drug(s) (dopamine antagonists)	4. Improvement of psychotic symptoms and possible development of EPSEs
	Dopamine / Acetylcholine		Acetylcholine / Dopamine
5. EPSEs (e.g., parkinsonism, akathisia)	6. An iatrogenic imbalance between ACh and dopamine has occurred	7. Add anticholinergic drug to treatment regimen	8. Continued improvement in psychotic symptoms and amelioration of EPSEs (restored balance between dopamine and acetylcholine)
			Dopamine / Acetylcholine

EPSEs, Extrapyramidal side effects; *ACh,* acetylcholine.

Environmental Considerations

Since the occurrence of the MPTP-related cases of PD, researchers have sought to identify environmental toxins as causative factors in the disease. Agricultural pesticides and herbicides are promising candidates, but firm links have yet to be established.

Drug-Induced Parkinsonism

Drug-induced parkinsonism, one of several related extrapyramidal side effects (EPSEs), is most often associated with the use of antipsy-

chotic or neuroleptic agents. Traditional antipsychotic drugs block dopamine receptors in the mesolimbic area of the brain; because of this biochemical characteristic, they are therapeutic in the treatment of psychosis (see Chapter 5). However, because dopamine receptor blockade is nonselective, the nigrostriatal pathway is also blocked, which leads to drug-induced movement disorders. Box 13.4 summarizes the theoretical neurochemical steps of the development and treatment of EPSEs in a patient who is taking antipsychotic medications.

Traditional antipsychotic medications can be

table 13.2
Efficacy of Anticholinergic Drugs*

EXTRAPYRAMIDAL SIDE EFFECTS	ANTICHOLINERGIC DRUGS
Akathisia: a subjective feeling of restlessness; occurs in approximately 50% of all patients taking long-term, high-potency neuroleptics	Diphenhydramine most effective; others equieffective
Akinesia: absence of movement	Amantadine, biperiden, and trihexyphenidyl most effective; ethopropazine least effective
Rigidity	Benztropine considered most effective; diphenhydramine least effective
Tremor	All anticholinergics basically equieffective

Modified from Bezchlibnyk-Butler KZ, Remington GJ: Antiparkinsonian drugs in the treatment of neuroleptic-induced extrapyramidal symptoms, *Can J Psychiatry* 39:74-84, 1994.
*Anticholinergic drugs include amantadine, benztropine, biperiden, diphenhydramine, ethopropazine, procyclidine, and trihexyphenidyl.

roughly divided into low- and high-potency categories. Low-potency drugs not only block dopamine receptors but also show an affinity for cholinergic, α-adrenergic, and histaminic receptors. High-potency neuroleptics possess a greater affinity for dopamine receptors. Therefore high-potency drugs such as haloperidol and fluphenazine are more likely to cause an imbalance between acetylcholine and dopamine and result in EPSEs. Because antipsychotic agents block dopamine receptors, they iatrogenically mimic the outcomes of neurodegeneration found in PD: tremors, bradykinesia, and rigidity. Akathisia, dystonia, and dyskinesia are also adverse responses to antipsychotic medications. Table 13.2 summarizes the efficacy of antiparkinson drugs for these EPSEs.

 Huntington's Disease

Choreas are hyperkinetic disorders that present with involuntary, unpredictable, random movements that eventually involve all muscle groups. Huntington's disease (HD) is a common form of chorea.

Formerly referred to as Huntington's chorea, HD is characterized by involuntary choreiform movements. Cognitive decline, personality alterations, and changes in social conduct occur and can have devastating effects on the family and other social support systems. Most cases can be traced from two English brothers who immigrated to the United States in 1630.

More than 100 years later, Dr. George Huntington, the son and grandson of Long Island physicians, was first to describe and report this disease process. By comparing his own observations with those of his father and grandfather, he established the inheritability of this disease among certain families in the New York area.

HD is an autosomal dominantly inherited neurodegenerative disease caused by a mutated gene on chromosome 4.[24] The disease typically strikes during the fourth or fifth decades of life, with children of an affected parent having a 50% chance of inheriting the disease. Before the modern era of testing for genetic markers, these children spent their lives wondering whether or not they would develop HD. Many of these individuals opted to remain childless rather than subject an offspring to this terrifying uncertainty. Unfortunately, even for those "missed" by the disease, childbearing was often no longer an option. In addition, many people who were unaware of their

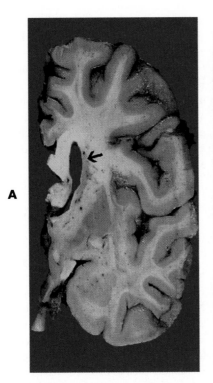
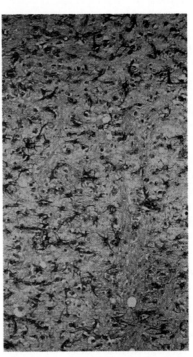

figure 13.4   **A,** A coronal section that demonstrates the caudate nucleus *(arrow)* in a patient with Huntington's disease. The severely atrophic caudate nucleus no longer bulges into the lateral ventricle, as seen in the normal brain (Figure 13.1). **B,** Microscopic section demonstrates the marked astrocytic gliosis found in the caudate nucleus in Huntington's disease. (See Chapter 2 for a discussion of gliosis.) *(Courtesy Dr. Richard E. Powers, Director, University of Alabama at Birmingham Brain Resource Program.)*

own risk for HD started families, which potentially expanded the gene pool for this disorder.

Epidemiology and Demographics

Because HD does not skip generations, unaffected parents cannot pass it on to their own children. Prevalence is approximately 5 per 100,000 population, with no gender preference.

Psychobiological Considerations

HD, a hyperkinetic disorder, is almost the polar opposite of PD. Instead of a paucity of movement there is overmovement; instead of a decrease in basal ganglia output there is an increase in basal

ganglia output; and instead of a deficiency of dopamine there is a relative excess of dopamine bioavailability.

Macroscopic Brain Alterations

On gross examination, the brain of a patient with HD may look normal, particularly in the early stages. The brain later becomes atrophic, with brain weight commonly less than 1100 g.[29] Atrophy of the caudate nucleus and putamen, as well as enlargement of the lateral ventricles are characteristic (but sometimes slight) (Figure 13.4, *A*). Neurodegeneration begins in the caudate nucleus and moves from the caudate tail to the lateral caudate; putamen destruction follows. Gross examination of the substantia nigra and the cerebellum is unremarkable. Because the macroscopic findings are equivocal, the diagnosis must be based on histological findings.

Microscopic Brain Alterations

Microscopic examination (Figure 13.4, *B*) reveals an extensive loss of neurons in the striatum (up to 90%), thalamus, hypothalamus, subthalamic nucleus, nucleus accumbens, SNpc (approximately 40%), and cortex.[27,29] A consequence of striatal degeneration is the loss of acetylcholine interneurons in the putamen and GABA-enkephalin projections from the indirect pathway of the GPe (see Figure 13.2) in the early stages of HD.[27] This loss reduces the activity of the subthalamic nuclei and their inhibitory effects on the GPi.

The neuronal deterioration in HD may be caused by a chain of neurophysiological events triggered by abnormalities of chromosome 4.[33] Although the pathogenetic mechanism is not understood, it is hypothesized that a defect in energy metabolism and the excessive activation of a specific glutamate receptor (*N*-methyl-D-asparate [NMDA]) leads to *glutamate excitotoxicity*, which causes cell damage and death.[23]

Neurophysiological Brain Alterations

The loss of acetylcholine interneurons and the subsequent decrease in cholinergic influence leads to a relative increase in dopaminergic activity in the indirect pathway. When coupled with the loss of GABA-enkephalin projections, an imbalance of the dopamine-acetylcholine-GABA system occurs. The overall effect is a loss of influence by the indirect pathway on the thalamus (thalamic disinhibition), resulting in involuntary movements. As the disease progresses, the direct pathway is affected and GABA–substance P neurons degenerate, which causes an underactive direct pathway and slowing of movement. This sequential destruction of GABAergic neurons—first GABA-enkephalin neurons of the indirect pathway and then GABA–substance P neurons of the direct pathway—does provide an explanation for the

somewhat paradoxical clinical observation that patients with HD experience both choreiform movements and bradykinesia.[26]

The deterioration in these neurotransmitter systems results from the atrophy of striatal nuclei and other nuclei previously mentioned and from the reduction of enzymes required for the formation of acetylcholine and GABA (choline acetyltransferase and glutamic acid decarboxylase, respectively).

Brain Imaging Techniques, Findings, and Research

Brain imaging techniques can be valuable in learning more about the disease process but currently do not have great diagnostic capability. MRI findings disclose caudate nucleus degeneration, and PET studies have revealed decreased glucose metabolism in some presymptomatic carriers and early-stage patients. Physiological imaging techniques such as PET may have greater research potential than the structural imaging techniques for presymptomatic and early-stage HD.

Clinical Applications

Clinical Findings and Course

HD is an incurable, progressive neurodegenerative illness. Early symptoms include absentmindedness, irritability, fidgeting, and occasional falls. Uncontrollable movements begin occurring but at first may be incorporated by the patient into a normal activity (e.g., an involuntary upward arm swing may be converted into a sweeping of the hand through the hair). As uncontrollable movements progressively worsen, falls begin to take a toll; eventually the patient is confined to a wheelchair and then to a bed with padded rails. In addition, speech dysfunction evolves from simple slurring to a total inability to communicate. Cognitive decline progresses to dementia, and psychologically the patient becomes depressed and psychotic. The course of the illness typically runs over a 15- to 20-year time span from diagnosis to death.[33] In that period of time the person with HD changes from a fully functioning human being to someone who is bedridden, unable to communicate, and demented.

Clinical Consequences

The inability to control muscles, the inability to communicate, and cognitive decline converge into a constellation of clinical consequences. Falls and other injuries resulting from lack of coordination and uncontrollable movements are persistent concerns. Choking and food aspiration present many problems. The inability to communicate culminates in frustration and anger. Changes in brain structure and neurophysiology cause dementia with associated memory loss, impaired impulse control, and paranoia. Depression, as a reaction to the diagnosis and the realization of what lies ahead, is not uncommon. Suicide as a response to hopelessness and helplessness is a major risk among patients in the early stages of HD. Psychotic symptoms, especially delusions and violent outbursts, are fairly common. Depression and psychosis should be aggressively treated, falls prevented, and angry outbursts managed without injury to the patient or others. Death usually results from heart failure or pulmonary complications caused by asphyxiation or aspiration of food.[35,38,54]

Clinical Management Implications

Psychosocial/Behavioral Implications

Patience with communication, ambulation, eating, and anger is a key behavior when working with the patient with HD. It is also important not to assume that a disability exists on the basis of another disability. For instance, an inability to communicate does not indicate an inability to understand and reason. Nursing strategies to prevent falls and injuries, aspiration of food, and bedsores/bed abrasions are imperative. However, decisions made to protect the patient must be balanced with extending autonomous function as long as possible and with maintaining dignity.

Support groups are available for families and other caregivers and are known to be helpful. Pro-

fessionals are best able to help the patient when alliances are built with caregivers and when families are treated with sensitivity and caring.

Genetic testing. Family members not only carry the brunt of caregiving but may also be uncertain about their own risk for developing HD. Genetic counseling and a presymptomatic diagnosis are available for those who wish to know if they are affected by this heritable disorder. This testing capability is particularly valuable for individuals with an unclear family history. Divorce, the untimely death of a parent, extramarital affairs, and uncertain parentage can contribute to this problem.

Psychopharmacology

The control of symptoms is the goal of drug treatment in HD. Dopamine antagonists such as haloperidol and clozapine help restore the dopamine-acetylcholine-GABA balance by blocking dopamine receptors in the striatum and increasing the production of enkephalins.[27] The net result is a reduction in choreiform movements but perhaps at the cost of function deterioration.[13] Theoretically, glutamate receptor blockers that prevent glutamate excitotoxicity would be beneficial, but studies are currently inconclusive.[47]

 ## Dyskinesias

Dyskinesias are *hyperkinetic* disorders characterized by involuntary movements similar to those observed in chorea. They affect muscles of the mouth and face, causing lipsmacking, teeth grinding, rolling or protrusion of the tongue, and other cosmetically disfiguring movements. Choreic movements of the extremities, truncal rocking, twisting, squirming, and pelvic gyrations can develop. Diaphragmatic involvement may impair breathing. Although the neuropathology is not known, the model proposed by Hallett[26] suggests an underactive indirect pathway and/or an overactive direct pathway, both of which cause choreiform movements. The majority of dyskinesias are iatrogenic. The most common dyskinesias are tardive dyskinesia associated with neuroleptic agents and L-dopa dyskinesia caused by levodopa therapy.

Tardive Dyskinesia

Tardive dyskinesia is a late-appearing neuro-muscular side effect that primarily results from neuroleptic drug therapy. It was first observed in the 1950s—soon after the introduction of an-tipsychotic drugs in large state hospital patient populations. Prevalence rates vary considerably between surveys (0.5% to 60%), but a rate be-tween 15% and 25% appears probable.[31, 32, 34, 37, 41] Demographic variables that increase susceptibility are age (elderly), ethnicity (African-American), and gender (female).[20,34,48]

Other risk factors may include a history of PD or epilepsy, duration of neuroleptic therapy (i.e., chronic therapy), high historical cumulative dosage, the use of high-potency neuroleptics, and the use of anticholinergics.[31,41,48]

Tardive dyskinesia typically occurs after chronic use of neuroleptic drugs or after neuroleptic with-drawal (emergent tardive dyskinesia). The former is associated with irreversibility, whereas tardive dyskinesia related to shorter-term use or neu-roleptic withdrawal may reverse. Etiologically, tar-dive dyskinesia is explained as dopamine receptor supersensitivity. After the chronic use of neurolep-tics, dopamine receptors in the striatum presum-ably become overly sensitive, thus creating a neu-rophysiological opposite of PD.

Unfortunately, treatment success has changed little over the past 40 years. When tardive dyski-nesia is diagnosed, neuroleptics are typically dis-continued. However, the available evidence is in-conclusive regarding whether doing so prevents worsening of symptoms. Two calcium channel blockers, nifedipine (Procardia) and verapamil (Calan) have produced statistically significant im-provements in patients with tardive dyskinesia.[3,14] The newer, atypical antipsychotic drugs, includ-ing clozapine (Clozaril), risperidone (Risperdal), olanzapine (Zyprexa), sertindole, and quetiapine (Seroquel) do not appear to cause tardive dyskine-sia and have been reported to improve dyskinetic symptoms.[7] Although calcium channel blockers

and atypical antipsychotics provide some opti-mism for treatment, prevention remains the most effective approach for tardive dyskinesia. Conser-vative treatment, including lower dosages when clinically realistic and the use of atypical agents, are approaches commonly used to reduce the inci-dence of this movement disorder.

L-Dopa Dyskinesia

L-Dopa dyskinesias occur in the treatment of PD and presumably are related to basal ganglia "overexposure" to dopamine. Technically, L-dopa dyskinesias are tardive (late-appearing) because they appear after 3 to 5 years of levodopa therapy; however, most clinicians reserve a diagnosis of tar-dive dyskinesia for the neuroleptic-induced disor-der. As previously noted, too much dopamine causes the indirect pathway to be underactive and the direct pathway to be overactive, thus releasing the thalamus from basal ganglia inhibition. Treat-ment approaches include adding a second med-ication. In newly diagnosed patients, the use of selegiline should slow symptom development and postpone the need for levodopa.

 ## Dystonias

The term *dystonia* implies lack or impairment of muscle tone and can be partially explained by co-contraction, or the simultaneous contraction of opposing muscle groups.[19] Dystonias can be roughly divided into idiopathic dystonias and drug-induced acute dystonic reactions.

Dystonia is characterized by involuntary move-ments that lead to persistent muscle contractions. These contractions are manifested by abnormal fixed postures and usually arise out of voluntary movements. These involuntary abnormal postures are embarrassing and painful, and can be terrify-ing. More common dystonic reactions include oculogyric crisis, blepharospasm, spasmodic torti-collis, and laryngeal-pharyngeal constriction. Spasmodic torticollis and laryngeal-pharyngeal constriction can cause a life-threatening breathing difficulty. Dystonia of the trunk, or dystonia mus-culorum deformans, can result in torsion so pronounced that sitting or standing is not possible. Ventilation can be impaired with this type of dystonia and lead to respiratory disease vulnerability. Voluntary movements in a patient with dystonia are slow and are characterized by overflow of movement (unneeded muscle movement).[26]

Psychobiological Considerations

The pathophysiology of dystonia is not well understood; neither macroscopic nor histological abnormalities have been documented on postmortem examination.[29] Bhatia and Marsden[5] propose that both the direct and indirect pathways (see Figure 13.2) are affected, with dysfunction of the indirect pathway predominating and being responsible for co-contraction of muscle groups. There is overactivity of the direct pathway, causing excessive and overflow movement, and overactivity of the indirect pathway, causing bradykinesia and rigidity. The model proposed in Figure 13.2 is inadequate to fully explain dystonia.

In addition to basal ganglia influence on thalamocortical neurons, a loss of inhibitory influence on the pedunculopontine nucleus (PPN) exists. The PPN mediates posture and reflexes and is inhibitory. When an unaffected person performs voluntary movement, the PPN inhibits reflexes; when that same person is at rest, the PPN liberates reflexes and allows such routine activities as sitting in a chair or standing (i.e., posture). When the PPN is released from inhibitory control of the basal ganglia, a reflex overresponsiveness develops, which causes rigidity. In other words, a dystonic reaction develops when a voluntary movement is burdened by reflexes that will not "turn off," resulting in bizarre postures and bradykinetic movements.[5,8,26] The role of the PPN in dystonia seems to be supported by animal studies in which thalamotomies reverse chorea but not dystonia in MPTP monkeys.[44]

Brain imaging results have not yielded conclusive evidence of predictable pathologic conditions. Various PET studies have demonstrated inappropriate overactivity of the basal ganglia and their projections to frontal areas during limb movement.[8] As Brooks states, "Whether the frontal association area overactivity is simply secondary to primary basal ganglia overactivity or represents an adaptive phenomenon in a conscious attempt to suppress the syndrome is unclear."[8]

Drug-Induced Acute Dystonic Reactions

Drug-induced acute dystonic reactions are most often the result of neuroleptic drug therapy. The dopamine antagonistic effects of neuroleptic agents cause a dysfunction in both the direct and indirect pathways. The incidence of acute dystonia related to neuroleptic drugs is high, with rates varying from 7% (with prophylaxis) to 50%.[17] Risk factors for developing acute dystonic reactions are young age, male gender, and taking high-potency agents.

Clinical Applications

The treatment of dystonia and drug-induced dystonic reactions begins with anticholinergic drugs. Tables 13.1 and 13.2 list anticholinergic agents and their relative efficacy for EPSEs. The prophylactic use of anticholinergics is debatable but less controversial in young men, the highest at-risk group. The following is a list of treatment protocols for EPSEs, including dystonic reactions:
1. Reduce neuroleptic dosage.
2. If changing dosage is not realistic, consider switching to a less potent neuroleptic.
3. Add an anticholinergic based on efficacy (Table 13.2).
4. If EPSEs continue, increase the amount of anticholinergic.
5. Continue use of the anticholinergic for several months; if treatment is stabilized, slowly decrease the amount until completely withdrawn.

Other drugs that have proven successful in the treatment of dystonic reactions include clonazepam (Klonopin) and carbamazepine (Tegretol).

Treatment of refractory idiopathic dystonia may be accomplished with botulinum toxin injections. Botulinum toxin interferes with acetylcholine at the neuromuscular junction, thus paralyzing the affected muscle and reversing the dystonic posture.[10] The paralysis remits within a

few months, with the biggest risk being overpara-
lyzing the area or causing paralysis too close to a
sensitive area (e.g., the larynx).[10]

•••

Summary

Disorders of movement are caused by dysfunction of the basal ganglia. The basal ganglia receive
input from the cortex and the SNpc and send
output to the thalamus. The movement loop is
complete when the thalamus sends output to the
cortex. The basal ganglia are part of the extrapyramidal system that supports voluntary movement
with unconscious background stability. A loss of
that stabilizing infrastructure causes three categories of movement disorders: hypokinetic, hyperkinetic, and dystonic. Degeneration of basal ganglia structures or changes in basal ganglia inputs
from the midbrain may alter the two major pathways in the basal ganglia—the direct pathway and
the indirect pathway—which results in a wide
range of movement disorders.

REFERENCES

1. Agid Y: Parkinson's disease: pathophysiology, *Lancet* 337:1321-1323, 1991.
2. Albin RL, Young AB, Penney JB: The functional anatomy of basal ganglia disorders, *Trends Neurosci* 12:336-375, 1989.
3. Barrow N, Childs A: An anti–tardive dyskinesia effect of verapamil, *Am J Psychiatry* 143:1485, 1986.
4. Bezchlibnyk-Butler KZ, Remington GJ: An-tiparkinsonian drugs in the treatment of neurolep-tic-induced extrapyramidal symptoms, *Clin J Psy-chiatry* 39:74-84, 1994.
5. Bhatia K, Marsden C: The behavioral and motor consequences of focal lesions of the basal ganglia in man, *Brain* 117(pt 4):859-876, 1994.
6. Borison R, Diamond B: Neuropharmacology of the extrapyramidal system, *J Clin Psychiatry* 48(suppl 9):7-12, 1987.
7. Borison R, Pathiraja A, Diamond B et al: Risperi-done: clinical safety and efficacy in schizophrenia, *Psychopharmacol Bull* 28:213-218, 1992.
8. Brooks D: The role of basal ganglia in motor con-trol: contributions from PET, *J Neurol Sci* 128(1):1-13, 1995.
9. Burkhardt CR, Weber HK: Parkinson's disease: a chronic, low-grade antioxidant deficiency? *Med Hypoth* 43:111-114, 1994.
10. Camicioli R: Movement disorders in geriatric reha-bilitation, *Clin Geriatr Med* 9(4):765-781, 1993.
11. Clough CG: Parkinson's disease: management, *Lancet* 337:1324-1327, 1991.
12. Cummings JL: Depression and Parkinson's disease, *Am J Psychiatry* 149(4):443-454, 1992.
13. Davis KL, Berger PA: Pharmacological investiga-tions of the cholinergic imbalance hypotheses of movement disorders and psychosis, *Biol Psychiatry* 13:23-49, 1978.
14. Duncan E, Adler L, Angrist B et al: Nifedipine in the treatment of tardive dyskinesia, *J Clin Psy-chopharmacol* 10(6):414-416, 1990.
15. Duvoisin RC: A brief history of parkinsonism, *Neurol Clin* 10(2):301-316, 1992.
16. Earle KM: Studies on Parkinson's disease including x-ray, fluorescent spectroscopy of formalin fixed brain tissue, *J Neuropath Exp Neurol* 27:1-14, 1968.
17. Gelenberg AJ: Treating extrapyramidal reactions: some current issues, *J Clin Psychiatry* 48(suppl 9):24-27, 1987.
18. Gibb WRG: Neuropathology of Parkinson's disease and related syndromes, *Neurol Clin* 10(2):361-376, 1992.
19. Gildenberg PL: Management of movement disor-ders: an overview, *Neurosurg Clin North Am* 6(1):43-53, 1995.
20. Glazer J, Morgenstern H, Doucette M: Predicting the long-term risk of tardive dyskinesia in outpa-tients maintained on neuroleptic medication, *J Clin Psychiatry* 54:133-138, 1993.
21. Goetz CG, Pappert EJ: Trauma and movement dis-orders, *Neurol Clin* 10(4):907-919, 1992.
22. Graybeil A: The basal ganglia, *Trends Neurosci* 18:60-62, 1995.
23. Gu M, Gash MT, Mann VM et al: Mitochondrial defect in Huntington's disease caudate nucleus, *Ann Neurol* 39(3):385-389, 1996.
24. Gusella JF, Wexler NS, Conneally PM et al: A poly-morphic DNA marker genetically linked to Hunt-ington's disease, *Nature* 306:234-238, 1983.
25. Guttman M: Dopamine receptors in Parkinson's disease, *Neurol Clin* 10(2):377- 386, 1992.
26. Hallett M: Physiology of basal ganglia disorders: an overview, *Can J Neurol Sci* 20(3):177-183, 1993.
27. Hartmann J, Kunig G, Riederer P: Involvement of transmitter systems in neuropsychiatric diseases, *Acta Neurol Scand* 87(suppl 146):18-21, 1993.

28. Hoehn MMM, Yahr MD: Parkinsonism: onset, progression, and mortality, *Neurology* 17(5):427-442, 1967.

29. Jellinger KA, Lantos PL, Mehraein P: Pathological assessment of movement disorders: requirements for documentation in brain banks, *J Neural Transm* 39(suppl):173-184, 1993.

30. Jenner P: What process causes nigral cell death in Parkinson's disease? *Neurol Clin* 10(2):387-403, 1992.

31. Jeste DV, Caligiuri MP, Paulsen JS et al: Risk of tardive dyskinesia in older patients: a prospective longitudinal study of 266 outpatients, *Arch Gen Psychiatry* 52(9):756-765, 1995.

32. Jeste DV, Eastham JH, Lacro JP et al: Management of late-life psychosis, *J Clin Psychiatry* 57(suppl 3):39-45, 1996.

33. Kandel E, Schwartz J, Jessell T et al: *Principles of neural science,* Norwalk, Conn, 1991, Appleton & Lange.

34. Kane JM, Smith JM: Tardive dyskinesia: prevalence and risk factors, 1959 to 1979, *Arch Gen Psychiatry* 39:473-481, 1982.

34a. Keltner NL, Folks DG: *Psychtropic drugs,* ed 2, St Louis. 1997, Mosby.

35. Kermis MD: Mental health in late life: the adaptive process, Boston, 1986, Jones & Bartlett.

36. Lannon MC, Thomas CA, Bratton M et al: Comprehensive care of the patient with Parkinson's disease, *J Neurosci Nurs* 18(3):121-131, 1986.

37. Lieberman J, Pollack S, Lesser M et al: Pharmacologic characterization of tardive dyskinesia, *J Clin Psychopharmacol* 8(4):254-260, 1988.

38. Matteson MA, McConnell ES: Gerontological nursing: concepts and practice, Philadelphia, 1988, WB Saunders.

39. Middleton F, Strick P: Anatomical evidence for cerebellar and basal ganglia involvement in higher cognitive function, *Science* 266:458-461, 1994.

40. Montgomery EB: Heavy metals and the etiology of Parkinson's disease and other movement disorders, *Toxicology* 97:3-9, 1995.

41. Mukherjee S, Rosen AM, Cardenas C et al: Tardive dyskinesia in psychiatric outpatients, *Arch Gen Psychiatry* 39:466-469, 1992.

42. Nolte J: *The human brain,* ed 3, St Louis, 1988, Mosby.

43. Olanow CW: Magnetic resonance imaging in parkinsonism, *Neurol Clin* 10(2):405-420, 1992.

44. Page RD, Sambrook MA, Crossman AR: Thalamotomy for alleviation of levodopa-induced dyskinesia: experimental studies in the 1-methyl-4-phenyl-1,2,3,6-tetrahydropyridine-treated parkinsonian monkeys, *Neuroscience* 55:147-165, 1993.

45. Parkinson J: *An essay on the shaking palsy,* London, 1817, Whittingham and Rowland.

46. Pletscher A, DaPrada M: Pharmacotherapy of Parkinson's disease: research from 1960 to 1991, *Acta Neurol Scand* 87(suppl 146):26-31, 1993.

47. Roberts GW, Leigh PN, Weinberger DR: *Neuropsychiatric disorders,* London, 1993, Wolfe.

48. Salzman GJ: Tardive dyskinesia: prevalence and risk factors in neuroleptic therapy, *Res Staff Phys* (2):59-65, 1985.

49. Scherman D, Desnos C, Darchen F et al: Striatal dopamine deficiency in Parkinson's disease: role of aging, *Ann Neurol* 26:551-557, 1989.

50. Silverstein PM: Moderate Parkinson's disease: strategies for maximizing treatment, *Postgrad Med* 99(1):52-54, 61-63, 67-68, 1996.

51. Stacy M, Jankovic J: Differential diagnosis of Parkinson's disease and the parkinsonism plus syndromes, *Neurol Clin* 10(2):341-359, 1992.

52. Tanner CM: Epidemiology of Parkinson's disease, *Neurol Clin* 10(2):317-329, 1992.

53. Tetrud JW, Langston JW: The effect of deprenyl (Selegiline) on the natural history of Parkinson's disease, *Science* 245:519-522, 1989.

54. Wills R: Cognitive changes of normal aging and the dementias. In Carnevali DL, Patrick M, editors: *Nursing management for the elderly,* ed 2, Philadelphia, 1986, JB Lippincott.

55. Zweig R: Functions of the basal ganglia, *Brain* 118(6):822, 1995.

chapter fourteen
Epilepsies

Among the common serious neurological disorders, epilepsy ranks second only to strokes and is associated with cognitive decline, behaviorial difficulties, and a mortality rate two to four times that of the nonepileptic population.[40] Epilepsy is a brain disorder characterized by a recurring excessive neuronal discharge and manifested by transient episodes of motor, sensory, or psychic dysfunction with or without unconsciousness or convulsive movements. The clinical manifestations of epilepsy range from minor staring spells that lack motor activity to life-threatening generalized seizures in which patients suffer bone fractures and require emergency medical intervention. The generic term **seizure** often refers to the motor activity only. The term **ictus** refers to the specific seizure event (e.g., post-ictal). A seizure can be broken into four clinical components: the **preictal, ictal** (or intra-ictal), **post-ictal,** and **inter-ictal** phases. The features and components of each phase vary according to the patient and the "type" of seizure disorder. Seizure disorders are associated with marked changes in recorded electrical brain activity.

The Neuroepidemiology Branch of the U.S. National Institute for Neurological Disorders and Strokes defines epilepsy as two or more afebrile seizures unrelated to acute metabolic disorders or to withdrawal from drugs or alcohol. Active epilepsy is defined as a seizure within the past 5 years or the current use of an antiepileptic drug (AED) on the basis of a correct diagnosis of epilepsy.[37] Individuals who have experienced only febrile or neonatal seizures are not included under this definition.

Epidemiology and Demographics

Epilepsy is one of the most common neurological disorders, but attempts to understand prevalence and incidence rates have been hampered historically by inconsistent definitions and classifications, diagnostic inaccuracies, and methodological problems in the field. Furthermore, underreporting has occurred because of the stigma attached to epilepsy and because some cultures view certain seizure types as annoyances rather than as serious neurological disorders (e.g., absence seizures).

The **incidence** of epilepsy in the United States is approximately 150,000 newly diagnosed cases per year out of approximately 300,000 people who seek medical intervention for seizures.[2,13,40] The **prevalence** of epilepsy in industrialized nations is thought to be between 0.5% and 1% of the population;[13,40] however, higher prevalence rates (2% to 3%) have been reported.[31,36] A higher prevalence rate exists in nonindustrialized countries, where as many as 57 people per 1000 population (5.7%) develop epilepsy.[37] Worldwide, as many as 50 million people are affected.[34] Currently, approximately 2 million patients have been diagnosed with epilepsy in the United States, 17% of whom are children under 17 years of age.[2] Approximately 1.5% to 2% of individuals over 75 years of age suffer from epilepsy in the United States.[15]

Epilepsy typically develops early in life (90 per 100,000 in the first year of life) or after age 65 (130 to 170 per 100,000), with the years in between relatively risk-free for idiopathic (cause unknown) seizures.[15] By age 20, almost 5% of all

box 14.1
Risk Factors for Epilepsy and Seizures

Early Life Variables

Genetic Factors

The risk of epilepsy increases by a factor of three when first-degree relatives are affected and is likely to be higher in cultures that permit marriage to relatives. Only 1% of epilepsies are thought to be genetically transmitted.

Perinatal Factors

Perinatal disease often causes epilepsy:
- Perinatal hypoxia and brain trauma: hippocampal damage is a common consequence of hypoxia/anoxia
- Prematurity
- Mother over 30 years of age
- Neonatal bilirubinemic encephalopathy

Febrile Seizures

Febrile seizures affect approximately 2% to 5% of children, with most recovering without long-term sequelae. Experiencing febrile seizures in childhood places an individual at a sixfold risk for developing epilepsy.

Infectious Processes

Parasitic Infections

Parasitic infections are much more common in developing regions of the world. The following are significant parasitic infections that lead to epilepsy and seizures:
- Cysticercosis: caused by the larvae of the pork tapeworm *Taenia solium* and a common cause of seizures in Africa, Latin America, and Asia
- Schistosomiasis: caused by *Schistosoma japonicum* and endemic in southeast Asia
- Paragonimiasis: caused by *Paragonimus westermani* and found in the Far East, southeast Asia, parts of Africa, and South America
- Toxoplasmosis: associated with AIDS, with epilepsy being a common consequence
- African trypanosomiasis (sleeping sickness): caused by *Trypanosoma brucei* and found in sub-Sarahan Africa
- American trypanosomiasis (Chagas' disease): caused by *Trypanosoma cruzi* and found in Central and South America
- Malaria: Found in tropical Africa, America, Asia, and the eastern Mediterranean region

Bacterial Infections
- Tuberculous meningitis: can cause epilepsy
- Pyogenic meningitis: found worldwide and probably the number-one cause in the United States; risk continues up to 20 years after infection

Viral and Other Infections
- Encephalopathies: can cause seizures and epilepsy (especially herpes simplex)
- Creutzfeldt-Jakob disease: a prion disease
- AIDS

Modified from International League Against Epilepsy: Guidelines for epidemiologic studies on epilepsy, *Epilepsia* 34(4):592-596, 1993.

box 14.1
Risk Factors for Epilepsy and Seizures—cont'd

Other Causes

Autoimmune diseases (e.g., lupus, multiple sclerosis)

Cerebrovascular accidents (e.g., stroke, intracerebral hemorrhage, subarachnoid hemorrhage)

Head injuries (e.g., fighting, motor vehicle accidents, bicycle accidents, brain surgery)

Metabolic abnormalities (e.g., metabolic diseases affecting the nervous system, such as hypoglycemia, hypocalcemia, hyponatremia, eclampsia, phenylketonuria, hypoxia)

Neoplasms (e.g., incompletely resected or unsuccessfully treated tumors)

Neurodegenerative disorders (e.g., Alzheimer's disease, Huntington's disease)

Toxic agents (e.g., chloroquine [used to treat malaria], prescription drugs [e.g., aminophylline, imipramine, bupropion], drug overdose, alcohol [acute ingestion and withdrawal], illicit drugs [e.g., cocaine], environmental exposure [carbon monoxide, lead, camphor, organophosphates])

children in the United States have experienced a seizure; however, only about one fourth of these children actually have epilepsy.[14] Most childhood seizures are febrile and self-limiting and cause no long-term sequelae. Neonatal seizures, particularly those occuring in the first week of life, are associated with negative outcomes, including death and neurological disorders (e.g., cerebral palsy and mental retardation).[14]

In the United States the diagnosis of epilepsy is roughly divided between partial and generalized epilepsy; in developing countries generalized seizures are more often diagnosed. This difference may reflect cultures that underreport what are perceived to be minor events. Men are more commonly affected by epilepsy than are women; this overrepresentation is probably a result of men's higher exposure to risk factors. Approximately 70% of epilepsies are idiopathic; 15% result from cerebrovascular problems, 6% result from tumors, another 6% result from alcohol, and 2% are caused by trauma.[33] The risk factors for epilepsy and seizures are found in Box 14.1.

Psychobiological Considerations

Most cases of epilepsy (70%) have an unknown etiology; gross anatomical examination therefore contributes little to the understanding of the neurological abnormalities related to epilepsy. However, Roberts, Leigh, and Weinberger[33] point out that, because of the continued refinement of neuropathological knowledge and technology, there is much to be learned about the cellular substrates associated with electrical misfirings in the brain. The percentage of idiopathic epilepsy may well diminish in the next quarter century as pathological bases are clarified.

Macroscopic Brain Alterations

Macroscopic brain alterations are found in any number of acquired epilepsies. Pathological conditions in the brain caused by trauma, tumor, stroke, or neurodegenerative disorders can be demonstrated by autopsy, brain imaging, or biopsy (Figure 14.1). Figure 14.2 depicts surgical procedures in the treatment of refractory epilepsy.

Microscopic Brain Alterations

With epilepsy, histological examination reveals changes at the cellular level. Nevertheless, after many years of study the relationship between brain pathology and epileptogenesis remains vague. Whether these changes follow the pattern of insult–seizure–neuronal destruction or seizure–neuronal destruction–insult is not clear. What is clear is that seizure activity causes some neuronal damage, and the neuronal damage can precipitate

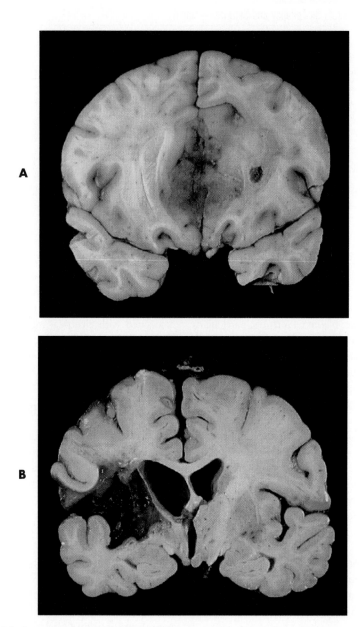

figure 14.1   Seizures can be caused by tumors and strokes. **A,** Coronal section of the brain demonstrates a midline glial tumor (malignant oligodendroglioma). **B,** Coronal section demonstrates old stroke on the left in the middle cerebral artery distribution. *(Courtesy Dr. Richard E. Powers, Director, University of Alabama at Birmingham Brain Resource Program.)*

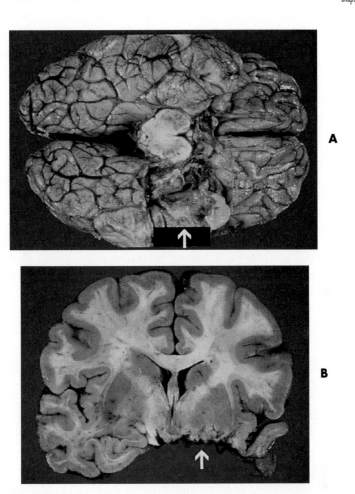

figure 14.2   Surgery is being used to control some refractory epilepsy. This photograph is of a
brain from a patient with intractable seizures. Arrows mark the surgery site. In both the ventral view **(A)**
and coronal view **(B)** the right hippocampus and parahippocampal gyrus have been removed, resulting
in a marked reduction in seizure frequency. *(Courtesy Dr. Richard E. Powers, Director, University of Alabama at Birmingham Brain Resource Program.)*

more seizures.[41,46] The pathological conditions of
the brain that are closely associated with epilepsy
include neuronal destruction related to seizure-
induced hypoxia, changes in cytoarchitecture, and
hippocampal abnormalities (mesial temporal sclerosis).

Status epilepticus can cause neuronal destruction. Neuronal loss is caused in part by hypoxia
and ischemia that occur after a time threshold

is passed. Changes in cytoarchitecture are expressed as changes in cellular configuration, size,
or density and have been confirmed by histological studies.[11,17]

Hippocampal Pathology

Seizures, especially status epilepticus, are believed to set in motion an excitotoxicity process
that broadly kills brain cells, with hippocampal

tissue being the most vulnerable.[17,26] Postmortem examinations reveal a shrunken and sclerotic hippocampus in many patients who suffer from idiopathic/cryptogenic temporal lobe epilepsy. One theory to explain the manner by which cell death occurs has been proposed by Wasterlain and Shirasaka[46] and involves the course shown in the box below.

This model is supported by case studies of domoic acid poisoning, in which many individuals became ill and suffered neurological symptoms after eating mussels. Domoic acid is an analogue of glutamate and binds with glutaminergic receptors. Cendes, Andermann, and Carpenter et al[4] describe the domoic acid poisoning of an 84-year-old man and his subsequent generalized seizures and complex partial status epilepticus. Postmortem examination revealed hippocampal atrophy.

Sloviter[41] proposes a slightly different model of hippocampal involvement in epilepsy. As noted in Chapter 1, the hippocampus and dentate gyrus contain three layers of neurons instead of six layers as in the cortex. The intermediate layer of the dentate gyrus is the *granule cell* layer; the intermediate layer of the hippocampus proper (Ammon's horn) is the *pyramidal cell* layer (Figure 14.3). Sloviter suggests that individuals with a history of status epilepticus, prolonged febrile seizures, head trauma, or encephalitis may experience deafferentation (interruption of sensory input) by inhibitory neurons projecting to the granule cell layer. This deafferentation leads to a cellular delamination of the granule layer cells and hence a loss of their inhibiting function. Without this inhibitory presence, responses to cortical stimuli may go awry, resulting in a seizure. Sloviter fur-

---

Seizures release glutamate (excitatory)→binds to NMDA and non-NMDA receptors→Ca^{++} floods cell→increasing intracellular Ca^{++}→activating Ca^{++} enzymes that irreversibly damage neurons

---

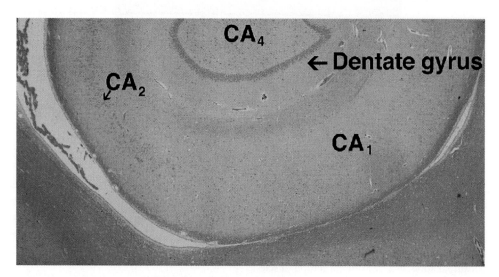

figure 14.3   Photomicrograph of the hippocampus that was surgically removed from the brain in Figure 14.2 reveals near-total neuronal loss in the CA1 region. CA2 and dentate gyrus are relatively spared. *(Courtesy Dr. Richard E. Powers, Director, University of Alabama at Birmingham Brain Resource Program.)*

ther suggests that a negative loop develops wherein hippocampal damage is both the cause and the effect of seizures that emanate from the hippocampus.[41]

The hippocampus proper of the hippocampal formation, or Ammon's horn, is not spared with epilepsy. Ammon's horn sclerosis is a common postmortem finding in patients with epilepsy.[48] Ammon's horn sclerosis appears to be associated with a history of febrile seizures, but because this sclerotic condition is not generally found in children, it is also thought to be a product of chronicity.

Neurophysiological Brain Alterations

Epileptic seizures are characterized by recurring excessive neuronal discharge. The process of neuronal discharge is mediated by neurotransmitters and their receptors. Excessive discharge is generated by an imbalance between excitatory and inhibitory neurotransmission. The excitatory neurotransmitters linked to seizures are glutamate and somatostatin. In addition to the role of glutamate excitotoxicity in neuronal destruction, there may be an increased density and sensitivity of glutamate receptors that contribute to the imbalance. Somatostatin may contribute to epileptogenesis by losing its ability to stimulate the inhibitory system.[33]

γ-Aminobutyric acid (GABA) is the major inhibitory neurotransmitter in the central nervous system (CNS) and is found in approximately 60% to 70% of all CNS synapses.[44] A reduction in GABA activity has been connected to a loss of local inhibition and to hyperexcitable clusters of neurons that lead to seizures.[49] Most pharmacological treatment approaches therefore focus on manipulating the GABAergic system.

The following box illustrates the synthesis of GABA:

Glutamic acid $\longrightarrow$ GABA
glutamic acid decarboxylase

The following box illustrates the metabolism of GABA:

GABA $\longrightarrow$ succinic semialdehyde
GABA aminotransferase

When GABA is released into the synaptic cleft, it attaches to a postsynaptic receptor and is either taken up into the presynaptic axon or taken up by neighboring glial cells.[44] Understanding the mechanism for GABA synthesis and metabolism provides a foundation for understanding the pharmacodynamics of AEDs, in which GABA receptors play a particularly significant role.

Two types of GABA receptors are found on the postsynaptic neuron: $GABA_A$ and $GABA_B$. $GABA_A$ receptors are of the most significance in treating epilepsy. $GABA_A$ receptor stimulation results in an increased inflow of chloride, which causes hyperpolarization of the cell (neuronal inhibition). The $GABA_A$ receptor has several distinct subtypes, including benzodiazepine and GABA subtypes. Measures that increase GABA synthesis, decrease GABA metabolism, decrease the reuptake of GABA into presynaptic and glial cells, or mimic GABA at the postsynaptic $GABA_A$ receptors increase GABA bioavailability and reduce seizure activity.

Brain Imaging Techniques, Findings, and Research

Magnetic resonance imaging (MRI) and computed tomography (CT) can detect some of the anatomical changes associated with epilepsy. They are particularly beneficial in detecting atrophy in the temporal lobes (Figure 14.4), hippocampal volume loss, and structural abnormalities such as dysplasias. This technique is less suited to identifying extratemporal lesions. Single photon emission computed tomography (SPECT) and positron emission tomography (PET) are two functional imaging procedures (see Chapter 4); they provide less anatomical resolution than MRI

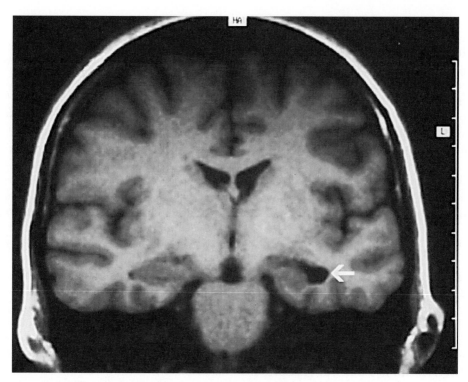

figure 14.4   T1-weighted coronal MRI reveals hippocampal atrophy and temporal horn enlargement *(arrow)*, which is a common result or cause of temporal lobe epilepsy. *(Courtesy Dr. Frank G.
Gilliam, Department of Neurology, University of Alabama at Birmingham.)*

but have demonstrated focal areas of reduced
blood flow and a decreased cerebral glucose metabolic rate.[43] SPECT is unique in that imaging can
occur during a seizure (an ictal SPECT). Although areas of increased and decreased perfusion
have been documented intra-ictally, interpretation
is difficult.[43] The diagnostic value of SPECT and
PET will grow as sensitivity and specificity for
identifying temporal and extratemporal epileptogenic sites improve.

Electroencephalography also plays a role in understanding epilepsy and seizures. An electroencephalogram (EEG) records the fluctuations in
electrical activity of large groups of neurons. It
also measures the extracellular current flow of
mostly cortical pyramidal neurons. The electrical
activity of pyramidal neurons can be measured because they are parallel to one another and because
their dendrites are always perpendicular to the
surface of the brain.[22] This configuration mini-

mizes attentuation of the electrical signal and allows "deeper" cortical layers to be measured.[22]
Studies of large numbers of people have resulted
in baseline "abnormal" EEGs against which comparisons of the EEGs of individuals with epilepsy
can be made. Specific seizure types have distinct
EEG patterns; these distinctions aid in diagnosis
and treatment.

Clinical Applications

Epilepsy is a condition that involves abnormal
electrical activity in the brain. Abnormal electrical
activity can be caused by any number of cerebral
or systemic diseases or disorders. These abnormal
occurrences have varying effects on the electrical
activity of the brain; hence several distinguishable
forms of seizures are recognized (Table 14.1). It
should be noted that seizures and epilepsy are not
strictly synonymous; many seizures are the re-

table 14.1
Seizure Classification and Description

SEIZURE TYPE	DESCRIPTION
Partial Seizures (focal or local)	More common than generalized seizures; 70% of adult seizures and 40% of childhood seizures are partial seizures; when partial seizures evolve to generalized seizures they continue to be classified as partial seizures
Simple partial seizures	Do not impair alertness; symptoms depend on area affected; *sensory* symptoms: visual, auditory, and gustatory hallucinations; *autonomic* symptoms: pallor, diaphoresis, vomiting, and flushing; *motor* symptoms: jacksonian; *somatosensory:* tingling
Complex partial seizures (also referred to as psychomotor or temporal lobe epilepsy)	Consciousness is impaired, amnesia is common, and confusion occurs; accounts for 50% of adult epilepsies
Partial seizures secondarily generalized	Simple partial onset with secondary generalization; complex partial onset with secondary generalization; simple partial onset to complex partial onset with secondary generalization
Generalized Seizures	Involve symmetrical distribution of abnormal electrical activity across the hemispheres of the brain; can include both convulsive and nonconvulsive seizures
Convulsive Seizures	
Clonic seizures	Occur mostly in childhood; generalized convulsive seizures lacking tonic component; characterized by clonic jerks; post-ictal phase typically short
Tonic seizures	Sustained contraction of large muscles; continuous tension of chest musculature impairs ventilation and causes pallor or more serious problems if prolonged
Tonic-clonic seizures	Consciousness lost abruptly; series of muscle spasms lasting 3 to 5 minutes from onset to recovery; post-ictal state may last from a few minutes to approximately half an hour; often characterized by confusion, dizziness, sleepiness, and a stunned look
Status epilepticus	Any seizure that occurs without intervals of non-ictal activity; most often applied to tonic-clonic convulsions occurring successively without restoration of consciousness or normal muscle movement for at least 30 mintues; brain damage is known to result from prolonged hypoxia and associated ischemia

table 14.1
Seizure Classification and Description—cont'd

SEIZURE TYPE	DESCRIPTION
Nonconvulsive Seizures	
Absence seizures	Abrupt, sudden loss of responsiveness; can be less than 10 seconds; a variant, true petit mal seizure; has a distinct EEG pattern; typically remits in adolescence
Myoclonic seizures	Characterized by single or multiple jerks that last 3 to 10 seconds; can be generalized or confined, synchronous or asynchronous
Atonic seizures	Sudden diminution of muscle tone, typically without loss of consciousness; injuries related to falls
Unclassified Epileptic Seizures	Includes all seizures that cannot be classified

sponse of a normal brain to a transient noxious insult.[9] Box 14.1 lists a variety of risk factors associated with epilepsy and seizures.

Clinical Findings and Course

Epilepsies and seizures may be broadly categorized as either **symptomatic** or **idiopathic**. Symptomatic seizures are considered to be the consequence of a known or suspected cerebral dysfunction.[18] In contrast, idiopathic epilepsies or seizures have no clearly detectable antecedent. Epilepsies and seizures are also categorized as **provoked** or **unprovoked**. Symptomatic versus idiopathic and provoked versus unprovoked are closely related dichotomies of epilepsy and seizures, but they do not completely overlap. For example, a symptomatic seizure can be considered unprovoked if an old and presumably stable (remote) insult causes a seizure to occur "out of the blue."

Provoked seizures occur in close time proximity to an *acute* systemic, metabolic, or toxic insult or occur in association with an *acute* CNS insult (e.g., infection, stroke, cranial trauma, intracerebral hemorrhage, or acute alcohol intoxication or withdrawal).[18] Unprovoked seizures are of unknown or remote etiology and can be divided between idiopathic epilepsies and **cryptogenic**

epilepsies. The Commission on Classification and Terminology of the International League Against Epilepsy[5] cautions against using the term *idiopathic* indiscriminately and reserves its use for seizures with a specific clinical history and EEG patterns.

Epileptic seizures are categorized according to characteristic physical and neurological signs. Each epileptic subtype has a characteristic EEG pattern.[20] Figure 14.5 displays the EEG patterns of a selected seizure type. Seizures are divided into broad categories: **partial (localization-related) seizures** and **generalized seizures.** If an aberrant electrical discharge is confined to a local area initially, the seizure is partial or focal. Even when the electrical aberration spreads from the focal area to the entire cerebrum (a secondarily generalized seizure), it remains classified as a partial seizure. A generalized seizure, on the other hand, has no clinical evidence of a focal onset. The diagnosis of each of these seizure types can be refined to include several subtypes.

Partial (Localization-Related) Seizures

Partial seizures are more common than generalized seizures and account for approximately 70% of all seizures in adults and 40% of all seizures in children.[8] They typically begin in a focal area. Abnormal brain activity can spread to other parts of

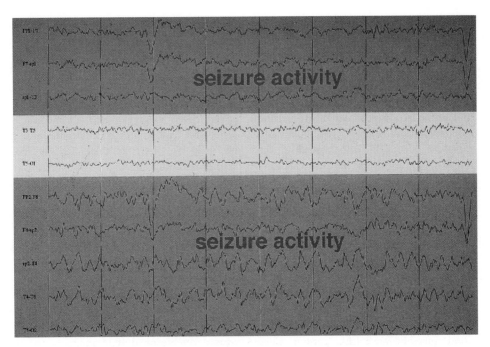

figure 14.5   A ten-channel EEG demonstrates temporal lobe spikes in a patient with epilepsy. *(Courtesy Dr. Frank G. Gilliam, Department of Neurology, University of Alabama at Birmingham.)*

that cerebral hemisphere or even to the other hemisphere. Partial seizure subtypes include simple partial seizures (no loss of consciousness), complex partial seizures (consciousness is impaired), and partial seizures that evolve to generalized tonic-clonic seizures.

Simple partial seizures. Simple partial seizures do not impair an individual's alertness or ability to respond to the environment. Because the electrical abnormality is localized, symptoms depend on the area affected. Motor symptoms include localized jerks, focal jerks that "march" to involve other muscles (i.e., jacksonian march), and speech problems. Sensory symptoms (visual, auditory, gustatory, and hallucinations) and somatosensory symptoms such as tingling may also develop. Autonomic symptoms such as pallor, sweating, vomiting, flushing, tachycardia, hypotension, and hypertension may be distressing to patients. Automatic behaviors can include lip smacking and repetitive movements.

Complex partial seizures. Complex partial seizures are also known as **psychomotor** or **temporal lobe epilepsy** and account for approximately one half of all patients with epilepsy.[48] Consciousness is impaired, amnesia is common, and confusion occurs during or after the seizure. Violent behavior (but not directed violence) may be a major component of seizure activity. Complex partial seizures typically begin as a perceived aura, which is that portion of a seizure that occurs before consciousness is lost and for which memory is retained.[12] A number of cognitive, affective, perceptive, and psychomotor symptoms can occur. Déjà vu, fear, anxiety, hallucinations, and automatic behaviors (automatisms) are commonly present. Between one third and one half of the patients with complex partial seizures are refractory to drug therapy.[48]

Generalized Seizures

Generalized seizures involve a symmetrical distribution of abnormal electrical activity across the hemispheres of the brain. A seizure is considered generalized when the clinical history reveals a lack of a focal onset or any evidence suggesting anatomical localization.[18] Generalized seizures can include both nonconvulsive and convulsive seizures. Nonconvulsive seizures primarily cause unresponsiveness and amnesia, whereas convulsive seizures cause unconsciousness, amnesia, and convulsions. Nonconvulsive seizures include absence seizures, myoclonic seizures, and atonic seizures. Major motor tonic-clonic seizures and generalized status epilepticus are important types of convulsive seizures.

Absence seizures. Absence seizures are characterized by a sudden loss of responsiveness. Often the loss of consciousness is so brief (<10 seconds) that those around the person are unaware of a change. A variant of an absence seizure is the true petit mal seizure, which produces a distinct three-per-second spike-and-wave EEG pattern. These seizures typically begin in childhood and remit during the teenage years.[29]

Myoclonic and atonic seizures. Myoclonic epilepsy is characterized by single or multiple jerks that typically last 3 to 10 seconds. Seizures can be generalized or confined, synchronous or asynchronous. Although underrecognized, juvenile myoclonic epilepsy is a relatively common disorder; it responds well to valproic acid.[38] Atonic seizures result in a sudden loss of muscle tone ("drop attacks"), typically without a loss of consciousness. Injuries related to falls are serious consequences of atonic seizures.

Tonic-clonic seizures. Tonic-clonic convulsions are historically referred to as *grand mal* seizures and are characterized by intense, repetitive tonic-clonic contractions of the entire body. Abnormal brain activity is symmetrical, and most brain pathways are involved. Seizures typically last between 3 and 5 minutes; prolonged seizure activity can result in brain hypoxia.

Status epilepticus. Status epilepticus is a condition in which seizures occur without intervals of non-ictal activity. The term is most often applied to tonic-clonic convulsions that occur successively without restoration of consciousness or normal muscle movements for at least 30 minutes. Brain damage is known to result from the prolonged hypoxia and ischemia associated with status epilepticus. Status epilepticus is a medical emergency and requires immediate attention; it has a mortality rate of 6% to 20%.[3] Because the successful resolution of status epilepticus is time-dependent, a diagnosis must be made early. Treatment must be initiated quickly to avoid serious consequences. Published reports indicate that from the time status epilepticus begins until it is successfully controlled, there is a 60-minute window in which to limit the neuronal necrosis and permanent cerebral injury that results from prolonged refractory status epilepticus.[21] After 60 minutes of status epilepticus, the following physiological problems develop: lactic acidosis, increased cerebrospinal fluid pressure, autonomic dysfunction (e.g., hyperthermia, excessive sweating, dehydration, hypertension followed by hypotension and shock), myolysis and myoglobinuria leading to nephrosis and renal shutdown, and cardiorespiratory failure.[7] Immediate intravenous medication is required for successful intervention. Jordan[21] emphasizes meticulous attention to ventilation and oxygenation, maintenance of adequate blood pressure, prevention of hyperthermia, and close monitoring of cardiac abnormalities as prerequisites to successful outcomes. Hippocampal and temporal lobe sites are primary targets for neuronal loss caused by ischemia; this neuropathological finding has been consistently linked to epilepsy on postmortem examination.[33]

It would be ethically inappropriate to study the natural course of untreated epilepsy. However, it is known that spontaneous remission occurs in significant numbers of people, who can then proceed in life without AEDs. The question of interest to health care professionals is whether the course of epilepsy is affected by AEDs. The obvious answer is that AEDs *do* affect the course, but there are voices that challenge this assumption. Keranen and Riekkinen[23] describe a group of people with untreated epilepsy in an underdeveloped country.

Half (total = 33) had complete remission after 20 years without treatment. Although absolute conclusions cannot be fashioned from such a small sample size, this phenomenon does raise the suggestion of a self-limiting process that proceeds with or without treatment.

Clinical Consequences

Many people with epilepsy lead normal, well-adjusted lives and are able to seek numerous career paths. For these individuals, educational goals are pursued and accomplished with the same success and failure rate as those without epilepsy. Socially, many people with epilepsy live and behave as well as their nonepileptic contemporaries. Others with epilepsy must adapt to a chronic illness that may require AEDs for the rest of their lives. Variables that influence social dysfunction include clinical factors related to epilepsy, the stigma and effects of AEDs, and psychosocial factors such as perceived shame, discrimination, and socioeconomic status.[19]

People with epilepsy are thought to be at greater risk for psychopathology and social dysfunction than is the general population. McKenna, Kane, and Parrish[27] reported a 7% incidence of persistent psychosis within this population; thus individuals with epilepsy are seven times more at risk for psychosis than those without epilepsy. However, a more exact study demonstrates that an increased susceptibility to a psychiatric disturbance occurs primarily when an individual suffers from both partial complex and major generalized seizures.[1] Anxiety and depression are other consequences of epilepsy and are common psychological disorders. Although epilepsy causes transient mental dullness and confusion, recurrent seizures do not result in a loss of intellectual viability. Mental retardation is associated with a higher prevalence of seizures, but the initial suspicion when finding mental slowness should be uncontrolled, subclinical seizures.[1]

Clinical Management Implications

Seizures vary widely among individuals. Some forms of epilepsy may be tolerated, whereas others cannot be tolerated and must be treated immediately. The first diagnostic questions are "What kind of seizure occurred?" "Was it a singular event?" and "Has this seizure been provoked?"

Epilepsy treatment typically begins with AED therapy and continues with one or more agents until remission occurs. An accurate diagnosis of seizure type drives the selection of an AED. An accurate diagnosis is aided by a careful history and an EEG. More than half of all patients with epilepsy suffer from more than one seizure type, which complicates their lives and effective treatment. Unfortunately, AEDs cannot control seizures in approximately 20% to 30% of the cases; individuals in this group are possible candidates for surgery (see Figure 14.2).[47]

By definition, epilepsy cannot be diagnosed until a second seizure occurs. If there has been no recurrence, the clinician must decide whether or not to treat. This decision would be much easier if AEDs were not associated with severe adverse physical reactions and high medical expenses. Adverse reactions range from annoying to life threatening. Medical expenses include the cost of the drug, blood-level determinations, and physician visits.[42] Other factors influencing the decision to treat or not treat after a single seizure are the potential debilitating effects of a second seizure, the amount of anxiety the patient can tolerate (i.e., "waiting for the next seizure"), and occupational implications. Etiology must also be considered. A provoked seizure (or acute symptomatic seizure) does not require an AED if the provoking factor can be identified and treated. If provoking factors cannot be eliminated, AED therapy must be initiated.

Psychosocial/Behavioral Implications

A number of psychosocial roles are affected in the patient with epilepsy. For example, epilepsy may affect the patient's work life, ability to drive, ability to drink alcohol, involvement in athletics, and decisions about becoming pregnant. Some jobs are inappropriate for a person with epilepsy, especially those that include responsibility for operating dangerous equipment. People with epilepsy experience twice the unemployment of nonepileptic individuals; those who do work are less likely to occupy professional and management positions.[2] In many areas of the country the ability to drive is the ability to work. Therefore taking away a person's privilege to drive is a life-changing decision that must be carefully weighed against exposing the public to unnecessary risk.[39] Driving prohibitions against individuals with epilepsy have been liberalized over the years, but restrictions rightfully remain. Although states differ in respect to these restrictions, a seizure-free interval of 1 to 2 years generally must occur before approval to drive is granted (see the section on environmental concerns later in this chapter).[10]

Psychopharmacology

The following are goals of AED therapy:
1. Control seizure activity.
2. Keep side effects to a minimum.
3. Use a single agent (monotherapy) whenever possible.

Five categories of AEDs and a large group of noncategorized AEDs provide the clinician with many options for treating patients. Unfortunately, many seizures are refractory to AEDs. The five major categories of AEDs are the hydantoins, the long-acting barbiturates, the succinimides, the oxazolidinediones, and the benzodiazepines. The AEDs that fall in the "other" category include

table 14.2
Seizure Types Matched Against Commonly Prescribed Antiepileptic Drugs*†

SEIZURE TYPES	AEDs FOUND TO BE EFFECTIVE
Partial Seizures (focal or local)	
Simple partial seizures	Clorazepate, gabapentin, lamotrigine, **phenobarbital,** primidone
Complex partial seizures	**Carbamazepine, phenobarbital, phenytoin,** primidone, valproic acid
Generalized Seizures	
Absence seizures	Clonazepam, **ethosuximide, valproic acid**
Myoclonic seizures	Clonazepam, **valproic acid**
Lennox-Gastaut syndrome	**Clonazepam**
Tonic-clonic seizures	**Carbamazepine, phenobarbital, phenytoin,** primidone, **valproic acid**
Status epilepticus	**Diazepam, lorazepam,** phenobarbital, phenytoin

Bold, first-line drug.

*A number of other AEDs can be used to treat seizures but should be categorized as second- to third-choice drugs or drugs of last resort. Those drugs and the seizures they affect follow:

Other hydantoins: ethotoin: tonic-clonic, complex partial; mephenytoin: partial, jacksonian

Other barbiturates: mephobarbital: tonic-clonic, absence

Other succinimides: methsuximide: absence; phensuximide: absence

Oxazolidinediones: trimethadione: absence; paramethadione: absence

Acetazolamide: absence, tonic-clonic, myoclonic

Lidocaine: status epilepticus

Paraldehyde: alcohol withdrawal

Phenacemide: complex partial

†The following seizure types and their treatment were not addressed in the table:

Magnesium: seizures related to magnesium deficiency (e.g., eclampsia)

Clonazepam: akinetic seizures

Carbamazepine: mixed seizures

proven agents such as valproic acid and carbamazepine, as well as newer, promising drugs such
as gabapentin and lamotrigine. Major considerations in AED therapy are patient size, cost of the
drug, history of allergic response (if any), childbearing potential, and tolerance to side effects.
When more than one drug is known to be effective
in the treatment of a specific seizure type, such criteria may help the clinician decide what to prescribe. Table 14.2 matches seizure type with AEDs
that have proven effective in their treatment. Tables 14.3 and 14.4 and Box 14.2 provide pharmacokinetic, dosage, and additional information
about the various types of AEDs. Dosage and other
specific information can also be found in the companion text, *Psychotropic Drugs*, second edition.[22a]

Hydantoins. Phenytoin (Dilantin) is the prototype hydantoin and is effective in the treatment of
tonic-clonic and complex partial seizures. It is active in the motor cortex, where it inhibits the
spread of abnormal electrical activity in the brain
by normalizing abnormal fluxes of sodium across
the cell membrane during or after depolarization.
This inhibitory effect stabilizes a state of hyperex-
citability. Phenytoin also decreases the activity of
the brainstem centers that are responsible for the
tonic phase of grand mal seizures.[30] Teratogenic

box 14.2
Drug Interactions for Most Antiepileptics

Drugs Affecting Antiepileptics

Alcohol
Antacids
Aspirin
Carbamazepine
Cimetidine (Tagamet)
Disulfiram (Antabuse)
Erythromycin
Fluoxetine (Prozac)
Phenobarbital
Phenytoin
Propoxyphene (Darvon)
Rifampin
Valproic acid

Drugs Affected by Antiepileptics

Folic acid
Meperidine (Demerol)
Oral anticoagulants
Oral contraceptives
Steroids
Theophylline
Vitamins D and K

Data from Ramsey RE, Graves NM, Rowan AJ et al: Clinical
issues in the management of epilepsy, Miami, 1993, University of Miami Press.

table 14.3
Pharmacokinetic Parameters of Major Antiepileptics

DRUG	STEADY STATE (DAYS)	THERAPEUTIC SERUM LEVELS (µg/mL)	TOXIC LEVEL (µg/mL)	HALF-LIFE (HOURS)	PROTEIN BINDING (%)
Phenytoin	7-10	10-20	>20	7-42	~90
Phenobarbital	16-21	15-40	>40	80*	40-60
Ethosuximide	5-10	40-100	>100	40-60	0
Clonazepam	3-7	20-80 ng	>80 ng	18-60	80
Carbamazepine	2-4	4-12	>12	12-17	76
Valproic acid	2-4	50-100	>100	6-16	90
Gabapentin		>2		5-8	<3
Lamotrigine		>2		25 (alone)	55

*Before increased hepatic metabolism is induced.

table 14.4

Side Effects Caused by Selected Antiepileptic Drugs*

AEDs	SIDE EFFECTS AND INTERVENTION STRATEGIES
Carbamazepine **Clonazepam** **Ethosuximide** **Phenobarbital** **Phenytoin**	**Central nervous system** effects, including drowsiness, dizziness, ataxia, sedation. Combination with other CNS depressants can cause a synergistic compounding of depressant effects. Monitor for and prevent falls; caution against driving or alcohol consumption.
Carbamazepine Clonazepam Ethosuximide Phenytoin	**Hematological disorders** are uncommon to rare but can be caused by these drugs and include agranulocytosis, aplastic anemia, thrombocytopenia, increased prothrombin time, and leukopenia. Carefully assess for fever, sore throat, malaise, and bruises.
Carbamazepine Clonazepam **Ethosuximide** Phenobarbital Phenytoin Valproic acid	**Gastrointestinal symptoms** such as nausea, vomiting, cramps, diarrhea, and anorexia occur with these drugs. Taking these medications with meals decreases GI upset.
Ethosuximide **Phenytoin**	**Gingival hyperplasia** can be caused by these agents. Meticulous oral hygiene practices are the best interventions.
Clonazepam Ethosuximide Phenobarbital **Phenytoin**	**Skin rashes** can be mild to life-threatening disorders such as exfoliative dermatitis. Typically the drug is discontinued when a rash appears.
Phenytoin	**Acne** develops in some teenagers. Change to another AED or other hydantoin.

Drugs in **bold** type commonly cause the corresponding side effect.
*This list should not be construed as an exhaustive list of the side effects caused by AEDs.

effects include cleft lip, cleft palate, and cardiac malformations.[6,25]

Long-acting barbiturates. Phenobarbital is the prototypical long-acting barbiturate. Its antiepileptic effect arises from its ability to alter ion movements across neuronal membranes and to inhibit neuronal transmission to the cerebral cortex. These effects slow the response of neurons to seizure-causing stimuli and slow the spread of abnormal electrical activity, which results in an increased seizure threshold. Phenobarbital is used in the treatment of tonic-clonic seizures and in both simple and complex partial seizures. Parenteral phenobarbital is used to stop status epilepticus when diazepam and phenytoin are ineffective or not available. Phenobarbital has been linked to congenital defects.

Succinimides. Ethosuximide (Zarontin) is the prototypical succinimide and is particularly effective in the treatment of absence seizures. Ethosuximide decreases absence seizures by depressing the motor cortex and raising the seizure threshold of the CNS. The distinct EEG pattern associated with absence seizures, the three-cycles-per-second spike-and-wave pattern, is also suppressed. Ethosuximide is a second-choice agent for absence seizures (behind valproic acid). Ethosuximide is one of the safer AEDs for use in women during pregnancy.

Oxazolidinediones. Oxazolidinediones are prescribed for absence seizures but typically are used only when other drugs have failed. These drugs cause serious side effects and are known to pose the greatest risk to the fetus.

Benzodiazepines. Diazepam (Valium) is the prototypical benzodiazepine used in the treatment of status epilepticus. Diazepam is effective in controlling these seizures approximately 95% of the time. It is also used adjunctively to treat other types of epilepsy. Lorazepam (Ativan), another benzodiazepine, is used as a first-choice agent in the treatment of status epilepticus.

An intravenous dose of 5 to 10 mg of diazepam stops most seizures within 5 minutes. Because the serum levels fall rapidly, it may be necessary to repeat the dose to maintain a seizure-free state. Repeated doses at 10- to 15-minute intervals are typically required. No more than 30 mg of diazepam should be given to treat a single episode.[30] If a second episode of status epilepticus occurs within 2 to 4 hours, this protocol can be repeated.[30]

Because of the short-lived effect of diazepam, a phenytoin infusion (18 mg/kg or less at a rate no faster than 50 mg/min) can be hung to follow the first dose of diazepam, thereby avoiding repeated doses of diazepam. If diazepam is used exclusively (up to 30 mg) and seizures persist, an IV phenytoin drip can be provided. A phenobarbital drip (at 100 mg/min) is the next option but should not follow diazepam because of the synergistic effect of the drugs in depressing respiratory drive.

Clonazepam (Klonopin) has proven effective in the treatment of Lennox-Gastaut syndrome, which is a combination of absence, akinetic, and myoclonic seizures. It may also be effective in treating absence seizures that do not respond to succinimides. Approximately one third of the patients who use clonazepam have breakthrough seizures, which indicates the development of tolerance to anticonvulsive effects.

Carbamazepine. Carbamazepine (Tegretol) is related to the tricyclic antidepressants and is indicated in the treatment of complex partial, tonic-clonic, or mixed seizures. It is not effective in controlling absence seizures. Carbamazepine may cause serious hematological side effects, but this occurrence is rare. Nevertheless, some clinicians are reluctant to prescribe this drug because of this possible reaction. Carbamazepine is not recommended during pregnancy or breast-feeding because an infant can achieve a serum level that is 60% of the mother's serum level.[45]

Valproic acid. Valproic acid (Depakene, Depakote) is a first-line drug for absence and tonic-clonic seizures. It is also used in the treatment of myoclonic and complex partial seizures. Valproic acid apparently inhibits the spread of abnormal discharges through the brain. Although the precise manner of this action is not known, it is thought that three mechanisms may contribute to its antiepileptic effect[30]: (1) an increase in GABA, (2) an increased postsynaptic response to GABA, and (3) an increase in the resting membrane potential. Lindhout and Omtzigt[25] report a 1% to 2% risk of spina bifida in the infants of mothers who take this drug during pregnancy. Some clinicians find this to be an acceptable level of risk and use both valproic acid and carbamazepine with caution.[16] Concentrations of valproic acid in breast milk have been found to be 1% to 10% of the mother's serum level.

Gabapentin. Gabapentin (Neurontin) is a relatively new AED and is used in the adjunctive treatment of partial seizures in adults and children over 12 years of age.[24] It is similar to GABA in structure but is more lipophilic because of molecular differences and therefore is better able to penetrate the blood-brain barrier.[32] Gabapentin is well tolerated and typically produces mild side effects. It does not have known interactions with other AEDs.

Lamotrigine. Lamotrigine (Lamictal) is used adjunctively for the treatment of partial seizures and may be effective in treating generalized seizures. In animal models, it blocks the sustained repetitive firing of neurons by prolonging the inactivation of sodium channels.[28] This effect may be its mechanism for suppressing seizure activity. Lamotrigine causes mild side effects.

Environmental Implications

Environmental concerns deal with safety for the patient and others. When possible, the offending or causative agent should be removed. Infectious processes should be treated, surgery for seizure-causing tumors or seizure types refractory to AEDs should be performed, and disturbances in the neuroendocrine system should be corrected (e.g., hypothyroidism with replacement therapy).[1] Issues such as driving, pregnancy, and employment have been addressed earlier in the chapter. Other environmental issues with safety implications are alcohol use, sports and recreation, bathing, and identification.[29] Alcohol use is discouraged because of its interactions with AEDs and because it aggravates seizures. Although a person with epilepsy need not abstain from alcohol, limited and cautious use is important. Certain sports such as swimming, mountain climbing, and bicycle riding may need to be avoided or closely supervised. For some individuals, showering may be preferable to bathing. To facilitate emergency treatment should it be needed, patients with epilepsy should wear identification bracelets such as those provided by Medic Alert.

Although these precautions and those mentioned earlier in the chapter are important, overcautiousness runs the risk of creating an invalid.[35] It is a grave injustice to guard against every risk factor and, in the process, immobilize a person.

Summary

Epilepsy is one of the most common neurological disorders; it affects approximately 2 million Americans and 50 million people worldwide. Most (70%) epilepsy is idiopathic, or of unknown etiology. Risk factors for the other 30% include
cerebrovascular accidents, tumors, alcohol use, and trauma. Histological examination reveals cellular level changes in the brain of a person with epilepsy. As neuropathological knowledge increases, it is thought that an identifiable etiology will be demonstrated in more cases. Most people with epilepsy are treated with antiepileptic drugs. Approximately 30% of all cases of epilepsy are refractory to drug therapy; surgery is often a recourse for these individuals. For many individuals, epilepsy will be a chronic disorder that lasts several years or a lifetime. Others will lead a relatively normal life without psychological or social problems.

REFERENCES

1. Adams RD, Victor M: *Principles of neurology,* New York, 1989, McGraw-Hill.
2. Begley CE, Annegers JF, Lairson DR et al: Cost of epilepsy in the United States: a model based on incidence and prognosis, *Epilepsia* 35(6):1230-1243, 1994.
3. Borgsdorf LR, Caldwell JW: *Clinical therapeutics: a disease-oriented approach to pharmacology and therapeutics,* Bakersfield, Calif, 1985, Kern Medical Center.
4. Cendes F, Andermann F, Carpenter S et al: Temporal lobe epilepsy caused by domoic acid intoxication: evidence for glutamate receptor–mediated excitotoxicity in humans, *Ann Neurol* 37:123-126, 1995.
5. Commission on Classification and Terminology of the International League Against Epilepsy: Proposal for revised classification of epilepsies and epileptic syndromes, *Epilepsia* 30:389-399, 1989.
6. Dalessio DJ: Seizure disorders and pregnancy, *N Engl J Med* 312:559-563, 1985.
7. Delgado-Escueta AV, Wasterlain C, Treiman DM et al: Management of status epilepticus, *N Engl J Med* 306(22):1337-1340, 1982.
8. Delgado-Escueta AV, Treiman DM, Walsh GO: The treatable epilepsies, *N Engl J Med* 308:1508-1514, 1576-1584, 1983.
9. Engel J, Starkman S: Overview of seizures, *Emerg Med Clin North Am* 12(4):895-923, 1994.
10. Fisher RS, Parsonage M, Beaussart M et al: Epilepsy and driving: an international perspective, *Epilepsia* 35(3):675-684, 1994.

11. Fried I, Kim JH, Spencer DD: Hippocampal pathology in patients with intractable seizures and temporal lobe masses, *J Neurosurg* 76:735-740, 1992.

12. Fried I, Spencer DD, Spencer SS: The anatomy of epileptic auras: focal pathology and surgical outcome, *J Neurosurg* 83:60-66, 1995.

13. Hauser WA: Recent developments in the epidemiology of epilepsy, *Acta Neurol Scand Suppl* 162:17-21, 1995a.

14. Hauser WA: Epidemiology of epilepsy in children, *Neurosurg Clin North Am* 6(3):419-429, 1995.

15. Hauser WA, Annegers JF, Kurland LT: Prevalence of epilepsy in Rochester, Minnesota: 1940-1980, *Epilepsia* 32:429-445, 1991.

16. Hiilesmaa VK: Pregnancy and birth in women with epilepsy, *Neurology* 42(suppl 5):8-11, 1992.

17. Honer WG, Beach TG, Ju L et al: Hippocampal synaptic pathology in patients with temporal lobe epilepsy, *Acta Neuropathol* 87:202-210, 1994.

18. International League Against Epilepsy: Guidelines for epidemiologic studies on epilepsy, *Epilepsia* 34(4):592-596, 1993.

19. Jacoby A, Baker GA, Steen N et al: The clinical course of epilepsy and its psychosocial correlates: findings from a UK community study, *Epilepsia* 37(2):148-161, 1996.

20. Jallon P: Electroencephalogram and epilepsy, *Europ Neurol* 34(suppl 1):18-23, 1994.

21. Jordan KG: Status epilepticus: a perspective from the neuroscience intensive care unit, *Neurosurg Clin North Am* 5(4):671-686, 1994.

22. Kandel ER, Schwartz JH, Jessell TM: *Principles of neural science,* ed 3, Norwalk, Conn, 1991, Appleton & Lange.

22a. Keltner N, Folks DG: *Psychotropic drugs,* ed 2, St Louis, 1997, Mosby.

23. Keranen T, Riekkinan PJ: Remission of seizures in untreated epilepsy, *Br Med J* 307:483, 1993.

24. Laxer KD: Guidelines for treating epilepsy in the age of felbamate, vigabatrin, lamotrigine, and gabapentin, *West J Med* 161(3):309-314, 1994.

25. Lindhout D, Omtzigt JG: Teratogenic effects of antiepileptic drugs: implications for the management of epilepsy in women of childbearing age, *Epilepsia* 35(suppl 4):S19-S28, 1994.

26. Masukawa LM, O'Connor WM, Lynott J et al: Longitudinal variation in cell density and mossy fiber reorganization in the dentate gyrus from temporal lobe epileptic patients, *Brain Res* 678:65-75, 1995.

27. McKenna PJ, Kane JM, Parrish K: Psychotic syndromes in epilepsy, *Am J Psychiatry* 142:895-904, 1985.

28. Meldrum BS: Lamotrigine: a novel approach, *Seizure* 3(suppl A):41-45, 1994.

29. Norman SE, Browne TR: Seizure disorders, *Am J Nurs* 81:984-994, 1981.

30. Olin BR, editor: *Drug facts and comparisons,* St Louis, 1995, Wolters-Kluwer.

31. Parks BR, Dostrow VG, Noble SL: Drug therapy for epilepsy, *Am Fam Physician* 59(3):639-648, 653-654, 1994.

32. Ramsey RE, Graves NM, Rowan AJ: Clinical issues in the management of epilepsy, Miami, 1993, University of Miami Press.

33. Roberts GW, Leigh PN, Weinberger DR: *Neuropsychiatric disorders,* London, 1993, Wolfe.

34. Rogawski MA, Porter RJ: Antiepileptic drugs: pharmacological mechanism and clinical efficacy with considerations of promising developmental state compounds, *Pharmacol Rev* 42:223-286, 1990.

35. Rowland LP: *Merritt's textbook of neurology,* ed 8, Philadelphia, 1989, Lea & Febiger.

36. Scheuer ML, Pedley TA: Current concepts: the evaluation and treatment of seizures, *N Engl J Med* 323:1468-1474, 1990.

37. Senanayake N, Roman GC: Epidemiology of epilepsy in developing countries, *Bull World Health Org* 71(2):247-258, 1993.

38. Sharpe C, Buchanan N: Juvenile myoclonic epilepsy: diagnosis, management and outcome, *Med J Aus* 162(3):133-134, 1995.

39. Shorvon S: Epilepsy and driving, *Br Med J* 310(6984):885-886, 1995.

40. Shorvon SD: The epidemiology and treatment of chronic and refractory epilepsy, *Epilepsia* 37(suppl 2):S1-S3, 1996.

41. Sloviter RS: The functional organization of the hippocampal dentate gyrus and its relevance to the pathogenesis of temporal lobe epilepsy, *Ann Neurol* 35(6):640-654, 1994.

42. So EL: Update on epilepsy, *Med Clin North Am* 77(1):203-214, 1993.

43. Spencer SS: The relative contributions of MRI, SPECT, and PET imaging in epilepsy, *Epilepsia* 35(suppl 6):S72-S89, 1994.

44. Suzdak PD, Jansen JA: A review of the preclinical pharmacology of tiagabine: a potent and selective anticonvulsant GABA inhibitor, *Epilepsia* 36(6): 612-626, 1995.

45. Vestermark V, Vestermark S: Teratogenic effect of carbamazepine, *Arch Dis Child* 66(5):641-642, 1991.

46. Wasterlain CG, Shirasaka Y: Seizures, brain damage and brain development, *Brain Dev* 16:279-295, 1994.

47. Wilder BJ: The treatment of epilepsy: an overview of clinical practices, *Neurology* 45(suppl 3):S7-S11, 1995.

48. Wolf HK, Campos MG, Zentner J et al: Surgical pathology of temporal lobe epilepsy: experience with 216 cases, *J Neuropathol Exp Neurol* 52(5): 499-506, 1993.

49. Zorumski CF, Isenberg KE: Insights into the structure and function of GABA-benzodiazepine receptors: ion channels and psychiatry, *Am J Psychiatry* 148(2):162-173, 1991.

appendix A

American Nurses Association Psychopharmacology Guidelines for Psychiatric–Mental Health Nurses*

This document describes the knowledge base psychiatric mental health nurses need in relation to one aspect of practice—psychopharmacology. It is intended only to inform and guide psychiatric mental health nursing education, practice, and research in this area. Thus this document should not be considered part of any state's nurse practice act, or viewed as a requirement for licensure, or construed as a legal standard by which to judge psychiatric nursing practice.

These guidelines will be evaluated and updated regularly. Psychiatric mental health nurses will demonstrate expanding expertise in psychopharmacology based on the state of the science, education, experience, practice setting, patient needs, and professional goals.

I. Neurosciences

Commensurate with level of practice, the psychiatric mental health nurse integrates current knowledge from the neurosciences to understand

*Reprinted with permission from *Psychiatric mental health nursing: psychopharmacology project,* Washington, DC, 1994, American Nurses Association.

etiological models, diagnostic issues, and treatment strategies for psychiatric illness.

Objectives. The psychiatric mental health nurse can:

- describe basic central nervous system structures and functions implicated in mental illness, such as the cerebrum, diencephalon, brainstem, basal ganglia, limbic system, and extrapyramidal motor system.
- describe basic mechanisms of neurotransmission at the synapse, such as neurochemical metabolism, role(s) of the presynaptic and postsynaptic membranes, reuptake, receptor binding, and autoregulation.
- describe the general functions of the major neurochemicals implicated in mental illness, such as serotonin, norepinephrine, dopamine, acetylcholine, GABA, and the peptides.
- describe the basic structure and function of the endocrine system, particularly as it is affected by the various hypothalamic-pituitary endocrine axes.
- identify the neurotransmitter system implicated in side-effect profiles of psychopharmacological agents, such as blockade of cholinergic receptors (blurred vision, dry mouth,

memory dysfunction), histaminic receptors (sedation, weight gain, hypotension), and adrenergic receptors (dizziness, postural hypotension, tachycardia).
- discuss the relevance of current biological hypotheses underlying major mental illnesses and the use of psychopharmacological agents.
- demonstrate a familiarity with the increased life-time risk of mental illness—for people who have a mentally ill first-degree (biological) relative—compared with the general population and based on genetic, epidemiological, family, adoption, and twin research.
- describe normal sleep stages and identify circadian rhythm disturbances, such as decreased REM latency and phase shift disturbances as evidenced by psychiatric disorders.
- demonstrate familiarity with recent research findings from neuroimaging techniques such as CT (computed tomography), MRI (magnetic resonance imaging), PET (positron emission tomography), and SPECT (single photon emission computed tomography), as well as the psychiatric uses of these techniques.
- discuss the purposes and limitations of current biological tests used in the diagnosis and monitoring of mental illness.

II. Psychopharmacology

The psychiatric mental health nurse involved in the care of patients who have been prescribed psychopharmacological agents demonstrates knowledge of psychopharmacological principles, including pharmacokinetics, pharmacodynamics, drug classification, intended and unintended effects, and related nursing implications.

Objectives. The psychiatric mental health nurse can:
- describe psychopharmacological agents based on the similarities and differences among drugs of the same and different classes.
- discuss the actions of psychopharmacological agents that range from global human behavioral responses to those at a cellular level, such

as the actions of lithium from mood stabilization to glomerular effects.
- differentiate the psychiatric symptoms targeted for psychopharmacological intervention from medication side effects and toxicities, and the appropriate interventions to minimize each.
- apply basic principles of pharmacokinetics and pharmacodynamics, such as half-life, steady state, absorption, and metabolism, in general and as they relate to age, gender, race/ethnicity, and organ system function.
- identify the appropriate use of psychotherapeutic agents related to the psychiatric needs of special populations.
- involve patients and their families and significant others in the design and implementation of the medication treatment plan, taking into account patient readiness, knowledge, environment, beliefs and preferences, and lifestyle.
- identify factors that may prevent the active collaboration of patients with medication regimens, and strategies to minimize these risks.
- describe nonpsychopharmacological interventions for target symptoms that are not responsive to psychopharmacological interventions, psychiatric symptoms unlikely to respond to drug treatments, and drug side effects that are not treated with drugs.
- discuss the use of standardized rating scales for measuring symptom severity and clinical response to psychopharmacological treatment, such as changes in target symptoms of illness and medication side effects.
- demonstrate the knowledge necessary to develop psychopharmacological education and treatment plans based on current neurobiological concepts and the patient's lifestyle and recovery environment.

III. Clinical Management

The psychiatric mental health nurse applies principles from the neurosciences and psychopharmacology to provide safe and effective management of patients being treated with psychopharmacological agents. Clinical management includes assessment, diagnosis, and treatment considerations.

A. Assessment

The psychiatric mental health nurse has the knowledge, skills, and ability to conduct and interpret patient assessments in relation to psychopharmacological agents. Assessments include physical, neuropsychiatric, psychosocial, and psychopharmacological parameters.

1. Physical Assessment

Objectives. The psychiatric mental health nurse can:

- collect health data related to past and present health problems and concurrent treatments for other psychiatric or medical problems the patient may have.
- collect health data related to current and past drug use (prescribed, over-the-counter, and illicit), current and past substance use (caffeine, nicotine, alcohol), and related health practices.
- conduct and/or interpret findings from a physical examination and laboratory studies to obtain information about pertinent organ system functioning.
- evaluate laboratory results that reflect drug effects on organ systems, drug blood levels and toxicities, and concurrent medical problems that may mimic or exacerbate psychiatric symptoms or drug effects.
- assess baseline and ongoing status of motor activity and sleep patterns, appetite, dietary practices and preferences, and functional status.

2. Neuropsychiatric Assessment

Objectives. The psychiatric mental health nurse can:

- conduct and/or interpret findings from a basic neuropsychiatric examination, including gross cranial and peripheral nerve function; gait; muscle strength, function, and range of motion; and mental status.
- identify chief neuropsychiatric complaints, presenting symptoms, and goals for psy-

chopharmacological interventions.
- make appropriate use of available informants and records to augment self-reports of neuropsychiatric assessment and premorbid patterns.
- demonstrate appropriate use of standardized rating scales to document mental status, drug effects on the core psychiatric symptomatology, and side effects such as those occurring on the extrapyramidal system.

3. Psychosocial Assessment

Objectives. The psychiatric mental health nurse can:

- utilize demographic and personal information for the development of a patient-centered medication treatment plan, considering the patient's ethnic/cultural background, developmental stage, cognitive ability, educational level, reading level and comprehension, socioeconomic status, and capacity to ask questions and seek answers.
- assess the effects of psychopharmacological interventions on the patient's quality of life, including the impact on interpersonal relationships, appearance, work and leisure functioning, diet, sleep, sexual performance, family planning, functional status, financial status, self-esteem, and perception of stigma associated with medication intervention.
- identify actual and potential sources of support for the patient such as significant others, household and family members, friendships and informal relationships, work relationships, and affiliations with community, social, and religious organizations.
- identify actual and potential barriers to treatment within the patient and the environment, such as impaired functional status, cultural/ethnic beliefs and practices, absence of a support system, limited cognitive abilities, stressors, financial hardships, deficient coping skills, impaired capacity to collaborate with treatment, limited transportation, and patient and family perceptions of illness and medication treatment.

4. Psychopharmacological Assessment

Objectives. The psychiatric mental health nurse can:

- identify patient-related variables pertinent to the risk/benefit assessment of psychopharmacological treatment such as demographic (age, general, ethnicity/race), physical (organ system function, concurrent illnesses), treatment (concurrent treatments), and personal (past history, self-care practices, goals for treatment, ability to pay, and quality of life) characteristics.
- identify drug-related variables important in the risk/benefit assessment of psychopharmacological agents, such as safety and efficacy, advantages and disadvantages compared with other drugs in the same class, therapeutic range, side-effect profile, toxicities, contraindications, potential interactions with other drugs or diet, polypharmacy considerations, safety in overdose, availability of information on long-term side effects, and cost.
- evaluate the appropriateness and least restrictive nature of psychopharmacological interventions for each patient.
- assess the ability and willingness of the patient and significant others to give informed consent for treatment with psychopharmacological agents.
- utilize standardized behavioral rating scales to assess and monitor drug effects and changes in target symptoms.

B. Diagnosis

The psychiatric mental health nurse has the knowledge, skills, and ability to utilize appropriate nursing, psychiatric, and medical diagnostic classification systems to guide psychopharmacological management of patients with mental illness.

Objectives. The psychiatric mental health nurse can:

- utilize standardized diagnostic systems as appropriate for making nursing (North American Nursing Diagnostic Association [NANDA], or other nursing systems) and psychiatric diagnoses (*Diagnostic and Statistical Manual* [DSM]), and interpreting medical diagnoses (*International Classification of Diseases* [ICD]).
- elicit information from the patient and other appropriate informants or records that is relevant to the diagnostic process.
- make nursing diagnostic judgments that include information about but are not limited to the psychiatric diagnosis, symptoms targeted for psychopharmacological intervention, clinical diagnoses, physical symptoms, coping responses, functional status, developmental level, learning capabilities, and the patient's quality of life and preferences.
- use these diagnostic judgments as the basis for setting treatment priorities and selecting and assessing nursing interventions, including management of psychopharmacological agents.
- communicate and integrate diagnostic impressions with other members of the health care team. This can include representatives of managed care enterprises.

C. Treatment

The psychiatric mental health nurse takes an active role in the treatment of patients with mental illness and integrates prescribed psychopharmacological interventions into a cohesive, multidimensional plan of care.

1. Initiation

Objectives. The psychiatric mental health nurse can:

- use information obtained during the nursing assessment to develop a medication treatment plan that considers target symptoms, side effects, concurrent treatments and health status, requirements of specific drugs, dietary and activity considerations, and patient-related variables.
- demonstrate an understanding of pharmacokinetic and pharmacodynamic principles that underlie safe and effective psychopharmacological management, such as how dosing and tapering schedules are adjusted and how patient-related variables are integrated.

- relate the length of time it may take a drug to have a therapeutic effect, the time it takes for expected side effects to occur and remit, early signs of unexpected or adverse effects, and nursing interventions to reduce side effects and facilitate therapeutic response.
- apply principles of health education and nursing ethics and legal parameters in informing patients about medication treatments, risks/benefits, concurrent and alternative treatments, and informed consent.
- apply least restrictive principles and advance directives to avoid the overuse or underuse of medications as chemical restraints, and to anticipate safety needs such as potential for harm to self or others, suicidality, aggression, assaultiveness, and violence.

2. Stabilization

Objectives. The psychiatric mental health nurse can:

- monitor target symptoms, acute medication effects, and functional status throughout the course of treatment.
- utilize information obtained from therapeutic drug monitoring, laboratory values, standardized rating scales, and patient and family reports to monitor progress.
- recognize indications for modifying dosing schedules and describe alternative medication strategies as needed.

3. Maintenance

Objectives. The psychiatric mental health nurse can:

- develop a plan of care—in collaboration with the patient, family, and other care providers as appropriate—that includes monitoring outcomes such as efficacy of treatment, changes in target symptoms, emergence of long-term side effects, laboratory values and physical findings relevant to specific medications, and occurrence of destabilizing stressors.
- identify possible barriers to maintenance care such as issues regarding transportation, finances, birth control, child care, support system, relocation, cultural/ethnic differences,

therapeutic relationship, and psychosocial stressors, as well as the patient's understanding of symptom reduction, symptom exacerbation, and side effects.

- facilitate the patient's transition from one treatment setting to another, such as from the hospital to the community, from one care provider to another, and from one treatment to another.
- develop a patient-education program for relapse prevention that can include self-monitoring techniques and teaching tools such as medication cards, handouts, diaries, bibliographies, and other materials to enhance ongoing education of patients, families, and significant others.
- enhance health promotion with restoration techniques that can be individualized for the patient and integrated with medication treatments, such as diet, exercise, leisure activities, and community, social, and religious affiliations.
- assist the patient, family, and significant others to establish advance directives regarding emergency interventions, including the use of psychopharmacological agents.

4. Discontinuation and Follow-Up

Objectives. The psychiatric mental health nurse can:

- relate current recommended practices regarding psychopharmacological maintenance requirements and duration of treatment for specific psychiatric disorders.
- discuss issues related to discontinuation of medication, including tapering schedules, and potential sequelae, such as withdrawal, dependence, rebound effects, and return of symptoms of illness.
- develop with the patient, family, and significant others a plan for self-care in a postmedication phase that considers assessments of quality of life, predisposing stressors, reemergence of symptoms, appropriate use of support systems, and contact sources for potential reevaluation of treatment status.
- assess the patient before, during, and after the course of treatment, clearly differentiating

between changes in the patient as a result of illness effects, drug effects, premorbid personality characteristics, effects of aging, and effects of the environment.

IV. Recommendations

These *Guidelines* are designed to be used as a tool for psychiatric mental health nurses to determine their knowledge and skill in psychopharmacology and to design a plan for their continued growth in this field. The *Guidelines* can also be used as the basis for the development of curricula and continuing education programs for psychiatric mental health nurses in psychopharmacology. New information in this field should be added to the *Guidelines* on a regular basis.

As a set of guidelines, this document should not be used in legal proceedings or as an evaluation of nurses' competence in this field by institutions or state or federal agencies.

Glossary of Neuroanatomy and Neurobiological Terms

abducens nerve The axons of CN VI pass through the pons and emerge from the brainstem at the junction of the pons and the pyramid. The nerve then passes through the cavernous sinus and exits the cranial cavity through the superior orbital fissure, where it supplies the lateral rectus muscle. Injury to one side prevents the patient from performing lateral eye movements. Over time, the affected eye turns inward.

abducens nucleus The nucleus for CN VI (the abducens nerve). It is situated beneath the facial colliculus in the floor of the fourth ventricle in the pons. It functions in lateral eye movement.

abuse A maladaptive pattern of substance use that causes clinically significant impairment.

acalculia The loss of ability to use numbers.

acetylcholine A neurotransmitter synthesized by choline acetyltransferase from acetyl-coenzyme A and choline. It is found in the peripheral nervous system at the myoneural junction, in autonomic ganglia for parasympathetic or sympathetic systems, and in the parasympathetic postganglionic synapses, including CNs III, VII, IX, and X. Acetylcholine is found in the spinal cord, basal ganglia, and numerous sites within the cerebral cortex. Cortical acetylcholine is synthesized primarily in the nucleus basalis of Meynert and in the septal area near the hypothalamus.

adenohypophysis The anterior portion of the pituitary gland.

adenylate cyclase An enzyme that synthesizes the second messenger cyclic adenosine monophosphate (cAMP).

agnosia The failure to recognize previously learned sensory inputs such as people's faces or the shape of doorknobs.

agraphia The loss of ability to write.

akathisia An inner sense of restlessness or compulsion to move (e.g., pacing) that is commonly induced by neuroleptic agents.

alexia The loss of ability to read.

allocortex (archicortex) "Old" cortex containing only three layers of neurons.

amnesia The inability to remember recent or remote facts or events. Hippocampal damage impairs recent memory.

amygdala A cluster of nuclei in the medial temporal lobe that is concerned with endocrine and behavioral functions and plays a role in food and water intake, drive behavior, and the emotions connected with those behaviors. In animal studies, electrical stimulation of the amygdala causes defensiveness, rage, and/or aggression.

amyloid Fibrillar proteinaceous material that accumulates within the brains of patients with Alzheimer's disease and other disorders. In amyloid angiopathy, the accumulated amyloid is located in the vessel walls. This accumulation can cause the vessels to rupture and result in a brain hemorrhage.

anaplastic astrocytoma Astrocytic tumor with a moderate degree of malignancy.

anergia The absence of energy caused by changes in brain biochemistry and/or anatomy. It is often a symptom in biologically mediated mental disorders such as schizophrenia and major depression.

GLOSSARY

angiography A neuroradiologic procedure that uses intravenous or intraarterial dyes to discover abnormalities of the vascular system, such as searching for aneurysms or arteriovenous malformations or assessing the extent of atherosclerosis.

anterior commissure White matter tract that connects the olfactory structures bilaterally, as well as the temporal lobes and the amygdala.

aphasia The inability to verbally communicate (i.e., expressive aphasia) or understand communication via spoken or written word (i.e., receptive aphasia).

apolipoprotein E (Apo-E) A recently identified protein that may play a role in the development of and possibly be a marker for Alzheimer's disease. It has been discovered that patients with Alzheimer's disease have a greater amount of Apo-E than patients without the disease.

apraxia The inability to perform previously learned motor tasks such as dressing, shaving, driving, and walking.

arachnoid The membranous middle covering of the meninges.

arachnoid granulations Collections of granular tissue located over the midline convexities that project into the superior sagittal sinus and reabsorb cerebrospinal fluid.

aspartate An excitatory amino acid neurotransmitter derived from the citric acid cycle.

association fibers White matter tracts that connect regions of the same hemisphere with each other.

astrocytes The major glial support cells of the central nervous system.

astrocytoma An astrocytic tumor with the lowest grade of malignancy.

auditory nerve A portion of CN VIII, along with the vestibular component. The auditory nerve arises from the spiral ganglia in the labyrinth of the inner ear. It enters the cranial vault through the internal acoustic meatus and enters the brainstem at the junction of the pons and medulla. The portion of the auditory nerve concerned with hearing travels to the two cochlear nuclei, which act as relay nuclei in the auditory pathway. Damage to CN VIII causes sensorineural deafness, such as occurs with an acoustic neuroma.

automatisms Automatic behaviors that occur in epilepsy and in some individuals during a hysterical state.

autonomic nervous system The division of the peripheral nervous system that is involuntary and innervates the viscera, heart, blood vessels, smooth muscle, and glands. It is divided into the parasympathetic (craniosacral system) and the sympathetic (thoracolumbar system).

autosomal A non–gender determining chromosome.

avolition Lack of motivation related to changes in brain biochemistry and/or anatomy. It is physiologically and psychologically related to anergia and is often a symptom in biologically mediated mental disorders such as schizophrenia and major depressive disorder.

axon The portion of the neuron that transmits signals.

basal ganglia Derived from the telencephalon, the basal ganglia are large masses of subcortical grey matter consisting of the caudate nucleus, putamen, and globus pallidus.

basilar artery The blood vessel formed by the fusion of the vertebral arteries; it divides into the posterior cerebral arteries. The basilar system perfuses the brainstem and cerebellum.

Bell's palsy Total paralysis of half of the face, including the brows. Because innervation of the face by the facial nerve has bilateral components, the lesion causing a Bell's palsy must be anatomically located after the bilateral input has been added.

Betz's cells The large neurons of the motor cortex.

Bielschowsky's stain A silver stain used in histology that enables the identification of axons, neurofibrillary tangles, and senile plaques.

blood-brain barrier (BBB) A structural division between the systemic circulation and the brain. The BBB is formed from specialized junctions in endothelial cells of vessels and from the disposition of astrocytic processes with perivascular end-feet. The BBB prohibits numerous substances from entering the central nervous system and causes a problem in drug delivery to the brain.

Bodian's stain A silver stain used in histology that enables the identification of axons, neurofibrillary tangles, and senile plaques.

brainstem The vital structure that carries all information to and from the cerebral cortex and spinal cord. Because the brainstem is also responsible for respiration, its function is essential for life. It consists of the midbrain, pons, and medulla.

Broca's area The motor speech region located in the left inferior frontal cortex for individuals with a dominant left hemisphere. Lesions of Broca's area produce an expressive aphasia.

calcarine cortex The primary visual cortex located in the occipital lobe.

catecholamines Derived from the amino acid tyrosine, these substances include dopamine, norepinephrine, and epinephrine. Catecholamines are a subcategory of the monoamines, which also include serotonin and histamine. Catecholamines and their synthesis products are widely distributed in the central and peripheral nervous system.

cauda equina The "horse's tail." The cauda equina consists of many spinal nerve roots invested in arachnoid and begins at approximately L1. The nerve roots branch off at their various levels as the structure descends.

caudal Toward the tail or downward.

caudate The basal ganglia nucleus that protrudes into the anterior horn of the lateral ventricle.

cell body The portion of the neuron that contains the nucleus.

cerebellar nuclei All portions of the cerebellar cortices project to the deep cerebellar nuclei, which consist of the dentate, emboliform, fastigial, and globose nuclei.

cerebellar peduncles Three pairs of white matter structures that connect the brainstem to the cerebellum. The inferior cerebellar peduncle connects with the medulla. The middle cerebellar peduncle connects with the pons, and the superior cerebellar peduncle connects with the midbrain.

cerebellum Involved with the coordination of muscle activity, regulation of muscle tone, and maintenance of equilibrium.

cerebral aqueduct The small passageway located in the midbrain that allows cerebrospinal fluid to flow from the cerebral hemispheres and down through the brainstem to the spinal canal.

cerebral peduncles Also known as the "crus cerebri," these white matter structures are found in the midbrain and contain the essential corticospinal (motor or pyramidal) tracts.

cerebrospinal fluid (CSF) A clear fluid produced by the choroid plexus that contains protein, sugar, and very few white blood cells. The CSF flows through the ventricular system and around the brain and spinal cord and is absorbed by the arachnoid granulations.

cholinergics Substances that stimulate the cholinergic system. In the peripheral nervous system, cholinergic drugs constrict the pupil, increase the production of saliva and respiratory secretions, slow the heart, and increase gastrointestinal peristalsis and urinary output.

chorea A Greek term for "dance." The choreas manifest as hyperkinetic disorders characterized by involuntary, unpredictable, and random movements of the trunk, head, face, and limbs.

choroid plexus Produces the majority of the cerebrospinal fluid and is located in the ventricles.

chromatin The genetic material in the nucleus of a cell.

chromatolysis Swelling of the neuronal cell body in reaction to injury of its axon.

chromogranin A substance commonly produced in neurons. If found in cells via immunohistochemistry, the cells are presumed to be neurons or neural crest derivatives.

cingulate gyrus A crescent-shaped convolution on the medial surface directly above the corpus callosum. The cingulate gyrus is part of the limbic system, makes valuable connections with the hippocampal complex and amygdala, and plays a role in the modification of visceral function.

circadian rhythms The day-to-day variance in some body functions influenced by light-intensity changes and regulated in the hypothalamus. Cycles include body temperature, steroid levels, and oxygen consumption.

circle of Willis The ring of interconnected arteries at the base of the brain composed of the anterior cerebral, anterior communicating, posterior communicating, and posterior cerebral arteries.

claustrum A thin layer of grey matter situated just beneath the insular cortex and separated from the more medial putamen by a thin lamina of white matter known as the external capsule. It contains discrete visual and somatosensory subdivisions with interconnections to the corresponding primary sensory areas of the neocortex.

commissural fibers White matter tracts that connect the two hemispheres.

computed axial tomography (CAT) scan A sophisticated x-ray examination of the brain that visualizes cortical structures. Commonly referred to as simply CT scan.

conduction deafness One of the two major subtypes of deafness. Conduction deafness is caused by an impairment in the conduction of sound through the external ear canal and ossicles to the endolymph.

conus medullaris The structure located at the caudal end of the spinal cord. It is found in adults at approximately the L1 level (range T12-L3).

cornu ammonis "Ammon's horn" of the hippocampus.

corpora amylacea Spherical bodies found in the grey matter. They increase with age and are without functional significance.

corpus callosum The largest white matter commissure connecting the right and left brain.

corpus striatum Basal ganglia that include the caudate, putamen, and globus pallidus.

cyclic adenosine monophosphate (cAMP) A second messenger that translates the neurotransmitter stimulation into a cellular response.

cytoarchitecture Refers to the pattern of neuronal arrangement typical for a particular brain region. Disruptions in cytoarchitecture may occur in schizophrenia and are related to neuronal migrational problems.

cytoskeleton The delicate meshwork of neurofilaments, microtubules, and associated molecules that is present in all neurons. Cytoskeleton is essential to cell shape and transport.

deafferentation The process of interrupting sensory (afferent) fibers.

delirium Abrupt onset. Temporary confusion and cognitive impairment from reversible causes.

delusion A fixed false belief with no basis in fact (e.g., a patient who claims to be the Messiah).

dementia The permanent loss of multiple intellectual functions from neuronal death or dysfunction.

dendrite The part of the neuron that accepts incoming signals.

dentate gyrus Part of the hippocampus. It contains three layers of neurons (archicortex).

dentate nucleus The largest of the deep cerebellar nuclei. It lies in the deep white matter of the cerebellum close to the vermis. In cross sections, it has "toothlike" convolutions (hence the term *dentate*).

dependence A maladaptive pattern of substance abuse that causes adverse clinical consequences.

diencephalon One of the secondary vesicles in fetal life derived from the prosencephalon. It eventually forms into the thalamus, epithalamus, hypothalamus, and subthalamus.

diurnal Occurring in the daytime.

dopamine A neurotransmitter primarily synthesized in the substantia nigra and the ventral tegmental area of the midbrain. Dopamine is derived from the amino acid tyrosine, and its immediate precursor is L-dopa. Decreased levels of dopamine are associated with parkinsonism, whereas excessive levels are present in schizophrenia.

dorsal Toward the posterior or back.

dorsal horn of the spinal cord Consists of grey matter and transmits information coming in and going out of the spinal cord and dorsal roots. It is volumetrically smaller than the ventral horns.

dorsal root ganglion (DRG) A swelling that contains nerve cell bodies and is located on the spinal dorsal roots. It is part of the system that helps disseminate sensory information to the entire central nervous system.

dura mater The thick, tough outer covering of the meninges.

dyskinesia Abnormal involuntary movements of muscles that commonly involve the face and mouth (e.g., lip smacking, teeth grinding, tongue protrusion, and tongue rolling). Dyskinesias are typically iatrogenic, with the two most common forms caused by neuroleptics (tardive dyskinesia) and dopaminergics (levodopa dyskinesia).

dysplasia Abnormal development of cells.

dystonia Disruption of muscle tone that is partially caused by the simultaneous contraction of opposing muscle groups. It results in persistent muscle contraction, with abnormal, fixed postures usually arising out of voluntary movements.

Edinger-Westphal nucleus Dorsal to the oculomotor nucleus, the Edinger-Westphal nucleus produces parasympathetic fibers to join the oculomotor nerve on its course to the eye.

electroencephalogram (EEG) A recording of the electrical activity of the brain. It identifies some types of epilepsy.

electron microscopy (EM) A procedure that enables the identification of much finer structural detail than light microscopy, such as the ability to view cellular organelles and junctions.

emboliform nucleus A wedge-shaped grey matter mass close to the hilum of the dentate nucleus. It is not recognizable during gross examination because of its small size.

encephalitis Infection of the brain parenchyma.

encephalopathy A temporary brain dysfunction with a variable mixture of clinical findings commonly caused by anoxia and liver or kidney failure.

endogenous opioid peptides Substances that exhibit opiate-like activity. These peptides are the natural ligands of the opiate receptors and include the endorphins.

enkephalins Widely distributed opioid-like neuropeptides that are part of the endorphin family. These substances mediate pain perception, taste, olfaction, arousal, emotional behavior, vision, hearing, neurohormone secretion, motor coordination, and water balance.

entorhinal cortex This region is regarded as a secondary olfactory cortical area and receives projections from the lateral olfactory tract fibers. It connects to the hippocampal formation, insula, and frontal cortices.

ependyma Cells that line the ventricular system.

ependymoma Neoplasm of ependymal cells located in the ventricles.

epidermal growth factor (EGF) One of the numerous growth factors involved in many brain processes. EGF is especially amplified in the progression of some brain tumors from a benign to a malignant state.

epithalamus Part of the diencephalon, it consists of the habenular commissure and the pineal gland.

excitotoxicity Destructive neuronal overstimulation produced by excitatory neurotransmitters such as glutamate.

extrapyramidal system Integrates automatic movements (e.g., postural adjustments and muscle tone) with the pyramidal or voluntary movement system. Blocking this system produces extrapyramidal side effects.

facial nerve (CN VII) Contains sensory components of taste and of sensation to part of the external ear, controls lacrimation (the parasympathetic portion), and contains motor components supplying the facial muscles of expression.

facial nucleus Three separate nuclei are associated with the facial nerve: the facial nucleus, the superior salivatory nucleus (parasympathetic), and the nucleus solitarius (shared by CNs VII, IX, and X). Blocking the superior salivatory nucleus with anticholinergic medications causes dry mouth.

falx cerebri The dural crescent-shaped sheath located in the interhemispheric fissure between the two hemispheres.

fastigial nucleus The most medial of the deep cerebellar nuclei. It lies near the midline in the roof of the fourth ventricle and receives fibers from the vestibular nuclei.

fibrous astrocytes Astrocytes largely confined to the white matter.

filum terminale The end of the spinal cord tapers into the filum terminale after all of the nerve roots have exited from the cauda equina. The filum contains pia and neuroglia but has no known functional role.

fissures Visible early in brain development, these deep channels separate large portions of the brain.

GLOSSARY

follicle-stimulating hormone (FSH) A hormone produced by the anterior pituitary that stimulates follicular growth in the ovary and spermatogenesis in the testes.

foramen of Luschka Contained in the lateral walls of the fourth ventricle and situated at the cerebellopontine angle, these foramina allow the lateral passage of cerebrospinal fluid to continue caudally to bathe the spinal cord.

foramen of Magendie Constituted by a deficiency in the membrane of the roof of the fourth ventricle, this is the principal communication between the ventricular system and the subarachnoid space.

foramen of Monro Also known as the intraventricular foramen, this is a small passageway that allows cerebrospinal fluid to exit the frontal horns of the lateral ventricle and enter the third ventricle.

fornix An arched white fiber tract that connects the hippocampus to the mamillary bodies.

gamma-aminobutyric acid (GABA) An inhibitory amino acid neurotransmitter formed during the citric acid cycle from its precursor glutamic acid. GABA receptors are widely distributed in the central nervous system and produce neuronal hyperpolarization through an influx of chloride ions. Drugs that increase GABA reduce anxiety and seizures.

ganglion cell tumor A low-grade neoplasia of the neurons.

glial cells Include astrocytes, oligodendroglia, and ependymal cells.

glial fibrillary acidic protein (GFAP) Cytoplasmic filaments that are the most reliable method for the histological identification of astrocytes.

glioblastoma multiforme The most malignant variety of astrocytic tumor.

gliosis An astrogliosis is a proliferation of reactive astrocytes, whereas a microgliosis is a proliferation of reactive microglial cells. Both of these conditions are nonspecific and can result from any pathological process in the brain.

globose nuclei Part of the deep nuclei of the cerebellum. These nuclei consist of one or more grey matter masses that lie between the fastigial and emboliform nuclei in the cerebellar white matter.

globus pallidus A grey matter structure located medial to the putamen. This portion of the basal ganglia is smaller and triangular in shape. It is subdivided into the globus pallidus externa and the globus pallidus interna.

glossopharyngeal nerve (CN IX) Mediates taste sensation from the posterior third of the tongue and innervates pain and temperature sensations in the pharynx. Cell bodies of CN IX terminate in the nucleus solitarius and nucleus ambiguus. Efferent fibers also supply motor innervation to skeletal musculature in the pharynx and neck. A parasympathetic component innervates the salivary glands along with the vagus nerve (CN X).

glutamate The major excitatory transmitter in the central nervous system with receptors throughout the brain. Glutamate stimulation of NMDA-activated channels permits excessive inflow of calcium ions and production of free radicals that may cause neuronal death.

glycine An inhibitory neurotransmitter formed during the citric acid cycle.

G-proteins Regulatory proteins coupled to opioid receptors, which are in turn coupled to second messenger systems or directly to ion channels.

granulovacuolar degeneration (GVD) A histological change seen almost exclusively in the pyramidal neurons of the hippocampus. Although a few neurons may be seen with this condition in normal aging, extensive GVD is usually seen only in Alzheimer's disease. The histological findings include vacuolation in the cytoplasm of the neurons, with small, darkly colored inclusions that are referred to as "granules."

gyrus (*pl* gyri) The folded outer surfaces of the brain where most of the neurons are located.

hallucination A false internal sensation perceived by the brain that lacks a corresponding external sensory stimulus (e.g., hearing voices or seeing people when no one is present).

hallucinogens Substances, both natural and synthetic, that alter perception.

hematoxylin & eosin stain The routine histochemical stain in most of pathology. Hematoxylin stains nuclei a bluish-purple color, and eosin stains cytoplasm and neuropil pinkish-red.

5-HIAA   5-hydroindole acetic acid. It is a metabolite of serotonin and can be measured in the urine and cerebrospinal fluid.

hippocampus   A cortical structure located in the mesial temporal lobe. It is the gateway for recent memory and is damaged in Alzheimer's disease.

Hirano bodies   Glassy, refractile, red bodies that are football-shaped. In Alzheimer's disease, they are found in greater numbers in the hippocampus. Among other substances, Hirano bodies contain actin, a muscle protein.

homeostasis   The maintenance of a physiological steady state.

homovanillic acid (HVA)   A metabolite of dopamine.

hydrocephalus   Marked dilation of the ventricular system caused by increased cerebrospinal fluid pressure or the loss of brain parenchyma.

hyperkinetic   Excessive movement, such as in choreas or dyskinesias.

hypoglossal nerve (CN XII)   Supplies motor components to the tongue and several extrinsic striated muscles. A unilateral lesion of the hypoglossal nerve can cause contralateral tongue weakness.

hypoglossal nucleus   Lies between the dorsal nucleus of the vagus and the midline of the medulla. It contains the cell bodies for the hypoglossal nerve.

hypokinetic   Abnormally decreased movement, such as that found in Parkinson's disease.

hypothalamus   A group of nuclei in the diencephalon that influences eating behavior, temperature regulation, emotional expression, and the autonomic system. Dopaminergic neurons in the hypothalamus control lactation.

immunohistochemistry   A process used in histology to localize and identify various substances in all types of cells. These substances can include neurotransmitters, enzymes, hormones, filaments, infectious agents, and numerous proteins. The procedure is analyzed by colorimetric methods.

incidence   The number of cases of a disorder per unit of population (e.g., 5 per 100,000) within a specific time interval.

infarction   The death of brain tissue resulting from the cessation of blood flow or the lack of oxygen to a specific brain region. Other similar terms include *stroke, cerebrovascular accident,* or *ischemic injury.*

inferior cerebellar peduncle   A white matter bundle also known as "restiform" and "juxtirestiform" bodies. This peduncle transmits information from the vestibular nuclei and spinal cord to the cerebellum.

inferior colliculus   A collection of neurons on the posterior aspect of the brainstem that along with the superior colliculus forms the tectum of the midbrain. It is a relay nucleus of the auditory pathway.

inferior frontal gyrus   Lesions in this area in the dominant hemisphere can cause a Broca's dysphasia.

insula   A cortical area buried deep inside the Sylvian fissure that can be seen when the temporal and frontal lobes are separated.

interhemispheric fissure   Separates the left and right hemispheres.

internal capsule   A broad band of myelinated fibers that separate the lentiform nuclei from the caudate nucleus and thalamus. Corticospinal (motor or pyramidal) tracts travel through the internal capsule, cerebral peduncles, and cerebral pyramids into the spinal cord, where they constitute the lateral corticospinal pathway. Damage to any of these structures can result in hemiparesis or hemiplegia.

intoxication   Reversible, substance-specific physiological and behavioral changes resulting from recent exposure to a psychoactive substance.

ion channels   Proteins traversing the cell membranes that recognize, select, and conduct specific ions, resulting in neuronal activity. These channels open and close in response to specific signals.

Korsakoff's psychosis   An alcohol-induced amnestic syndrome with severe impairment of recent memory. Patients with this condition are not truly psychotic.

Lafora bodies   Rounded intracytoplasmic bodies seen in Lafora disease, a type of myoclonic epilepsy.

lateral geniculate body   A small collection of neurons that is shaped like a jockey cap and lies beneath the thalamus. They provide a thalamic relay for visual information. These neurons send fibers back to the calcarine cortex in the occipital lobe.

lentiform nuclei   The putamen and globus pallidus of the basal ganglia.

leptomeninges A term for the surface coverings of the brain, including the arachnoid and pia mater.

Lewy bodies Eosinophilic cytoplasmic inclusions seen in neuromelanin-containing neurons in Parkinson's disease.

limbic system An interconnected system of brain regions. It functions in feeding behavior, aggression, and the expression of emotion.

lipofuschin A muddy brownish color in neurons that accumulates with increasing age.

locus ceruleus A small nucleus ("blue spot") in the pontine tegmentum whose neurons are the major source of norepinephrine in the brain; present bilaterally.

lumbar puncture (spinal tap) A procedure in which a needle is inserted via the L5–S1 interspace through the dura of the spinal canal and into the arachnoid space. It is performed to withdraw cerebrospinal fluid.

luteinizing hormone (LH) An anterior pituitary hormone that stimulates both epithelial and interstitial cells in the ovary. Together with FSH, it induces follicular maturation and the formation of corpora lutea.

Luxol fast blue (LFB) stain Used in histology to stain myelin and reveal the major fiber tracts (except for the few that consist completely of unmyelinated axons).

macrophages Phagocytic cells transformed from microglial cells.

magnetic resonance imaging (MRI) Specialized, high-resolution structural images of brain that use magnetic fields.

mamillary bodies Rounded, grey matter structures that lie beneath the floor of the third ventricle between the cerebral peduncles. The most important connection of the mamillary bodies are efferent fibers known as the mamillothalamic tract. These fibers project to the anterior nucleus of the thalamus, then to the cingulate gyrus, and then back to form a vital closed limbic system loop.

medial Toward the midline.

medial geniculate body A small nucleus located in the diencephalon that functions in the auditory pathway.

medulla Approximately 3 cm long and the most caudal portion of the brainstem. It controls respiration and supplies innervation to the tongue and palate.

medulloblastoma A malignant cerebellar tumor composed of neurons.

meningiomas Generally benign tumors of meningothelial cells.

meningitis Infection or inflammation of the outer covering of the brain.

meningothelial (arachnoid) cells Maintain the dura, arachnoid, and pia.

mesencephalon A primary fetal brain region (vesicle) developed by the end of the fourth week of fetal life. It eventually forms the midbrain.

mesocortical tract A dopaminergic tract that projects from the ventral tegmental area near the substantia nigra to the neocortex, particularly the prefrontal cortex. It is involved in motivation, planning, behavior, attention, and social behavior.

mesolimbic tract Catecholaminergic neurons (mostly dopaminergic) with cell bodies located in the ventral tegmental area of the midbrain and axons that project to the hippocampus, entorhinal cortex, amygdala, anterior cingulate gyrus, nucleus accumbens, and other limbic regions.

metencephalon One of the secondary vesicles derived in fetal life from the rhombencephalon, which eventually forms the pons and cerebellum.

3-methoxy-4-hydroxyphenylglycol (MHPG) A metabolite of norepinephrine.

microglial cells Small, rod-shaped cells that function as the major "scavenger cells" of the brain.

midbrain The most rostral division of the brainstem. It contains important structures such as the cerebral aqueduct, superior and inferior colliculi, red nuclei, substantia nigra, cerebral peduncles, and oculomotor and trochlear cranial nerve nuclei.

middle cerebellar peduncle Also known as the "brachium pontis," it is the largest of the three cerebellar peduncles. The most important connection transports information from the cortex to the cerebellum by way of the pontine nuclei.

middle frontal gyrus Contains the frontal eye fields and plays a role in voluntary eye movements.

migrational abnormality The abnormal location or connection of neurons within the central nervous system.

monoamine oxidase (MAO) An enzyme found within most tissues that catalyzes the breakdown of monoamines such as dopamine, norepinephrine, and serotonin.

monoamine oxidase inhibitors (MAOIs) Drugs that inhibit the breakdown of MAO, thus leading to the accumulation of monoamines.

monoamines A system of neurotransmitters that contain one amino group and are derived from amino acids. Subcategories of monoamines include the catecholamines (dopamine, norepinephrine, epinephrine), which are derived from tyrosine, and the indolamine serotonin, which is derived from tryptophan. Histamine is categorized as a monoamine but is biochemically different. Monoamine-synthesizing neurons are found primarily in the brainstem but have a wide net of influence because of the ubiquitous distribution of their axonal projections.

mortality rate The death rate.

multimodal association cortex Neocortical regions that interpret information from multiple sensory modalities and provide sophisticated integration of incoming information (e.g., the temporal pole).

myelencephalon One of the secondary vesicles derived in fetal life from the rhombencephalon. It eventually forms the medulla.

neocortex (isocortex) "New" cortex containing six neuronal layers.

neostriatum The caudate and the putamen (the "new" corpus striatum).

nervus intermedius (CN VII) The sensory root of the facial nerve.

neural groove Formed from the neural plate by the eighteenth day of fetal life.

neural plate Appears by the sixteenth day of fetal development. It is the first step in the developing nervous system.

neural tube Formed in the fetal central nervous system by the end of the third week.

neuroblastoma A malignant neuronal tumor usually seen in children.

neurocytology The study of cells in the nervous system.

neurofibrillary tangle A mass of abnormal filamentous material located within the cell body of neurons. Tangles occur in several brain disorders and are composed of cytoskeletal components.

neurohypophysis The posterior portion of the pituitary gland.

neuromelanin A rich, deep-brown pigment that is found in neurons of the substantia nigra and locus ceruleus.

neuronophagia Dead or dying neurons that become phagocytized by lymphocytes and microglial cells.

neurons Function as the fundamental sensory and motor unit of the brain. They are composed of the cell body, perikaryon, axon, and dendrites.

neuropeptides Proteins that act as neurotransmitters or neurohormones. These highly diverse proteins have excitatory or inhibitory neuronal activity and include enkephalins, endorphins, and substance P.

neuropil The woven fabric of brain tissue composed of astrocytic processes, axons, and dendrites.

neurotransmitter A chemical found in nervous tissue. Stimulation of specific receptors by these chemicals produces changes in the target neuron or organ.

nicotinic acetylcholine receptors Ganglionic and neuromuscular receptors for acetylcholine.

nigrostriatal tract A dopaminergic system with neurons in the substantia nigra that project to the corpus striatum. The degeneration of these neurons produces Parkinson's disease. Neuroleptic blockade of this system causes extrapyramidal side effects.

Nissl stain Assists in the identification of Nissl substance in neurons.

Nissl substance Produces neurotransmitters essential to proper signal transduction of the neuron.

N-methyl-D-aspartate (NMDA) A glutamate receptor that triggers cellular depolarization.

norepinephrine A catecholamine neurotransmitter that is primarily synthesized in neurons of the locus ceruleus in the pons. Deficiencies of norepinephrine are linked to depression.

nucleus accumbens   At the level of the septum pellucidum, this nucleus is adjacent to the medial and ventral portions of the caudate and putamen. The neurons in this nucleus project to both the globus pallidus and the substantia nigra.

nucleus basalis of Meynert   Located bilaterally directly beneath the anterior commissure, it is the major brain site for the production of acetylcholine. Fibers from this nucleus project diffusely to the cerebral cortex.

obex   The apex of the V-shaped boundary at the inferior portion of the fourth ventricle.

oculomotor nerve (CN III)   Formed in the midbrain from axons of the oculomotor nucleus. The oculomotor nerve emerges along the sides of the interpeduncular fossa. It travels through the cavernous sinus and leaves the cranial cavity via the superior orbital fissure.

oculomotor nucleus   The nucleus of the oculomotor nerve (CN III). It lies in the periaqueductal grey matter of the midbrain, ventral to the aqueduct at the level of the superior colliculus. The parasympathetic portion of CN III is located in the Edinger-Westphal nucleus.

olfactory bulb   The flattened portion of the olfactory system that lies immediately lateral to the hemispheric fissure beneath the frontal lobe. It is the termination of the olfactory nerves. Neural impulses travel from the olfactory bulb, down the olfactory tract, and to the olfactory areas of the cerebral cortices.

olfactory cells   Neurons found in the bone and epithelium of the nasal cavity. These neurons give off unmyelinated axons that constitute the olfactory nerves.

olfactory nerves   Formed from the olfactory cells of the nasal epithelium. They pass through the bone of the cribriform plate beneath the frontal lobes and enter the olfactory bulbs. The olfactory system mediates the sense of smell.

oligodendrocytes   The myelin-forming cells of the central nervous system.

oligodendrogliomas   Neoplastic tumors of oligodendrocytes.

opioid receptors   Receptors that mediate the various pharmacological effects of the opiate drugs. Multiple receptors are designated as mu, kappa, delta, and lambda, which subserve different physiological functions.

optic chiasm   A fusion point for the optic nerves. Some fibers cross at this point and provide visual input to both sides of the calcarine cortex in the occipital lobe.

optic nerve (CN II)   A nerve composed of fibers that originate in ganglion cells in the retina and extend to the optic chiasm.

optic tracts   Nerve fibers from the optic chiasm that extend to the lateral geniculate nuclei.

paired helical filaments (PHFs)   The abnormality that comprises the tangles located in neurons in Alzheimer's disease. They are visible only under the electron microscope.

parahippocampal gyrus   Neocortex located immediately adjacent to the hippocampus that processes incoming and outgoing information.

parasympathetic nervous system   The craniosacral division of the autonomic nervous system. It is also called the cholinergic system because it is driven by acetylcholine. Blockage of this system by anticholinergic drugs causes many annoying symptoms (e.g., dry mouth and blurred vision).

parenchyma   The tissue substance of the brain, including neurons, astrocytes, oligodendrocytes, and blood vessels.

pathognomonic   Specific characteristics of a disease that enable its recognition and differentiation from other diseases.

periaqueductal region   The grey matter that surrounds the cerebral aqueduct in the midbrain.

perikaryon   The neuronal cell body, not including the processes.

periventricular areas   Largely composed of white matter, these areas of the brain border the ventricular system, including the lateral, third, and fourth ventricles.

phencyclidine (PCP)   A synthetic hallucinogen traditionally used as an animal tranquilizer. Although a euphoric state is sought, wild and frightening effects often occur within the abuser.

pia mater   The thin inner covering of the meninges investing the brain.

Pick's bodies   Circular neuronal intracytoplasmic inclusions seen in Pick's disease. Pick's bodies are stained with silver preparations and contain cytoskeletal components.

planum temporale   The triangular-shaped, flattened surface of the superior temporal gyrus that lies immediately posterior to the transverse temporal gyrus and is buried within the lateral sulcus. This cortex provides sophisticated language skills.

pons   The middle portion of the brainstem. The pons consists of two functionally different areas: the basis pontis and the dorsal pons (pontine tegmentum). The basis pontis contains the corticospinal tracts and the pontine nuclei, and the pontine tegmentum houses the fourth ventricle, locus ceruleus, and several cranial nerve nuclei and tracts.

positron emission tomography (PET)   Specialized functional images of brain that depict metabolic or receptor activity. PET radiolabels are high-intensity, short–half-life compounds that require a cyclotron (atom smasher) for production.

postcentral gyrus   The primary sensory area located in the parietal lobe immediately posterior to the central (rolandic) sulcus.

posterior fossa   The posterior inferior regions of the cranial vault that house the cerebellum and brainstem.

precentral gyrus   The primary motor area in the frontal lobe located immediately anterior to the fissure of Rolando.

prevalence   The frequency of occurrence.

projection fibers   White matter tracts that connect distant areas with the cortex.

prosencephalon   A primary vesicle developed by the end of the fourth week of fetal life that eventually forms the forebrain. It is composed of the telencephalon and diencephalon.

protoplasmic astrocyte   Astrocytes largely confined to grey matter.

psychosis   A nonspecific brain disorder manifested by failure to distinguish an internal perception from external reality. Hallucinations and delusions are common manifestations of psychosis and may result from many types of brain dysfunction (e.g., trauma, drugs, and schizophrenia).

putamen   The largest grey matter region of the basal ganglia. It is situated lateral to the globus pallidus.

pyramidal system   The motor system that controls voluntary movement of voluntary muscle groups. Neurons in the motor strip (the precentral gyrus) project to the spinal cord via the internal capsule and corticospinal pathways.

raphe nuclei   Properly part of the pontine tegmentum, the raphe nuclei are associated with the reticular formation and synthesize serotonin.

red nucleus   A rounded grey matter structure located below the midbrain tectum. It receives input from the cerebellum and sends fibers to the thalamus and spinal cord via the rubrospinal tract.

reticular formation   Consists of interconnected regions in the brainstem tegmentum, lateral hypothalamus, and thalamus. It functions in arousal, consciousness, and the sleep-wake cycle.

reuptake   The physiological process that occurs when a neurotransmitter is taken up into the presynaptic neuron after having been released into the synapse. Some psychotropic drugs are designed to prevent the reuptake of a specific neurotransmitter in order to increase the synaptic presence of that neurotransmitter.

rhombencephalon   A primary vesicle developed by the end of the fourth week of fetal life. It forms the metencephalon and the myelencephalon.

Rosenthal fibers   Eosinophilic structures present in the processes of astrocytes. They imply chronicity of a process.

rostral   Toward the head or upward.

schizophrenia   A neurodevelopmental brain disorder with onset in late adolescence. It is characterized by hallucinations, delusions, and deterioration of psychosocial function. Most cases of schizophrenia occur spontaneously, but some result from brain injury.

Seiver-Munger stain   A silver stain used in histology that enables the identification of axons, neurofibrillary tangles, and senile plaques.

senile plaque   A circular collection of microscopic debris that disrupts the normal woven appearance of brain tissue. Low numbers of plaques are present in aging, but high numbers are diagnostic of Alzheimer's disease.

sensorineural (nerve) deafness   One of the two major subtypes of deafness patterns. It can be caused by the interruption of cochlear nerve fibers from the ear to the brainstem nuclei, such as by acoustic neuromas.

serotonin (5HT)   A monoamine neurotransmitter from the indolamine family. It is derived from the amino acid tryptophan. Deficiencies of serotonin are linked to depression.

shunt   A catheter inserted through the skull and brain and into the lateral ventricle to drain cerebrospinal fluid.

single photon emitted computed tomography (SPECT)   Brain scans that assess metabolic or receptor activity. SPECT radiolabels are stable and do not require production by a cyclotron.

spinal accessory nerve (CN XI)   Motor neurons of CN XI supply the trapezius and sternocleidomastoid muscles and have their cell bodies in the spinal accessory nucleus (which is located in the ventral horn of spinal cord segments C1-C5). Lesions of the spinal accessory nerve or nucleus cause contralateral weakness of the sternocleidomastoid or trapezius muscles.

striatum   Basal ganglia that include the caudate and putamen.

subarachnoid space   Separates the arachnoid from the pia mater and contains numerous blood vessels and abundant CSF.

subdural space   Separates the dura from the arachnoid. It normally contains only minute amounts of CSF.

subiculum   The transition zone between the hippocampus and the neocortex. It contains a 4- or 5-layer cortex and is essential to the transmission of information.

substance P   A neuropeptide composed of a chain of 11 amino acids. It is involved in the pain pathway and has been found in the brainstem, pituitary gland, hypothalamus, striatum, and ventral horn of the spinal cord.

substantia nigra   A thin dark line of melanin-containing neurons, which are located adjacent to the cerebral peduncles of the midbrain. The substantia nigra receives afferent fibers from the cortex and basal ganglia. The efferent pathways from the substantia nigra are dopaminergic tracts to the basal ganglia (the nigrostriatal tract).

subthalamic nucleus   In the shape of a thick, biconvex lens, the subthalamic nucleus lies below the thalamus and above the substantia nigra. It is part of the diencephalon.

sulcus (pl sulci)   Small trenches on the exterior surface of the brain that separate the gyri. Sulci allow for more "coastline" of grey matter.

superior cerebellar peduncle   A small collection of fibers that is also known as the "brachium conjunctivum." It receives and sends cerebellar impulses to and from the thalamus and spinal cord, with relays in the red nuclei.

superior colliculus   Along with the inferior colliculus, the superior colliculus forms the tectum of the midbrain. It is involved with voluntary control of ocular movements.

superior temporal gyrus   A long gyrus (5 to 7 cm) that forms the inferior margin of the Sylvian fissure. Lesions in the dominant hemisphere (usually the left hemisphere) cause a Wernicke's dysphasia.

Sylvian fissure   A sulcus that separates the temporal lobe from the frontal and parietal lobes.

sympathetic nervous system   The thoracolumbar division of the autonomic nervous system. It is also called the adrenergic system because it is driven by adrenergics. This system provides immediate adaptation for fight or flight.

sympathomimetic drugs   A drug that, by acting on adrenergic receptors, can cause physiological changes similar to those produced by the sympathetic nervous system.

synaptic space   A specialized junction between neurons where neurotransmitters are released.

synaptophysin   A protein used in immunohistochemistry that is abundant in neurons and thus enables their identification.

tectum of midbrain   The tectum (or roof) of the midbrain is formed by the two pairs of colliculi (superior and inferior) and their accompanying white matter tracts.

telencephalon   One of the secondary vesicles in fetal life that is derived from the prosencephalon. It eventually forms the cerebral hemispheres.

tentorium cerebelli   The posterior leaflets of dura that lie above the cerebellum and separate the occipital lobe from the cerebellum.

thalamus   A large collection of nuclei in the diencephalon. It is located on either side of the third ventricle.

thought disorder   A nonspecific brain disorder in which patients are unable to organize thoughts into paragraphs and think and speak in disconnected sentences or phrases. Patients lose the ability to maintain a consistent theme in their thoughts.

transverse temporal gyrus   Located in the temporal lobe, this structure is the segment of the superior temporal gyrus that is buried in the Sylvian fissure and extends from the lateral surface to the insular cortex (i.e., transverse). This region includes the primary auditory cortex and is often called Heschl's gyrus.

trigeminal nerve (CN V)   The principal sensory nerve of the head and the motor nerve for the muscles of mastication. Several different nuclei are integrated into the trigeminal system, including the chief sensory nucleus, the spinal nucleus of CN V, the mesencephalic nucleus, and the motor nucleus.

trochlear nerve (CN IV)   Innervates the superior oblique muscle of the eye and is the only crossed cranial nerve. The trochlear nucleus is immediately caudal to the oculomotor nucleus at the level of the inferior colliculus in the midbrain, and its fibers compose the only cranial nerve to emerge from the dorsal aspect of the brainstem. This nerve emerges caudal to the inferior colliculus, traverses the cavernous sinus, and exits via the superior orbital fissure into the orbit.

tuberoinfundibular tract   A dopaminergic system with neurons in the arcuate nucleus of the hypothalamus that project to the pituitary stalk. This tract controls the secretion of prolactin.

ultrasonography   A neuroradiologic test that does not expose the patient to ionizing radiation. Mechanical waves are introduced over the surface of the body with a video probe to provide information concerning the structures below. It is quite useful as a noninvasive procedure to determine the degree of atherosclerosis in the carotid arteries and therefore assess the need for angiography.

unimodal association cortex   Neocortical regions that interpret sensory inputs originating from a single sensory modality (e.g., the superior temporal gyrus interprets auditory information).

vagus nerve (CN X)   Involved with many brainstem nuclei, including the nucleus ambiguus, nucleus solitarius, inferior and superior salivatory nuclei, and dorsal nucleus of the vagus. The vagus nerve provides sensory mediation of fibers of the tongue and pharynx and mediates the gag reflex. It also provides afferents from the thoracic and abdominal viscera, efferents to motor fibers for neck striated musculature, and a large component of parasympathetic efferents.

vein of Galen   In the midline, this vein lies beneath the splenium of the corpus callosum. The interior veins of the cerebrum (the internal cerebral veins), and the basal veins of Rosenthal drain into the vein of Galen. This blood eventually travels to the venous sinus system of the brain and ultimately is drained into the internal jugular vein.

ventral   Toward the anterior or front.

ventral tegmental area (VTA)   Located in the midbrain, this region is dorsomedial to the substantia nigra and ventral to the red nuclei. The nuclei in this area produce dopamine. The efferent pathways from the VTA include the mesocortical and mesolimbic tracts.

ventricle   The system of connected brain cavities that are filled with cerebrospinal fluid, including the lateral ventricles (in the central portion of the telencephalon), the third ventricle (which runs between the thalami), the fourth ventricle (in the pons and medulla), and the connecting cerebral aqueduct (in the midbrain).

vermis of cerebellum   Connects the two lateral cerebellar hemispheres. Vermal lesions, which are commonly caused by the chronic ingestion of alcohol, cause gait ataxia and broadening of the base of the gait.

vestibular nerve   The vestibular portion of CN VIII. It arises from the vestibular ganglia in the labyrinth of the inner ear. The nerve enters the cranial vault through the internal acoustic meatus and enters the brainstem at the junction of pons and medulla. The vestibular portion of CN VIII mediates the system of body equilibrium and terminates in the vestibular nuclear complex, which consists of four nuclei and is situated in the rostral medulla.

GLOSSARY

Wallerian degeneration   Degeneration of an axon distal to a site of axonal injury. The cell body can compensate for Wallerian degeneration by growing new axons.

Wernicke's area   The sophisticated auditory association cortex that is located within the planum temporale and interprets spoken language.

Wernicke's encephalopathy   Confusion and ophthalmoplegia caused by thiamine deficiency; most common in alcoholics. It results in necrosis and hemorrhage in the mamillary bodies and periventricular structures of the brainstem.

withdrawal   A syndrome that develops following the cessation of or abrupt reduction in dosage of a regularly used substance.

index

notes

notes

notes

Don't miss these other outstanding psychiatric nursing titles from Mosby!

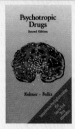

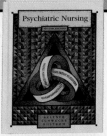

The latest DSM-IV-based data on side effects and interactions!

How psychiatric nursing is practiced today...

PSYCHOTROPIC DRUGS, 2nd Edition
By Norman L. Keltner, RN, CRNP, EdD, and David G. Folks, MD

Now provides up-to-date, DSM-IV-based data on mood, anxiety, seizure and sleep disorders, schizophrenia and other psychotic disorders, and substance abuse disorders, including alcoholism.

♦ Includes in-depth discussions of SSRI medications and covers the newest psychopharmaceuticals, such as Luvox and Risperdal.

♦ Includes 100 drug profiles that list significant parameters for specific drugs such as dosages, pharmacokinetics, and side effects.

1997. ISBN: 0-8151-4968-9 (28187)

PSYCHIATRIC NURSING, 2nd Edition
By Norman L. Keltner, RN, CRNP, EdD; Lee Hilyard Schwecke, EdD, MSN, RN; and Carol E. Bostrom, MSN, RN

♦ Accurately reflects contemporary practice, with chapters on timely topics such as psychobiology, family, culture, rehabilitation, case management, sexual disorders, and dual diagnosis.

♦ Includes cutting-edge content on ANA psychiatric nursing standards, psychotropic drugs, drug side effects, DSM-IV criteria, DSM-IV diagnoses and related NANDA diagnoses.

♦ Reformatted nursing care plans include the six-step nursing process, NANDA diagnoses, and expanded nursing interventions.

1995. ISBN: 0-8016-8069-7 (08069)

To order, ask your bookstore manager or call toll-free: 800-426-4545, 24 hours a day.
Be sure to visit the Mosby Web Site at http://www.mosby.com
We look forward to hearing from you soon!

Mosby

PMA-030